INSTRUCTOR'S MANUAL TO ACCOMPANY CLINICAL DECISION MAKING

Case Studies in Psychiatric Nursing

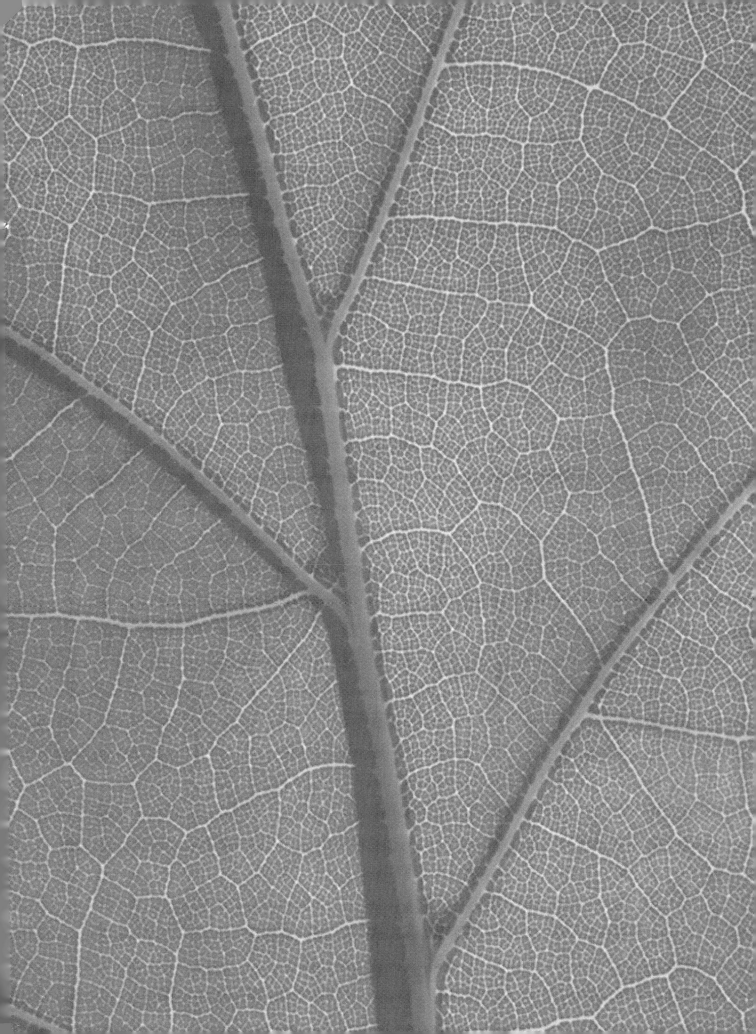

INSTRUCTOR'S MANUAL
TO ACCOMPANY
CLINICAL ~~DECISION MAKING~~

Student Learning Division

Assign Reading-Case Study for next wk. Anxiety, Depression, Bipolar, Schizophrenia

in Ps~~ychiatric Nur~~sing

Betty Kehl Richardson
PhD, RN, CNS-MHP, BC, LPC, LMFT

THOMSON
★
DELMAR LEARNING

Australia   Canada   Mexico   Singapore   Spain   United Kingdom   United States

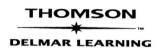

THOMSON
DELMAR LEARNING

Instructor's Manual to Accompany Clinical Decision Making: Case Studies in Psychiatric Nursing

by Betty Kehl Richardson, PhD, RN, CNS-MHP, BC, LPC, LMFT

Vice President,
Health Care Business Unit:
William Brottmiller

Director of Learning Solutions:
Matthew Kane

Acquisitions Editor:
Maureen Rosener

Product Manager:
Elizabeth Howe

Editorial Assistant:
Chelsey Iaquinta

Marketing Director:
Jennifer McAvey

Marketing Manager:
Michele McTighe

Marketing Coordinator:
Danielle Pacella

Production Director:
Carolyn Miller

Content Project Manager:
Jessica McNavich

ISBN-13: 978-1-4018-3846-1
ISBN-10: 1-4018-3846-4

Notice to the Reader

Contents

Reviewers

Ann K. Beckett, PhD, RN
Assistant Professor
Oregon Health and Science University School of Nursing
Portland, Oregon

Jane E. Bostick, PhD, APRN, BC
Assistant Professor of Clinical Nursing
University of Missouri–Columbia
Sinclair School of Nursing
Columbia, Missouri

Kimberly M. Gregg, MS APRN, BC
Adult Mental Health Clinical Nurse Specialist
Altru Health Systems
Instructor
University of North Dakota
Grand Forks, North Dakota

Bethany Phoenix, RN, PhD, CNS
Associate Clinical Professor
Coordinator, Graduate Program in Psychiatric/Mental Health Nursing
University of California, San Francisco
San Francisco, California

Charlotte R. Price, EdD, RN
Professor and Chair
Augusta State University Department of Nursing
Augusta, Georgia

Linda Stafford, PhD, RN, CS
Division Head, Psychiatric Mental Health Nursing
The University of Texas Health Science Center at Houston
School of Nursing
Houston, Texas

Preface

The *Instructor's Manual to Accompany Clinical Decision Making: Case Studies in Psychiatric Nursing* provides all of the cases from the book with their accompanying questions, answers, and rationales. Answers and rationales allow the instructor to facilitate discussion of the critical thinking questions while using the answers as a guide. Each case includes the table of variables and references.

Thomson Delmar Learning's Case Studies Series was created to encourage nurses to bridge the gap between content knowledge and clinical application. The products within the series represent the most innovative and comprehensive approach to nursing case studies ever developed. Each title has been authored by experienced nurse educators and clinicians who understand the complexity of nursing practice as well as the challenges of teaching and learning. All of the cases are based on real-life clinical scenarios and demand thought and "action" from the nurse. Each case brings the user into the clinical setting, and invites him or her to utilize the nursing process while considering all of the variables that influence the client's condition and the care to be provided. Each case also represents a unique set of variables, to offer a breadth of learning experiences and to capture the reality of nursing practice. To gauge the progression of a user's knowledge and critical thinking ability, the cases have been categorized by difficulty level. Every section begins with basic cases and proceeds to more advanced scenarios, thereby presenting opportunities for learning and practice for both students and professionals.

All of the cases have been expert reviewed to ensure that as many variables as possible are represented in a truly realistic manner and that each case reflects consistency with realities of modern nursing practice.

Praise for Delmar Learning's Case Study Series

"These cases show diversity and richness of content and should stimulate lively discussions with students."

—Linda Stafford, PhD, RN
Division Head, Psychiatric Mental Health
Nursing, School of Nursing, The University of
Texas Health Science Center at Houston

"The use of case studies is pedagogically sound and very appealing to students and instructors. I think that some instructors avoid them because of the challenge of case development. You have provided the material for them."

—Nancy L. Oldenburg, RN, MS, CPNP
Clinical Instructor, Northern Illinois University

"[The author] has done an excellent job of assisting students to engage in critical thinking. I am very impressed with the cases, questions, and content. I rarely ask that students buy more than one . . . book . . . but, in this instance, I can't wait until this book is published."

—Deborah J. Persell, MSN, RN, CPNP
Assistant Professor, Arkansas State University

"[The case studies] are very current and prepare students for the twenty-first-century mental health arena."

—CHARLOTTE R. PRICE, EdD, RN
Professor and Chair, Augusta State University
Department of Nursing

"One thing I always tell my students is that they will encounter mental health issues in all the various areas of nursing that they practice. Often they don't grasp this concept. . . . Many mental health nursing books focus on mental health settings and miss the other settings. I appreciate the fact that different settings were used in this reading . . . inpatient and outpatient, as well as med-surg, plastic surgery, etc."

—KIMBERLY M. GREGG, MS APRN, BC
Adult Mental Health Clinical Nurse Specialist,
Altru Health Systems, Instructor, University of
North Dakota

"This is a groundbreaking book. . . . This book should be a required text for all undergraduate and graduate nursing programs and should be well-received by faculty."

—JANE H. BARNSTEINER, PhD, RN, FAAN
Professor of Pediatric Nursing, University of
Pennsylvania School of Nursing

How to Use this Book

Every case begins with a table of variables that are encountered in practice, and that must be understood by the nurse in order to provide appropriate care to the client. Categories of variables include age, gender, setting, ethnicity, cultural considerations, preexisting conditions, coexisting conditions, communication considerations, disability considerations, socioeconomic considerations, spiritual considerations, pharmacological considerations, psychosocial considerations, legal considerations, ethical considerations, alternative therapy, prioritization considerations, and delegation considerations. If a case involves a variable that is considered to have a significant impact on care, the specific variable is included in the table. This allows the user an "at a glance" view of the issues that will need to be considered to provide care to the client in the scenario. The table of variables is followed by a presentation of the case, including the history of the client, current condition, clinical setting, and professionals involved. A series of questions follows each case that ask the user to consider how she would handle the issues presented within the scenario. Suggested answers and rationales are provided for remediation and discussion.

Organization

Cases are grouped according to psychiatric disorder. Within each part, cases are organized by difficulty level from easy, to moderate, to difficult. This classification is somewhat subjective, but they are based upon a developed standard. In general, difficulty level has been determined by the number of variables that impact the case and the complexity of the client's condition. Colored tabs are used to allow the user to distinguish the difficulty levels more easily. A comprehensive table of variables is also provided for reference, to allow the user to quickly select cases containing a particular variable of care.

The cases are fictitious; however, they are based on actual problems and/or situations the nurse will encounter. Any resemblance to actual cases or individuals is coincidental.

Acknowledgments

For the invitation to write this book, the author wishes to express her appreciation to Erin Silk and Matt Kane of Thomson Delmar Publishers. A number of product managers and staff were involved over time, and the author thanks them for their help. The author is most indebted to Elizabeth (Libby) Howe, the final product manager, who provided guidance, feedback, ideas, and encouragement to keep the project alive and get the book into print. Another special thanks goes to Nora Armbruster, who managed the final production stage and made it possible to meet the print deadline. The author wants to especially thank the reviewers and copy editors of this book, for their time, expertise, critical comments, and suggestions, which resulted in changes to make the book much better.

A number of colleagues at Austin Community College, Austin, Texas; Austin State Hospital; and Seton Shoal Creek Psychiatric Hospital, as well as other psychiatric and medical facilities, were consulted about selected aspects of the cases to verify accuracy and currency. The author recognizes and appreciates the important contributions of these colleagues: Sally Samford, Marita Peppard, Donna Edwards, Kris Benton, Kitty Viek, Jane Luetchens, and many others.

Teachers and school nurses were consulted, as were parents of children with special issues. The author wishes to recognize their important contributions, especially Edna Nation, who teaches high school students in Liberty Hill, Texas, for her dedication to helping all students—including those with medical and mental health problems—achieve their maximum potential and for sharing her ideas with the author.

The author thanks her family and friends for their patience and understanding during the long months of research and writing. This project could not have been finished without their encouragement and cooperation.

Dedication

This book is dedicated to my son Mark, who has battled cancer throughout most of the time this book was in progress. Sharing with me some of his innermost thoughts, fears, and struggles has reinforced for me that what student nurses, family, and others see on the surface in a brief interaction with a client can be a very different picture than what is going on inside the client. Compassion, empathy, and therapeutic communication do help us understand that inner person. I am indebted to Mark for all he has taught me.

Additionally, this book is dedicated to all the good nurses in various fields of nursing, not just psychiatric mental health nursing, who apply psychiatric techniques and principles when working with clients who have mental health diagnoses and/or issues.

Note from the Author

These case studies were designed to help nursing students at all levels to not only fine tune their critical thinking skills and their therapeutic communication skills, but to develop a deeper understanding of, and empathy for, clients who have what we currently refer to as psychiatric problems. The mind and body are inseparable, so physical health problems are interwoven with mental health problems within the cases. The student nurse, and anyone else who reads these case studies, is encouraged to ask themselves: "What is the most therapeutic approach or response to this client in this situation?" as they answer the questions within the cases.

About the Author

Dr. Richardson began a nursing career in 1959 as a new diploma graduate. She worked five years in obstetrical nursing at Memorial Medical Center, Springfield, Illinois; much of this time she worked in the labor rooms and applied nearly everything she learned in psychiatric nursing to emotionally support laboring women, new mothers, and grieving parents who lost babies. She next worked as an office nurse for Dr. Tom Masters, a general internist who specialized in Diabetes. The following several years she worked for the Illinois Department of Mental Health Mental Retardation, working on an outpatient team serving three rural counties. The team followed the blurred role concept in which every member did intake evaluations and did counseling with people having the full range of diagnoses and issues possible in mental health work. This work stimulated a return to school for a bachelor's in nursing and a master's in administration from the University of Illinois at Springfield, a master's degrees in adult nursing from the Medical College of Georgia, and a PhD in psychiatric mental health nursing from the University of Texas at Austin, Texas. Her dissertation was "The Psychiatric Inpatient's Perception of the Seclusion Room Experience." She published the results of this study in *Nursing Research.* Dr. Richardson has taught in an RN to BSN program, two ADN programs, and a licensed vocational nursing program. She received the NISOD teaching award for teaching excellence from the University of Texas.

Throughout the years, volunteer work has been a passion. Dr. Richardson made fifteen trips to Honduras and Nicaragua with MEDICO, a nonprofit organization taking medical, eye, and dental care to remote areas that are medically underserved. She co-led trips to the Moskito Coast of Nicaragua and Honduras and volunteered for several months in a program to take boys off the streets of LaCeiba, Honduras. Additional volunteer work has been with the homeless in Austin, Texas.

Dr. Richardson is also a licensed professional counselor and a licensed marriage and family therapist and has done therapy for over thirty years (full time and part time). She has worked as a therapist in a residential program for children and adolescents and as a service administrator and therapist on a child/adolescent unit in a private psychiatric hospital. She led weekend groups in a private psychiatric hospital for many years while teaching full time. She was Director of Nursing of Austin State Hospital, Austin, Texas, for six years. Over the years, Dr. Richardson has had training with a number of the great theorists such as Bettleheim, Azrin, Frankl, Ellis, and others. She has had training in a variety of therapies from Psychoanalytic Theory to Play Therapy to Brief Psychotherapy. She is a board-certified clinical specialist in child adolescent psychiatric nursing (certified by the American Nurses Association). She continues in her private practice, works part time in a drug study clinic, freelances for publishers, and has written a monthly column for parents in the newsmagazine *Austin Parent* since 1992. Dr. Richardson has lived in Austin, Texas, for over twenty-five years, and she can be contacted there by e-mail at bkrich@sbcglobal.net.

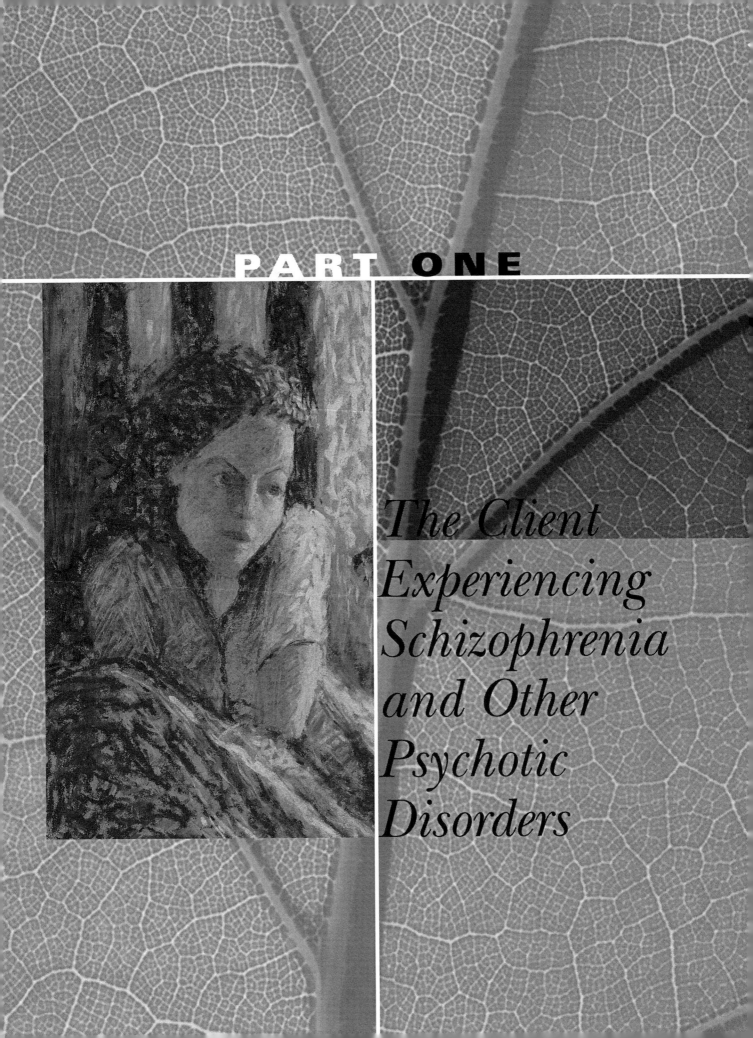

PART ONE

The Client Experiencing Schizophrenia and Other Psychotic Disorders

Sarah

GENDER

Female

AGE

34

SETTING

- Psychiatric hospital

ETHNICITY

- Hungarian American

CULTURAL CONSIDERATIONS

- Hungarian customs

PREEXISTING CONDITION

COEXISTING CONDITION

COMMUNICATION

DISABILITY

SOCIOECONOMIC

SPIRITUAL/RELIGIOUS

PHARMACOLOGIC

- Valproic acid (Depakote)
- Risperodone (Risperdal) liquid
- Venlafaxine hydrochloride (Effexor XR)

PSYCHOSOCIAL

LEGAL

- Confidentiality
- Consent
- Client's rights
- Release of information

ETHICAL

ALTERNATIVE THERAPY

PRIORITIZATION

DELEGATION

MODERATE

SCHIZOAFFECTIVE DISORDER, BIPOLAR TYPE

Level of difficulty: Moderate

Overview: Requires familiarity with the current diagnostic requirements for Schizoaffective Disorder and approaches to the psychotic client, including checking the client's mouth to prevent cheeking of medications. Requires critical thinking about accepting gifts from clients.

Client Profile

Sarah is a 34-year-old female. Born in Hungary, she married an American and came to this country when she was 25 years old. About a year later, Sarah began a series of admissions to psychiatric facilities. She was diagnosed with major depression and later with Schizoaffective Disorder. About a month ago, Sarah stopped keeping outpatient appointments, stopped taking her medication, stopped bathing, and stopped eating, but was sleeping all the time. Sarah's mood symptoms suddenly became less noticeable, and she began wandering her yard after dark, saying the neighbors were in the trees. Sarah began to carry a gun to protect herself against the neighbors, who she thought were out to kill her. When she started to fire the gun into the trees, her brother got a court order to have Sarah committed for treatment.

Case Study

Two deputies, one male and one female, and her brother have brought Sarah to the psychiatric hospital to be admitted. The nurse does an assessment on Sarah and discovers Sarah has been on risperodone (Risperdal) liquid, valproic acid (Depakote), and venlafaxine (Effexor XR). The psychiatrist orders these medications to be continued. At first the nurse is unable to get Sarah to sign consent forms to take the medication, but after a few days, she does sign the forms. By this time, her pregnancy test has come back negative, and she is started back on her usual medication.

The nurse finds Sarah to be somewhat tangential with loose associations. When the nurse assigns Sarah to attend a medication class, she refuses. When asked to interpret a proverb, she refuses.

Sarah begins to talk about her food being poisoned and being "king" of the hospital. She claims to have subjects to take care of the food and those who try to poison it.

Sarah tells the nurse that she has been hospitalized eight times previously at another psychiatric facility. The nurse sends a signed release of information form to the designated psychiatric facility requesting copies of Sarah's latest psychosocial assessment, treatment plan, and discharge summary. The requested information reveals that Sarah's discharge diagnosis at that facility was Schizoaffective Disorder, Bipolar Type.

After three weeks on medication, Sarah no longer seems to have hallucinations and delusions. The psychiatrist is ready to discharge Sarah, but her Depakote level comes back low. A nurse discovers Sarah has been cheeking her morning dose and sometimes her evening dose of Depakote and has been putting the medicine in a pair of shoes.

Sarah hands the nurse an envelope with two hundred dollars and the words "Thank-you nurse" written on the outside. About this time the nurse notices that Sarah has suddenly become hyperverbal, hyperactive, intrusive, and sexually suggestive to peers and staff.

Questions and Suggested Answers

1. **What is Schizoaffective Disorder?** The term *schizoaffective* was introduced in the 1930s and was included in the *American Psychiatric Association Diagnostic and Statistical Manual* for the first time in 1980. The symptoms defining Schizoaffective Disorder have changed with each revision of the manual (Frisch and Frisch, 2006). Currently the diagnosis of Schizoaffective Disorder requires an uninterrupted period of illness during which the client experiences a major depressive episode, a manic episode, or a mixed episode, concurrent with symptoms for schizophrenia such as disorganized speech, grossly disorganized or catatonic behavior, lack of motivation, scarcity of speech, or flattened affect. During the same illness the client must have at least two weeks without prominent mood symptoms, having instead delusions or hallucinations. Schizoaffective disorder is divided into the following types: Bipolar Type and Depressive Type. In Bipolar Type the person

must have either a manic or a mixed episode and can also have a major depressive episode. In the Depressive Type the client has only a major depressive episode (APA, 2000).

2. **Do Sarah's symptoms match those of Schizoaffective Disorder, and if so, how?** It appears that Sarah had a period of illness in which she had a major depressive episode. She was then delusional and hallucinatory for over two weeks, during which her mood symptoms were not predominant. Since she has had a depressed episode and a manic episode in this illness, she probably meets the criteria for Schizoaffective Disorder Bipolar Type.

3. **On what basis do you think Sarah was court committed?** Sarah's court commitment, by a judge, is based on her being a danger to others, as evidenced by firing a gun into the trees. A bullet may accidentally find its way into a neighboring home and kill or wound a neighbor.

4. **Why was Sarah's medication delayed? Why did the nurse not start it on admission?** There are at least two reasons the medication was not started on admission. The first reason is the necessity to obtain a negative pregnancy test prior to starting antipsychotic and mood-stabilizing medication. Some medications are not given if a client is pregnant to avoid harming the fetus. Second, the client had not yet signed the consent forms for the specific medications. However, if a court-committed client refuses to sign a consent form for the prescribed medications, these medications can be court ordered by a judge for a given period of time according to the law in the state where the client is being treated.

5. **Why does the nurse ask Sarah to interpret a proverb?** The nurse is assessing if Sarah is capable of abstract thinking. If she cannot think abstractly, then she is a concrete thinker. The nurse will select a proverb such as "A rolling stone gathers no moss." A concrete thinker will interpret in a way similar to this: "If a rock rolls down a hill, there will be no sign of green on the stone at the bottom." An abstract thinker will say something like: "If a person moves or changes jobs all the time, they won't collect friends or build retirement funds." If the nurse determines that Sarah cannot think abstractly, then the nurse will communicate in a concrete way.

6. **Does Sarah have hallucinations and/or delusions? What makes you think so?** Yes, she does. A hallucination is seeing, hearing, smelling, feeling, or tasting something that is not there. Sarah sees the neighbors in the trees and hears them talking. Ongoing assessment could reveal other hallucinations at various times. The nurse can respond therapeutically to a client who is hearing a voice by acknowledging that she or he (the nurse) does not hear anything but realizes that the client does hear it.

   A delusion is a false fixed belief that cannot be dislodged by reasoning. Sarah comes to believe that she is king of the hospital. Even if someone tells her that she is a woman and kings have to be men, she will persist in believing she is king. Sometimes delusions are grandiose and clients believe they are a famous or important person or have an important job or are wealthy, while other times they believe they are being persecuted. The delusional client will not give up the delusion because of logic; however, he or she will more likely give up the delusion or at least act on it less when his or her mental health improves through rest, cognitive therapy, change in environment and interactions, and/or medication. The nurse can respond to the client's delusional content by changing the subject or distracting the client to other activities rather than reinforcing the delusion by encouraging the client to discuss it. While it is helpful for the nurse to hear the client's delusions, once this content is known, discussion should be avoided.

7. **What is the age of onset, the male to female ratio, and the prevalence of Schizoaffective Disorder?** Early adulthood is the typical age of onset of Schizoaffective Disorder, though onset can occur at any time between the start of adolescence and the last years of life. The depressive type may be more common in the older adult while the bipolar type may be seen more often in young adults. The incidence of Schizoaffective Disorder is more common in women. Schizoaffective Disorder may be less common than schizophrenia (APA, 2000).

8. **Discuss the current theories of etiology, treatment, and prognosis of Schizoaffective Disorder.** Work done on the human genome suggests genetic makeup as an etiological factor in Schizophrenia, Bipolar Disorder,

and Schizoaffective Disorder. A current popular belief is that people with these disorders have vulnerabilities such as poor environment, limited recourses, and others, as well as strengths such as talent, wealth, and good parenting. One theory of causation is that when the vulnerabilities are too much for the strengths, then mental illness surfaces. Many researchers theorize that the cause is multifactorial.

Psychosocial therapies as well as drug therapies are used to treat Schizoaffective Disorder. Drugs alone cannot manage the problems of unemployment, homelessness, and/or poverty, which often are seen in clients with Schizoaffective Disorder. Clients need social and occupational rehabilitation therapy. These clients also need family and community support as many clients with Schizoaffective Disorder experience loneliness (www.mentalhealth.com).

In regard to drug treatment, currently most clinicians are targeting the mood symptoms with one or more mood-stabilizing medications (e.g., lithium carbonate, lithium citrate, venlafaxine, and Inderol), an antipsychotic medication to target the positive and negative symptoms of schizophrenia, and an antidepressant for depressive episodes.

Some clinicians think that Schizoaffective Disorder has an anxiety component as well as a thought and mood component and speak of it almost as a triad of disorders (www.mentalhealth.com; Cossoff and Hafner, 1998). These clinicians may add an antianxiety medication to the client's prescribed medications.

For the client who is medication noncompliant, the clinician may order long-acting depot antipsychotic medication injections (e.g., haloperidol [Haldol] fluphenazine decanoate or enanthate [Prolixin]) or the newer atypical antipsychotic risperodone (Risperdal), which comes in a long-lasting depot injection.

Some clinicians disagree with the current etiological studies in the area of neurotransmitters and disagree with the treatment of Schizoaffective Disorder (www.schizoaffective.org).

The prognosis of Schizoaffective Disorder is believed to be better than that of Schizophrenia, but not as good as that for a mood disorder. It is also thought that people with a diagnosis of Schizoaffective Disorder, Bipolar Type would have a better outcome than those with Schizoaffective Disorder, Depressive Type (APA, 2000). Keltner et al. (2002) points out that prolonged delusions and/or hallucinations experienced by clients with Schizoaffective Disorder may make it more difficult to treat these clients. This may be a factor in the occupational and social dysfunction that often translates to major difficulty keeping a job or personal relationships.

9. **What nursing diagnoses would you most likely write for Sarah?** Possible nursing diagnoses include but are not limited to:

- Risk for other-directed violence
- ~~Disturbed thought processes~~ *Impaired Sensory perception (delusions, hallucinations)*
- Risk for medication noncompliance *R/T biochemical imbalances*

10. **What goals and interventions do you suggest for Sarah for one of these nursing diagnoses?** For the diagnosis of risk for other-directed violence, goals could include:

- A short-term goal: No incidence of violence during the next week.
- A longer-term goal for discharge: Will verbalize that the neighbors are not out to harm her and she has no intent to harm the neighbors.

Interventions will address such things as keeping harmful objects away from client, doing medication education, working on medication compliance strategies, building trusting relationships, finding recreational and occupational activities, and working on Ericksonian stage of life tasks.

For the diagnosis of disturbed thought processes, interventions will address activities to decrease isolation, to help the client to realize the voices are not real, and to ignore delusions to keep from reinforcing them.

Interventions for medication noncompliance will include checking client's mouth after medication administration, assigning client to medication education class, discussing medications with client, providing positive reinforcement for taking medication, and contracting with client to take medications.

11. **What are the possible explanations for the client giving the nurse an envelope with money in it? How would you respond to this gift offer if you were the nurse?** In the manic state clients will often be gregarious and overly generous (e.g., giving a hundred dollar tip to a waitress who served them only a cup of coffee). Sarah has displayed some manic behaviors, and her offering the nurse money may be a manifestation of mania. On the other hand, in the client's native country, Hungary, it is the custom to give tips to the nurses and doctors as the pay is quite low. Some treatment facilities in this country have policies against accepting gifts from clients while others do not, leaving the decision to accept or not up to the individual nurse. Accepting the gift would change your nurse-client relationship from a therapeutic professional relationship to one in which you are ingratiated and may be expected by the client to provide a different and better standard of care compared to that provided to other clients.

References

American Psychiatric Association. (2000). *Diagnostic and Statistical Manual of Mental Disorders, 4th ed.* Text Revision. Washington, DC: American Psychiatric Association.

Cossoff, S.J., and Hafner, R.J. (1998). "The Prevalence of Comorbid Anxiety in Schizophrenia, Schizoaffective Disorder and Bipolar Disorder." *Australian and New Zealand Journal of Psychiatry* 32(1): 61–71.

Frisch, N.C., and Frisch, L.E. (2006). *Psychiatric Mental Health Nursing, 3rd ed.* Albany, NY: Thomson Delmar Learning.

Keltner, N.L., L.H. Schwecke, and C.E. Bostrom. (2000). *Psychiatric Nursing, 4th ed.* St. Louis: C.V. Mosby.

———.(1996). "Schizoaffective Disorder." *Harvard Mental Health Letter* 13(4): 1–5.

www.mentalhealth.com. Accessed June 20, 2006.

www.schizoaffective.org. Accessed June 20, 2006.

Dean

GENDER

Male

AGE

48

SETTING

- Community clinic for low-income clients

ETHNICITY

- American Indian and White American

CULTURAL CONSIDERATIONS

- Pima Indian culture

PREEXISTING CONDITION

- Diabetes

COEXISTING CONDITION

- Cough, fever

COMMUNICATION

DISABILITY

SOCIOECONOMIC

- Homeless

SPIRITUAL/RELIGIOUS

PHARMACOLOGIC

- Metformin (Glucophage)
- Risperodone (Risperdal)
- Trihexyphenidyl (Artane)
- Benztropine (Cogentin)

PSYCHOSOCIAL

- Isolating

LEGAL

- Confidentiality
- Consent for release of information

ETHICAL

- Respect for client's lifestyle choices (paternalism vs. autonomy)

ALTERNATIVE THERAPY

- Medicine man to overcome sources of evil influence on his life

PRIORITIZATION

DELEGATION

MODERATE

SCHIZOPHRENIA

Level of difficulty: Moderate

Overview: Requires the nurse to self-assess feelings about working with a homeless mentally ill client with diabetes and symptoms of Tardive Dyskinesia. The nurse must consider the client's Native American culture.

Client Profile

Dean, a 48 year-old male, grew up on a Pima Indian reservation in Arizona. He left the reservation after high school to serve in the army but was diagnosed and treated for Schizophrenia at age 21 and was discharged early. He has been in and out of psychiatric facilities for several years. He periodically takes a bus back to the reservation to see a medicine man, but he does not stay as he has no work and only distant, poor family there.

Case Study

Dean has come to the community health center. While he is sitting in the lobby, the nurse observes Dean without him being aware of this. The nurse notices that at times he seems to be talking to the air around him. She also notices that Dean is smacking his lips, his tongue protrudes at times, and he periodically coughs without covering his mouth.

When it is time for the nurse to do an assessment on Dean, the receptionist notifies the nurse that Dean has not filled out the intake form. The nurse tries to help him by asking him for his address. Although his speech is somewhat disorganized at times, the nurse finds out from Dean that he is homeless and currently living on the streets. His chief complaint is "not feeling well." The nurse takes Dean's vital signs, which are: T. 100.4, R. 22, P. 100, BP 152/98. He is 5 foot 8 inches tall and weighs 235 pounds. When weighed he says he has recently lost thirty pounds.

When the nurse asks Dean what medications he is on, he shows her some empty medicine bottles, saying he has run out of his medication and does not have the money to buy more. The labels on the bottles indicate he is on metformin (Glucophage), an oral antidiabetic medication, and risperodone (Risperdal). The nurse asks him why he takes Risperdal and also inquires about other medication he has taken in the past. He replies that he was diagnosed with Schizophrenia at age 21 and that he was on Thorazine for several years, then Haldol, then Prolixin injections, and maybe some he forgot before the current Risperdal. He explains that he has gone to the community mental health center twice to get more Risperdal samples and waited most of the day each time without being seen by the psychiatrist. Dean says he either lost, or someone stole, his last supply of Risperdal, so he has not been taking it for about a month. The nurse suspects Dean is hearing voices.

When asked about any health problems, he says he has diabetes, which he is supposed to "keep under control with diet and pills." He also complains of a cough, something the nurse noticed earlier. After the nurse develops some rapport with Dean, he tells her about seeing and hearing an owl that frightens him. He talks about needing to see a medicine man.

Questions and Suggested Answers

1. **What are some feelings that nurses could have about working with people who are homeless and mentally ill, and why would it be important for a nurse to think about his or her feelings toward this population?** It is important for a nurse to think through his or her feelings about the homeless and especially those in this population who have a mental illness, because in order to be effective in working with this group a nurse must be respectful and empathetic, project a caring manner, be therapeutic and professional, and set limits firmly but compassionately when necessary. Some health care professionals have had disturbing experiences with parents, relatives, and/or others who are mentally ill and/or homeless. Some nurses have stereotypical ideas or biases about these populations. Some nurses have mental health diagnoses themselves and work hard to keep their own mental health in balance and then are called to work with people who may not have worked as diligently. Any of these issues and perhaps others need to be worked through in order to be therapeutic with homeless mentally ill clients.

2. **Discuss the possible significance of Dean's appearance and observed behaviors.** Dean seems to be talking to the air, which could mean he is hearing voices and responding to them. He has some lip smacking and a protruding tongue, which could be associated with Tardive Dyskinesia.

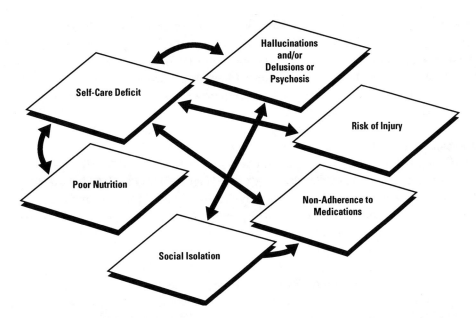

Concept map of issues and problems associated with schizophrenia.

Dean is coughing and has a fever, symptoms that could be associated with any number of conditions including, but not limited to: allergies, the common cold, dry mouth, upper respiratory infection, smoking and alcohol use, or tuberculosis. The fever could be symptomatic of some problem separate from the cough. It could be due to an infection anywhere in the body. The nurse needs to do a head to toe assessment and get a good health history.

Dean is unkempt, which could be due to lack of motivation associated with Schizophrenia and/or lack of access to shower facilities. Dean is overweight, which may lead to health problems associated with diabetes (e.g., circulatory problems and neurological problems).

3. **What screening tests and/or lab procedures seem to be indicated?** A screening test for Tardive Dyskinesia (TD), such as the AIMES test, needs to be done. In some facilities psychiatrists do a baseline screening test for TD on all clients, and the nurses are trained to do screening tests at regular intervals after the baseline is obtained. A blood glucose level needs to be determined. Hemoglobin A1c may be helpful in determining the degree of diabetic control. This client also needs to be screened for tuberculosis.

4. **What is Tardive Dyskinesia, how common is it, and what is the treatment for it? What did the nurse observe about Dean that would suggest Tardive Dyskinesia?** Tardive Dyskinesia is a neurological disorder characterized by involuntary purposeless movements. The most common movements are of the tongue and lips and include: grimacing, lip smacking and puckering, and pursing movements of the lips and protrusion of the tongue. There may also be involuntary movements of arms, legs, and trunk and fingers (www.ninds.nih. gov/disorders/tardive/tardive.htm).

Tardive Dyskinesia has mainly been associated with the long-term use of neuroleptic drugs, especially the older typical neuroleptics also referred to as antipsychotics. Frisch and Frisch (2006) point out that TD occurs in at least 5 percent of persons who continue on antipsychotic medication for more than a year and its incidence increases significantly with longer durations of treatment.

When symptoms of TD occur, the dosage of the neuroleptic medication is often minimized or in some cases the client is placed on one of the newer atypical neuroleptic medication, such as risperodone, at lower doses.

The nurse has some clues that suggest Dean may have Tardive Dyskinesia. Dean has been on neuroleptic medication since he was 21 years old. The nurse saw lip smacking behaviors and a protruding tongue when observing Dean.

5. **Is diabetes common among persons with a diagnosis of Schizophrenia? Is diabetes more common among Native American Indians? Discuss the possibility of persons with Schizophrenia having medical problems.** Studies of persons with Schizophrenia, including one reported by Subramaniam, Chong, and Pek (2003) involving 194 subjects, support the idea that having Schizophrenia brings with it an increased risk of developing Diabetes Mellitus as compared to the general population.

   In addition to diabetes being more common among persons with Schizophrenia, it is also more common among Native American Indians. The highest rate of diabetes in the world is found among American Indians. "One-half of adult Pima Indians have diabetes and 95% of those with diabetes are overweight" (http://diabetes.niddk.nih.gov/dm/pubs/pima/obesity/obesity.htm). A "thrifty gene" theory was proposed by geneticist James Neel to explain why large percentages of Pima Indians are overweight. This theory describes the Pima as relying on hunting, fishing, and farming for food for thousands of years and experiencing periods of feast and famine. To adapt to these extremes, Neel proposes that the Pima developed a gene that permitted greater storage of fat during times of plenty so they would not starve during times of famine. "The traditional Pima Indian diet consisted of only about 15 percent fat and was high in starch and fiber, but currently almost 40 percent of the calories in the Pima diet is derived from fat. As the typical American diet became more available on the reservation after the war, people became more overweight" (http://diabetes.niddk.nih.gov/dm/pubs/pima/obesity/obesity.htm). Being overweight brings slower metabolism, which, when combined with a high fat diet and a genetic tendency to retain fat, puts the Pima Indian at high risk for diabetes. Researchers from the National Institute of Diabetes and Digestive and Kidney Disease of the National Institutes of Health have been doing research on the Pima Indians for more than thirty years.

   People with a diagnosis of Schizophrenia have just as many medical problems as the general population and perhaps more due to not getting annual health check-ups. Nurses in all health care settings will encounter persons presenting with medical problems as well as psychiatric mental health problems.

6. **What precautions should the nurse take with the homeless population?** Universal precautions are to be taken with all clients, and the homeless population is no exception. The homeless may have sexually transmitted diseases or hepatitis in greater percentages than in the general population. The homeless may be exposed to and contract tuberculosis, including drug-resistant TB. The nurse needs to provide tissues to coughing clients and advise them how and where to cough and how to safely dispose of the tissues. It is necessary to follow up on all symptoms of tuberculosis with the homeless population and to screen for tuberculosis. This screening is especially important in this client's case because the tuberculosis rate is significantly higher (nearly six times higher in 2003) in Native American Indian populations (www.lungusa.org/site/pp.asp?c=d vLUK900Egb=35804) than among non-Hispanic White Americans. This client has some symptoms found in tuberculosis (e.g., cough, fever, and weight loss).

7. **What additional information about Dean would be helpful, and how could this be obtained? What reason can you think of for Dean wanting to see a medicine man?** Dean has shared with the nurse that he is seeing and hearing an owl that frightens him. The nurse needs to assess the significance of this owl and why it scares this client. The nurse can assess what seems to make this hallucination appear and lessen. The nurse must assess for delusional thinking, as well as any thoughts of self-harm or harming others. Had Dean not mentioned his hallucinations, the nurse could have approached him directly, asking if he is hearing voices, or indirectly by mentioning that sometimes people hear or see things.

   A possible reason for Dean wanting to see a medicine man from the Pima Indian reservation may be associated with his hearing and seeing the owl repeatedly. The Pima believe that the owl's hooting is ominous and signals approaching death. Some Pima Indians attribute death, illness, and misfortune to sorcery and may want to employ a medicine man to overcome the influence of sorcerers (www.accessgenealogy.com/native/tribes/pima/pimaindianhist.htm).

   A release of information form, signed by the client, will permit the nurse and/or the health care provider to talk with the psychiatrist at the community mental health center about what medication Dean has been on in the past and the best plan for medicating and treating him now. Information about the results of any recent screening for Tardive Dyskinesia can be obtained, as well as any necessary copies of Dean's past mental health records.

The nurse needs to know the results and location of Dean's last TB skin test or chest X-ray. If he had a negative test for TB recently, confirmation from the agency where this was done can be obtained with a signed release of information form. If a recent test for TB was positive and Dean was diagnosed with TB, he needs to be treated. If a test for TB has not been done recently, he needs to be screened.

It would be helpful to learn from Dean what a typical day is like for him on the streets, especially in terms of managing his diet, medication, and hygiene. Hwang and Bugeja (2000) reported that a group of homeless people with diabetes had identified the following problems in managing their diabetes: the type of food served in shelters, inability to make dietary choices or to coordinate medicines with meals, difficulty obtaining diabetic supplies, and problems with theft of supplies. Dean may experience similar problems.

The nurse needs to be alert to any clues, and to question the client, about why he thinks he has a fever and about any history of elevated blood pressure. Expect the health care provider to order laboratory tests and do an examination to gather additional data about Dean's symptoms. Weight loss can be from many causes, including tuberculosis, cancer, or change in diet. Do not assume low weight is from living on the streets.

The nurse needs to learn if this client has any supportive people in his life. Craig and Timms (2000) point out that there are subgroups of homeless, with the mentally ill making up about a third of this group. One major difference from the other subgroups is that the homeless mentally ill tend to have only "fragmentary ties" to family and anyone of a supportive nature. Reducing isolation is a major focus for the nurse and the health care team.

8. **What findings by the health team would be sufficient to get Dean hospitalized in a psychiatric facility, and what opportunities might hospitalization present?** If the health care team finds that Dean is a danger to himself and/or others, this finding could be sufficient to get him hospitalized in a psychiatric facility. Depending on what beds are available and what admission policies are in place locally, he may or may not have to go through a community mental center for admission or be court committed by a judge. Admission to a psychiatric hospital would provide close observation and evaluation by trained mental health professionals who could follow up on psychiatric symptoms and assess the client's need for neuroleptic (psychotropic, antipsychotic) medication. There would most likely be access to a multidisciplinary team including nurses, social workers, chaplains, recreational therapists, and occupational therapists that can do a holistic assessment of needs and help him with a variety of issues, including obtaining any benefits he is entitled to that he is not now receiving (e.g., social security disability payments, Medicare, Indian benefits, veterans' benefits, and housing such as a group home or a rent subsidized apartment).

9. **What findings might get this client hospitalized in a general hospital, and what opportunities might that present?** If this client's blood sugar level is determined to be high enough to need intervention or if he has foot or leg ulcers or any major health problem, he could be hospitalized in a general hospital. This would present an opportunity for nurses to do further assessment and intervention, such as assessing his knowledge about diabetic self-care. Most hospitals have social workers who could work with Dean to assess his sources of income and his means of access to health care, as well as to help him with housing if he wants to get off the street. The social worker may be able to access sources of funds available to the native Indian population and may be able to work with Dean to get him to the reservation to see a medicine man after discharge. General hospitals often have counselors that work with clients in regard to mental problems and spiritual counselors.

Hospitalization, whether it is in a psychiatric unit or hospital or a medical hospital, provides an opportunity to integrate mental health and medical care.

10. **If you were the nurse in this case, would you want to get Dean off the street and into some other type of living situation? Why or why not? What reasons could he have for wanting to continue living on the streets?** Although you may think it would be safer for Dean and easier for him to control his diet and medications and manage his diabetes if he were in a stable living situation, Dean may not want to stop living on the street. Timms and Borrell (2001) discuss the ethical dilemma of paternalism versus autonomy. It is important to give the homeless mentally ill information about resources but to recognize their right to autonomy. If Dean does not want to leave the streets, you will have to accept this and work with him to do some problem solving about how to manage his diabetes on the street.

    Kasprow and Rosenbeck (1998), in a study involving 36,938 veterans, found that Native American Indians are overrepresented in the homeless population by about 19 percent. Little or nothing is known about why Native American Indian veterans prefer the streets; however, in general clients who prefer to live on the street often do so because of control issues as well as for financial reasons. When these clients try to stay with family or friends, live at the Salvation Army, or live in a group living facility, they usually find there are rules to follow and people to interact with about the rules. In these situations, others often control when and what the client eats or drinks, when they can leave or must leave, and what time the client must be in bed. American Indians and others may prefer living in nature to living with people who control or try to control their lives.

11. **Discuss resources likely to be available in the community for the homeless mentally ill, such as food, clothing, shelter, and medical care.** Many communities have churches or other organizations that provide facilities for the homeless to bathe and shave in, temporary assistance in paying for prescription medication, health clinics for those unable to pay for health care, and places where the homeless can go to get their meals. The Salvation Army is often a community resource for meals and shelter. Libraries usually provide free Internet services, raising the possibility of teaching the homeless to make clinic appointments by e-mail and to chat with the nurse regarding treatment regimen problems and concerns. Beebe (2002) suggests that telephone contact could help stabilize these clients; however, the nurse is more likely to reach a homeless client by e-mail than by telephone.

12. **What nursing diagnoses and interventions would you write for this client?** Possible nursing diagnoses include:

    - Imbalanced nutrition: more than body requirements but recent unexplained weight loss. This needs further assessment for cause, and interventions will be based on cause, although a dietary consult from the dietitian would be helpful.
    - Ineffective therapeutic regimen management. The client has not been taking his medication although he has made efforts to get it. Interventions include: building a trusting relationship, identifying causes for client not taking medication in the past and problem solving to develop a plan to assure he has medication, providing a method to help client remember pills, contracting informally with client to take his medication 100 percent of the time, and teaching client to keep a simple log of medications and responses to medications and to present this log to prescribing health care provider especially if problems arise.
    - Risk for impaired skin integrity: related to complications of diabetes. It is important to assess the skin and to carry out and teach good foot and skin care. Diabetics are known to not heal as well as nondiabetics, so maintaining skin integrity is important for this and other reasons.
    - Risk for peripheral neurovascular dysfunction. Interventions include teaching the client about this problem and prevention through keeping diabetes in control.
    - Disturbed thought processes. Interventions include administering of neuroleptic medication, not challenging delusions, providing earphones and radios to ascertain if listening to the radio reduces disturbed thought processes, and reducing isolation.
    - Social isolation. Interventions include building a trusting relationship and starting with interactions with one other person then building up to small group interactions, teaching leisure skills, teaching how to approach others, and teaching communication skills (assign to communication class if one available).

Develop a follow-up plan to keep contact with the client and evaluate progress toward meeting goals. Explore possible extended family that the client could reestablish contact with.

References

Beebe, L.H. (2002). "Problems in Community Living Identified by People with Schizophrenia." *Journal of Psychosocial Nursing* 40(2): 38–45.

Craig, T. and P. Timms. (2000). "Facing Up to Social Exclusion: Services for Homeless Mentally Ill People." *International Review of Psychiatry* 12(3): 206–212.

Frisch, N.C. and L.E. Frisch. (2006). *Psychiatric Mental Health Nursing, 2nd ed.* Albany, NY: Thomson Delmar Learning.

http://diabetes.niddk.nih.gov/dm/pubs/pima/obesity/obesity.htm. Accessed January 29, 2006.

Hwang, S.W. and Ann L. Bugeja. (2000). "Barriers to Appropriate Diabetes Management among Homeless People in Toronto." *Canadian Medical Association Journal* 163(2): 161–166.

Kasprow, W.J. and R. Rosenbeck. (1998). "Substance Use and Psychiatric Problems of Homeless Native American Veterans." *Psychiatric Service* 49:343–350. Available online at http://ps.psychiatryonline.org/cgi/content/full/49/3/345.

Subramaniam, M., S. Chong, and E. Pek. (2003). "Diabetes Mellitus and Impaired Glucose Tolerance in Patients with Schizophrenia." *Canadian Journal of Psychiatry* 48(5): 345–348.

Timms, P. and T. Borrell. (2001). "Doing the Right Thing: Ethical and Practical Dilemmas in Working with Homeless Mentally Ill People." *Journal of Mental Health* 10(4): 419–427.

www.accessgenealogy.com/native/tribes/pima/pimaindianhist.htm. Accessed January 29, 2006.

www.lungusa.org/site/pp.asp?c=dvLUK900E&b=35804. Accessed September 27, 2005.

www.ninds.nih.gov/disorders/tardive/tardive.htm. Accessed September 27, 2005.

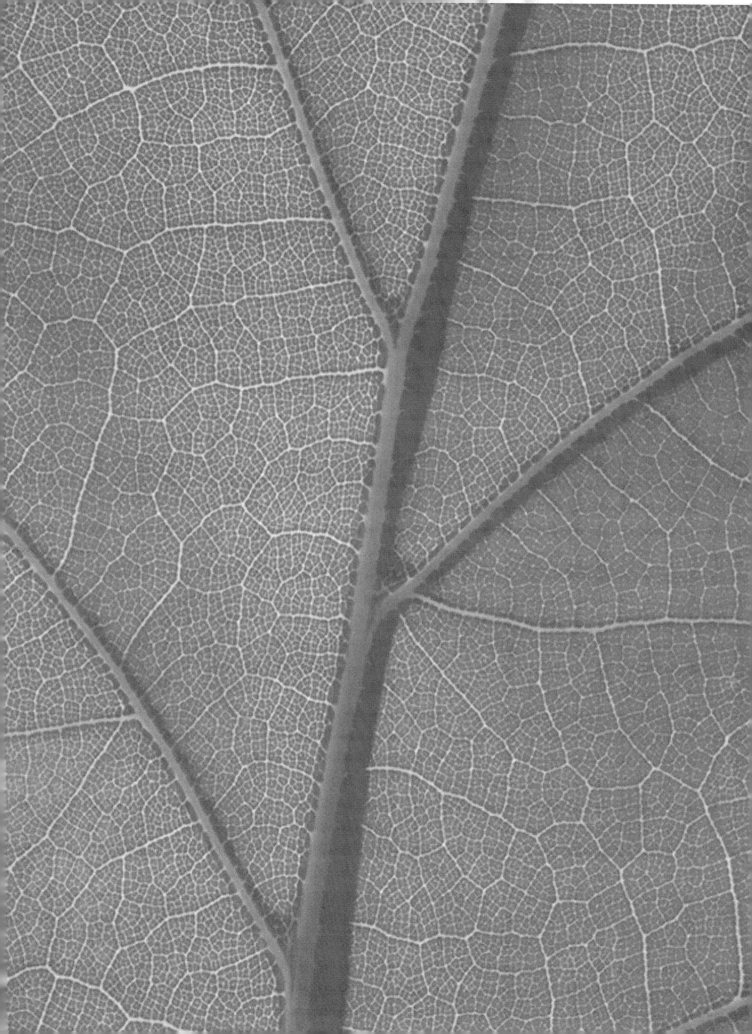

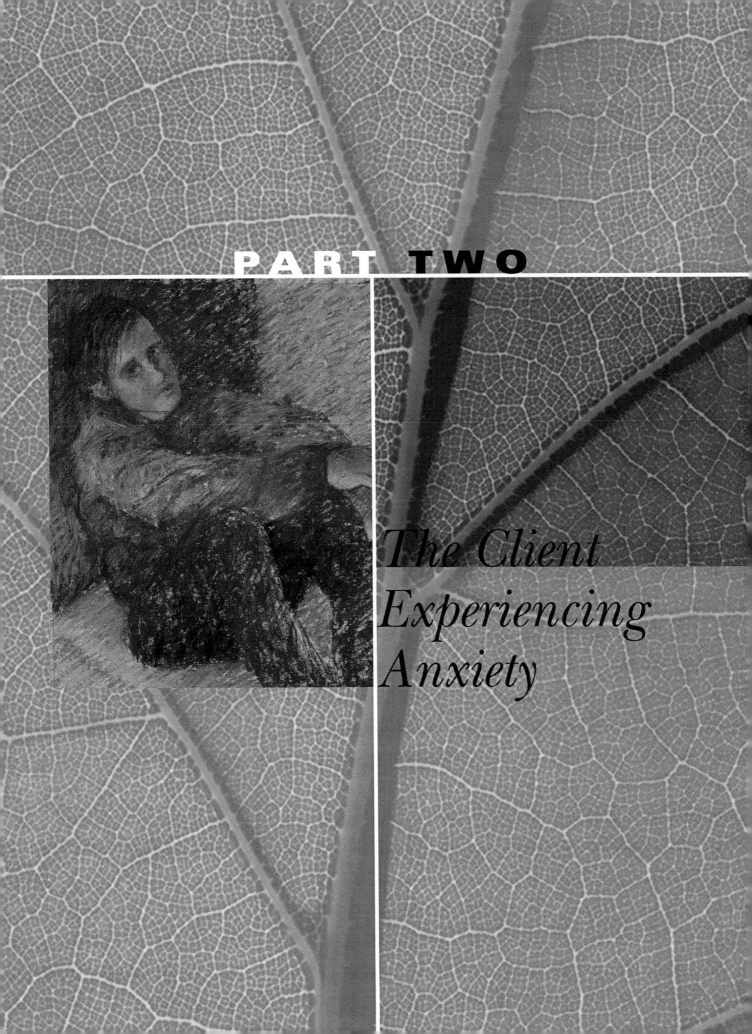

PART TWO

The Client Experiencing Anxiety

Jim

GENDER

Male

AGE

26

SETTING

- Evening outpatient treatment program

ETHNICITY

- White American

CULTURAL CONSIDERATIONS

PREEXISTING CONDITION

COEXISTING CONDITION

- Alcoholism

COMMUNICATION

DISABILITY

SOCIOECONOMIC

SPIRITUAL/RELIGIOUS

PHARMACOLOGIC

- Refusal to eat with or in front of others limits socialization
- Socialization revolves around alcohol

PSYCHOSOCIAL

LEGAL

- Confidentiality
- Informed consent
- DWI

ETHICAL

ALTERNATIVE THERAPY

PRIORITIZATION

DELEGATION

SOCIAL PHOBIA (SOCIAL ANXIETY DISORDER)

Level of difficulty: Moderate

Overview: Requires nurse to use therapeutic communication techniques. The nurse must also use critical thinking to identify her own thinking errors, teach the client and peers to recognize and correct thinking errors, and develop a care plan for a client with dual diagnosis: Social Phobia and Alcohol Abuse.

Client Profile

Jim is a 26-year-old husband and father of a preschool child. He lives and works in a small town in the finance department of an automobile dealership. The main places to gather socially in this small town are churches and bars. Jim prefers the bars where he can watch sports on T.V., talk to people, and drink "a couple of beers" with coworkers and friends. Jim's plan to drink a couple of beers usually turns into a dozen or more beers.

Jim never eats with anyone from work and usually turns down all social engagements that he and his wife are invited to. If he has to attend a work-related social event, he has a feeling that others are looking at him and judging him and he experiences tremors, palpitations, and sweating. Jim never accepts anything to eat at these events. Friends have stopped inviting Jim and his wife to dinner as the invitations are always declined. Jim tells his best friend: "I just don't feel comfortable eating in front of other people. I am afraid I will do something embarrassing and humiliate myself. This sounds unreasonable, even to me; but that is just the way that I am." Jim has been offered a job that pays more money and has better hours, but he would have to take clients to lunch and dinner. He has turned this job down due to his extreme discomfort with eating in public or with anyone other than his immediate family.

Case Study

Jim is attending a nightly outpatient chemical abuse treatment program as part of his follow-up after an inpatient program for substance abuse, a deal his lawyer worked out after he was found guilty of driving while intoxicated. The nurse at the treatment program notices that Jim does not go to the cafeteria with the rest of his group for the evening meal but sits alone in the lobby watching sports on television. The nurse wonders if Jim has enough money to buy dinner and begins to worry that he will be hungry when she does the medication education group later. She thinks about offering him half of her sandwich she brought from home, but stops herself from doing this as she recognizes she has committed a thinking error. The nurse has begun to wonder about Jim and why he seems so reticent, so hesitant to answer questions or share in group sessions or the community meetings. Last time she asked him a question in the community meeting, his face flushed and peers teased him, saying he was blushing like a girl and accusing him of having a crush on the nurse.

The nurse approaches Jim and says: "I notice you did not go to eat with your group."

Questions and Suggested Answers

1. **Was the nurse's decision not to offer Jim half of her sandwich a good idea or not? Give a rationale for your answer. What else could the nurse do?** Yes, this was a good decision. The nurse recognized that she had jumped to a conclusion about Jim being hungry and yet not eating because he has no money. Jumping to a conclusion is one of several thinking errors described by Dr. David Burns (1999). The nurse realized she needs to check with Jim to find out why he is not eating with his peers.

   It could be nontherapeutic for the nurse to offer to share her sandwich as Jim could interpret the sandwich gift in any number of ways. The client could, for example interpret this as the nurse being sexually attracted to him and wanting a social relationship. An appropriate alternative action by the nurse would be to order a sandwich from the cafeteria for the client to eat later in private.

2. **What do you think is the rationale for the nurse's opening remark: "I notice you did not go to eat with your group"? What therapeutic communication techniques are you familiar with that could be used in communication with Jim?** The nurse is making an observation, one of several therapeutic communication techniques that are nonthreatening to clients and designed to facilitate communication. The remark is neither approval nor disapproval. This is a good opening remark that may elicit some comments from the client about his discomfort about eating in front of others.

In addition to the technique of observation, therapeutic communication techniques include using broad openings (e.g., "Where would you like to begin?"); encouraging (e.g., "Tell me more" or "Go on"); refocusing (e.g., "Lets go back to when you said _____"); summarizing (e.g., "So far we have talked about _____ and _____"); offering self (e.g., "I have some time to talk with you this morning"); and using silence (i.e., sitting with the client in silence and waiting as long as it takes for the client to say something).

3. **How do you think the nurse could best deal with the peers' comments about Jim blushing?** One of many ways to handle this situation is to point out to the peer who attributed Jim's blushing to a crush on the nurse that this is jumping to a conclusion and to direct him to check with Jim about what is going on. The nurse can work with the group in terms of recognizing Burns's (1999)"thinking errors." Thinking errors include magnifying, minimizing, catastrophising, and "hop-overs" (pointing the finger at someone else's behavior to avoid confronting one's own behavior). The nurse needs to encourage members to call each other on "thinking errors and to identify when they are making thinking errors themselves."

4. **What is Social Phobia? Do you think this client has signs and symptoms that match those of Social Phobia (Social Anxiety Disorder)? Give a rationale for your answer.** Social Phobia involves a persistent, high level of fear about a social or performance situation or situations where others could judge or evaluate the person, leading to embarrassment. It can be about a fear of speaking in public, taking tests, meeting new people, performing in public, eating in public, or interacting with others in some way in a social situation. See the table on Social Phobia criteria that this client meets and the rationale.

Criteria for Social Phobia	Client
Marked and persistent fear of at least one social or performance situation where there are unfamiliar people who may judge or evaluate. The person fears their actions or their anxiety symptoms will be embarrassing or humiliating.	Yes, the client has a fear of eating in front of people outside his immediate family. He fears he will do something to embarrass himself and others will judge him.
Anxiety almost always occurs when exposed to the dreaded social situation. Anxiety can take the form of a situationally bound or predisposed panic attack.	Yes, the client had tremors, palpitations, and sweating on the rare occasions when he has sat down to eat in public.
Client recognizes fear as excessive or unreasonable.	To be assessed. The client has made a statement that this fear of eating in public sounds unreasonable even to himself, but that this is just the way he is. He probably realizes that his fears are different and excessive, knowing that other people do not turn down jobs because of a fear of eating in public, but this is to be assessed with an open mind.
Client avoids feared social or performance situation or endures it with extreme anxiety or distress.	Yes.
There is significant interference with the client's normal routine, academic or occupational functioning, social activities or relationships because of the avoidance, anxious anticipation, or distress regarding feared social or performance situations. The client exhibits marked distress about having the phobia.	Yes, the fear interference with the client's ability to eat socially with others and limits him to jobs where social dining with others is not required.
Fear or avoidance not due to physiological effects of a substance or medical condition or mental disorder.	Even though client uses/abuses alcohol, it is reasonably clear that his fear of eating in public is not caused by the alcohol use.

(Adapted from APA, 2000)

5. **Are there any differences in the signs and symptoms of children with Social Phobia compared to those of adults?** There are a few differences in the signs and symptoms of children with this disorder and in the criteria for children to meet the diagnosis of Social Phobia. Children with this disorder may not recognize the fear as excessive or unreasonable. For children to be diagnosed with Social Phobia they must have the capacity to have age-appropriate social relationships with persons who are familiar to them and their anxiety must be not just with adults but in peer settings. Clients under age 18 have to have duration of signs and symptoms for at least six months to receive a diagnosis.

6. **What are some theories of causation of Social Phobia?** The cause of Social Phobia is unknown. It has been suggested by some researchers that this disorder is hereditary based on family and twin studies. Tilfors (2004) reviewed the literature on Social Phobia and found that "studies suggest that Social Phobia does have a neuroanatomical basis in a highly sensitive fear network centered in the amygdaloid-hippocampal region, i.e. 'the alarm system' of the brain and encompassing the prefrontal cortex."

   A theory proposed in the 1970s by Mussen suggests that some children have hypersensitive nervous systems at birth and low thresholds for anxiety and fear. How much support and nurturance the parents give this child in early life is then an important factor in whether they develop Social Phobia (Curtis, Kimball, and Stroup, 2004). It has been suggested that children learn anxious behaviors from anxious parents modeling anxious responses in given situation. It has also been suggested that parents' warnings and excessive instructions may contribute to development of Social Phobia.

   There are some studies and speculation about ethnic/cultural factors in the development of Social Phobia, for example, some Asian ethnic/cultural groups have an emphasis on humility and avoiding embarrassment and shame (Okazaki, 2003).

   The most common theme of various researchers is that a combination of factors is involved. Curtis, Kimball, and Stroup (2004, 5) state: "It appears that genetics, the type, and amount of nurturance and parental instructions received as a child and societal trends all interact to play a role in developing and maintaining this disorder." The reality is that we really don't know what causes Social Phobia and it may be different combinations of factors in different clients.

7. **What is the incidence of Social Phobia?** Social Phobia (Social Anxiety Disorder) is currently thought to be the most common phobia. The lifetime incidence of this disorder is estimated to be about 14 percent in the population of the United States. At any one time it is estimated to affect 2–13 percent of the population in the United States. Various studies have found that only about 20 percent of the people who report Social

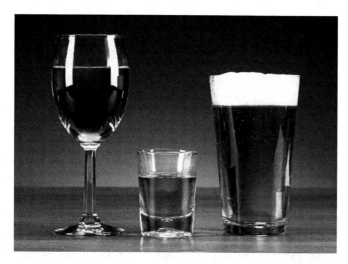

About 20 percent of clients with social anxiety disorder also have an alcohol use disorder.

Phobia say that it interferes with their lives and seek professional help, and only 6 percent use medication to treat Social Phobia (Curtis, Kimball, and Stroup, 2004).

8. **What other disorders or problems are common in the population experiencing Social Phobia? Could there be a connection between this client's drinking and Social Phobia (Social Anxiety Disorder)? If so, how would you assess for a connection?** About 20 percent of clients with Social Anxiety Disorder also have an alcohol use disorder (AUD). An AUD is either alcohol dependence or abuse (Book and Randall, 2002). Other common comorbidity problems include depression and obsessive-compulsive disorder.

There could be a connection between the client's drinking and Social Phobia. People with high levels of social anxiety have typically reported thinking that alcohol helps them to feel more comfortable and to cope in social settings (Book and Randall, 2002). While alcohol is a depressant, it also lowers inhibitions and may initially tend to increase a person's socialization level. Alcohol, for some clients, may represent a form of self-medicating.

In assessing this client, questions would be designed to determine if the Social Phobia came before the drinking and if the pattern of drinking suggests using alcohol to relieve stress and/or anxiety. After rapport is built the nurse can ask the client about his fear of eating in public and encourage him, through therapeutic communication techniques, to describe when this fear began, what he is thinking about and experiencing when he is in a feared situation, and what he does to relieve his anxiety/fear. Jim may have had this fear of eating in public since he was a child. This client could have discovered early on that drinking seemed to help him deal with his anxiety, he could have an inherited genetic predisposition to addiction, or he could simply have fallen into a pattern of heavy social drinking. The nurse needs to get a good family history of alcoholism as well as a history of the client's use/abuse.

Clients often minimize their alcohol intake, so check with others to see if the client is being truthful. If a client fears embarrassment, he might fear disclosing the true amount of his alcoholic beverage consumption.

9. **What is the current thinking about heredity and alcohol abuse? What are some current treatments for those with early onset alcoholism?** A recent Harvard Mental Health Letter from the Harvard Medical School ("Drug Treatment for Alcoholism Today," July 2005) announced that researchers have possibly found a new treatment for early onset alcoholism in an anti-nausea drug used in the treatment of cancer, ondansetron (Zofran). The same article mentions a new blood test used in the study of ondansetron for treating alcoholism, which may soon be given to clients in alcohol abuse treatment centers, presumably to identify an inherited form of early onset alcoholism. Researchers have long suspected that there is a biochemical difference in people who have early onset alcoholism (an inherited form of alcoholism usually exhibited before age 25) compared to those who become addicted later in life and/or drink to treat their depression and/or anxiety.

Traditional treatments for alcohol abuse include: the twelve-step program, Alcoholics Anonymous (AA), confrontation, psychodrama, transactional analysis, education about the disease, assertiveness training, self-esteem building, Cognitive Behavioral Therapy (which includes thinking errors mentioned earlier), and others.

The Harvard Mental Health Letter ("Motivational Interviewing," March 2005) describes Motivational Enhancement Therapy (MET) for treatment of alcohol abuse. This therapy became popular in the 1990s and continues to be used not only for alcohol abuse but other conditions as well. About ten years ago the National Institute of Mental Health sponsored researchers who conducted Project MATCH, a large clinical trial comparing three treatments for alcohol abuse: Cognitive Behavior Therapy, twelve-step programs, and MET. All three were found to be equally effective; however, MET cost less and took less time. One part of MET is Motivational Interviewing (MI), which is based on four principles: 1. express empathy; 2. develop discrepancy; 3. roll with resistance; and 4. support self-efficacy. In MI the therapist works as a partner, not an expert. Graham (2004), a nurse who uses MI with clients, casts doubt on whether MI is for every client with alcohol problems. She suggests that no one treatment fits all.

10. **What are some of the current treatments being used to treat Social Phobia?** Exposure therapy is a common treatment modality for Social Phobia. The therapist develops a rapport with the client and sets up situations in which the client is helped to gradually face his or her feared situation. The client who fears riding in an airplane could begin by role-playing riding in a plane, followed by going to the airport, followed by a short plane ride with a trusted relative or friend, followed by a short trip without a companion. The person who fears public speaking might stand at the podium, then give a two-minute talk at the podium to the therapist, and gradually increase the exposure. It is helpful if the person is taught some relaxation techniques such as relaxation breathing, biofeedback, or guided imagery.

    Cognitive Behavioral Therapy (CBT) is a therapy commonly used to treat Social Phobia. This therapy recognizes three cognitive stages (three thinking steps) that a person with Social Phobia goes through. First there is anticipatory processing. The client perceives negative feedback from others or imagines that it will occur. The person worries excessively and becomes very apprehensive about an upcoming social interaction. The second stage is in-situation processing during which the self-talk increases and the client is acutely tuned to the early warning signs of anxiety. The person may begin to take safety precautions like looking often at the nearest exit, drinking alcohol, and not giving eye contact to others. At this time the person with Social Phobia is so focused on their anxiety that they may make social mistakes like not remembering names or talking or laughing excessively. The third stage is postmortem, in which the person scrutinizes the past interaction (Curtis, Kimball, and Stroup, 2004). The therapist works with the client to recognize these stages and change the thoughts at each stage. The client learns to say things like "I will put food on my plate and I will put a bite in my mouth and eat it successfully." This is referred to as guided self-dialog.

    Pharmacotherapy may be helpful. Medications prescribed for clients with Social Phobia includes SSRIs. Sometimes benzodiazepines such as alprazolam (Xanax), Lorazepam (Ativan), and clonazepam (Klonopin) are prescribed (Book and Randall, 2002). These benzodiazepines are controlled substances and although helpful in alleviating symptoms of social phobia, they are cautiously prescribed and may not be advisable when there is alcoholism or other substance addiction.

    Virtual Reality Therapy is also used in the treatment of Social Phobia in settings where professionals have the training and equipment to carry it out. Rothbaum of Emory University and Hodges at the University of North Carolina introduced this therapy in the 1990s to treat a variety of fears such as fear of public speaking, fear of spiders, PTSD, and others. In this therapy the client is exposed to the feared situation gradually in a virtual reality setting using specially created software. There are sound effects to mimic an actual situation. The participant may wear a glove that tracks the position of their hand, they may use a joystick to move through a program, or in some cases scenes are presented through a special helmet. Programs can be individually developed to fit the client's feared situation, such as public speaking before a virtual audience. Through this method the therapist exposes the client gradually to stimuli that activate emotions and teaches the client to modulate their fear response to a healthier response. "Patients can get relief from pain or overcome their phobias by immersing themselves in computer generated worlds" (Hoffman, 2004).

11. **What nursing diagnoses would you likely write for this client?** Nursing diagnoses could likely include some of the following diagnoses:

    - Impaired social interaction
    - Altered role performance
    - Dysfunctional family processes: alcoholism
    - Ineffective coping
    - Deficient diversional activity
    - Chronic or situational low self-esteem
    - Anxiety

12. **Discuss possible goals and interventions for this client. Is it possible to treat the alcoholism and the Social Phobia concurrently?** The goals need to be set with the client as a participant in goal setting. The client will be more motivated to achieve goals if they are his or her goals. One possible goal for this client would be to eat at least 50 percent of a meal while eating with one staff member that the client trusts. When this is

accomplished, a new goal could be to eat a meal with a peer and gradually increase this to two, then three peers.

Goals can also relate to the client's problem with alcohol. Even if he is using alcohol to self-medicate, it has gotten him into legal trouble and his outpatient program is likely teaching abstinence. Goals may include finding alternative ways to deal with stress, doing the twelve-step work of Alcoholics Anonymous, or finding an AA sponsor who has been clean and sober for some designated period of time. Another goal could be related to finding at least one friend who does not drink alcoholic beverages and to scheduling some social event with this friend each week.

Interventions might include role-playing a dinner party with a guest, saying no to friends who offer alcoholic drinks, communication group, work on self-esteem, substance abuse education groups, journaling, and activity sessions to teach and encourage hobbies and ways to have fun without drinking. Many of the interventions mentioned above relate well to relieving both the alcoholism and Social Phobia.

References

American Psychiatric Association. (2000). *Diagnostic and Statistical Manual of Mental Disorders, 4th ed.* Text Revision. Washington, DC: American Psychiatric Association.

Book, S.W. and C.L. Randall. (2002). Social Anxiety Disorder and Alcohol Use. *Alcohol Research and Health* 26(2): 130–136.

Burns, D. (1999). *Feeling Good: The New Mood Therapy.* Rev. ed. New York: Harper and Collins.

Curtis, R.C., A. Kimball, and E.L. Stroup. (2004). "Understanding and Treating Social Phobia." *Journal of Counseling and Development* 82(1): 3–10.

"Drug Treatment for Alcoholism Today." (July 2005). *Harvard Mental Health Letter* 22(1): 3–5.

Graham, J. (2004). "Motivational Interviewing: A Hammer Looking for a Nail." *Journal of Psychiatric and Mental Health Nursing* 11(4): 494–497.

Hoffman, H.G. (2004). "Virtual-Reality Therapy." *Scientific American* 291(2): 58–65.

"Motivational Interviewing: An Approach to Counseling for Behavioral Change Attracts Growing Interest." (March 2005). *Harvard Mental Health Letter* 21(9): 5–6.

Okazaki, S. (2003). "Expressions of Social Anxiety in Asian-Americans." *Psychiatric Times* 20(10): 76–79.

Tilfors, M. (2004). "Why Do Some Individuals Develop Social Phobia? A Review with Emphasis on the Neurobiological Influences." *Nordic Journal of Psychiatry* 58(4): 267–276.

MODERATE

GENDER

Female

AGE

50

SETTING

- Community mental health center

ETHNICITY

- Mexican American

CULTURAL CONSIDERATIONS

- Hispanic

PREEXISTING CONDITION

COEXISTING CONDITION

COMMUNICATION

DISABILITY

SOCIOECONOMIC

- Daughter of migrant farmers; currently middle class

SPIRITUAL/RELIGIOUS

PHARMACOLOGIC

- Calcium
- Vitamins
- Hormone replacement
- Buspirone (BuSpar)

PSYCHOSOCIAL

- Impaired social isolation

LEGAL

ETHICAL

ALTERNATIVE THERAPY

- Herbal treatments containing Kava and Passaflora obtained from a curandara

PRIORITIZATION

DELEGATION

GENERALIZED ANXIETY DISORDER

Level of difficulty: Moderate

Overview: Requires critical thinking to understand and manage the common Hispanic practice of extended family being with a client for health care visits. The nurse must also identify behaviors common in clients with a diagnosis of Generalized Anxiety Disorder (GAD) and become knowledgeable about treatment modalities, including the antidepressant BuSpar.

Client Profile

Betty, a 50-year-old woman, came to this country with her parents when she was 7 years old. The family members worked as migrant farm workers until they had enough money to open a restaurant. Betty married young. She and her husband worked in the family restaurant and eventually bought it from the parents. They raised seven children, all grown and living on their own. Betty and her husband live in a mobile home close to the restaurant. She does not work in the family restaurant anymore because she worries excessively about doing a poor job. Betty no longer goes out if she can help it. She stays at home worrying about how she looks, what people think or say, the weather or road conditions, and many other things. Betty is not sleeping at night and keeps her husband awake when she roams the house. She keeps her clothing and belongings in perfect order while claiming she is doing a poor job of it. She does not prepare large family dinners anymore, though she still cooks the daily meals; one daughter has taken over the family dinners. This daughter has become concerned about Betty being isolated at home and worrying excessively and calls the community mental health center for an appointment for Betty.

Case Study

Betty presents at the community mental health center accompanied by her husband, her children and their spouses, several grandchildren, and a few cousins. When Betty's name is called and she is told that the nurse is ready to see her, she frowns and says: "What will I say? I don't know what to say. I think my slip is showing. My hem isn't straight."

Betty says she wants her whole family to go in to see the nurse with her. The nurse notices that Betty is extremely well groomed and dressed in spite of concerns she has been voicing about her appearance. Before the psychiatric nurse interviews Betty alone, she hears from the daughter that Betty "worries all the time" and although she has always been known to be a worrier, the worrying has become worse over the past six or eight months. The husband shares that his wife is keeping him awake at night with her inability to get to sleep or stay asleep.

The nurse interviews Betty alone. The nurse notices that Betty casts her eyes downward, speaks in a soft voice, does not smile, and seems restless as she taps her foot on the floor, drums her fingers on the table, and seems on the verge of getting out of her chair. Themes in the interview include: being tired, getting tired easily, not being able to concentrate, not getting work done, trouble sleeping, worrying about whether her husband loves her anymore and whether she and her husband have enough money, and not having the energy to attend to the housework or her clothing.

The nurse has the impression that Betty's anxiety floats from one worry to another. There is no convincing Betty that she looks all right. Any attempt to convince her that she need not worry about something in particular leads to a different worry before coming back to the earlier worry.

The community mental health psychiatrist examines Betty and, after a thorough physical examination and lab studies, finds nothing to explain her fatigue and difficulty sleeping other than anxiety. Betty produces her medicine bottles and says she is currently taking only vitamins, hormone replacement, and calcium. The psychiatrist asks the nurse to contact Betty's family health care provider to get information on any medical or psychiatric conditions he is treating her for; the report comes back that she has no medical diagnoses and the family health care provider thinks she suffers from anxiety. The psychiatrist prescribes buspirone (BuSpar) for Betty.

Two weeks later, during a home visit to Betty, the nurse learns, with some probing, that Betty is upset with her husband for loaning all their savings to the daughter and her husband to build a new home, while they continue to live in an older mobile home. At the end of the nurse's home visit, Betty's daughter arrives and tells the nurse that she wonders if Betty is making any progress. Betty also worries she is not getting better and asks the nurse about taking some herbal medicines containing Kava and Passaflora that her sister got from a curandara (folk healer); her sister wants to take her to see the curandara and have her do a ritual to cure the evil eye that was placed on Betty and made her sick.

Questions and Suggested Answers

1. **What behaviors does this client have that match the criteria for a diagnosis of Generalized Anxiety Disorder?** In order to meet the criteria for a diagnosis of Generalized Anxiety Disorder (GAD), a person must have "excessive anxiety and worry" and "apprehensive expectation" occurring on more days than it does not occur for at least six months and involving a variety of worries about various events or activities. The person has to find it difficult to control the anxiety and worry. In addition, the person must have at least three other symptoms from a list including restlessness, fatiguing easily, concentration difficulties, irritability, muscle tension, and sleep problems, which include difficulty getting asleep, difficulty staying asleep, or feeling as if the sleep has not satisfied their needs (APA, 2000). Betty has had excessive worry most days for over six months. The nurse observed this client's restless behavior and heard her complaints of fatigue. The client's husband described her failure to sleep at night.

   In addition to the criteria already mentioned, the person diagnosed as having GAD must experience significant distress or impairment in some area of functioning, such as social or occupational, as a result of the anxiety, worry, or physical symptoms. Betty has experienced impairment in both social and occupational areas of her life as a result of her anxiety and worry.

2. **How common is the diagnosis of Generalized Anxiety Disorder? Is it common for clients with GAD to have comorbidity, and should this client be assessed for any particular condition?** According to Mason and Jacobson (1999), Generalized Anxiety will affect one in twenty adults sometime during their lives and most of those affected will be women. This is congruent with the DSM IV-TR statement that the lifetime prevalence rate of GAD was 5 percent based on a community sample.

   A large percentage of people with GAD are believed to have a comorbid diagnosis. Wells (1999) describes one national comorbid survey that found more than 90 percent of those with a diagnosis of GAD had a comorbid diagnosis, with 22 percent experiencing dysthymis and 39–69 percent experiencing depression. This client needs to be screened for symptoms of mood disorders.

3. **What explanation do you have for the number of family members coming to the community mental health center with this client? If you were the nurse, how would you deal with Betty's request for her whole family to accompany her to see you?** Hispanic and Hispanic Americans are often part of a large extended family system. It is not unusual for extended family members to accompany a Hispanic or Hispanic American person to the office of health care providers or to a health care facility.

   You need to build some rapport with the family, and this involves respecting the family and their culture, acknowledging each family member, and accepting any input given voluntarily from family members. When the client has medical problems, the nurse can perform most if not all procedures with family members present. When the client has mental health problems, it is important to observe interactions with others, but it is also exceedingly important to talk with the client alone so the client's issues can be explored in a therapeutic environment with a professional and without the distraction of family members.

4. **Before the nurse, or any other staff at the community mental health center, can talk with Betty's family health care provider, what do they need to do?** Before talking with the family health care provider about Betty's case, the nurse needs to get a release of information form signed by Betty.

5. **What does the nurse need to know about buspirone? What teaching needs to be done with the client in regard to buspirone? What medications other than buspirone are being used in the treatment of GAD, and how effective are they?** The nurse needs to know the following information about buspirone:

   • It binds to serotonin and dopamine receptors increases norepinephrine metabolism in the brain.
   • It is contraindicated in hypersensitivity and severe hepatic or renal impairment.
   • Usual dose is 20–30 mg/day and is not to exceed 60mg/day.
   • Concurrent use with itraconazole or erythromycin increases blood levels and dosage reduction may need to occur if using these drugs.

- Patients changing from other antianxiety drugs to BuSpar should be gradually tapered off their other antianxiety meds before being placed on BuSpar.
- While some improvement may occur in seven to ten days, optimal improvement takes three to four weeks.

Teaching about buspirone needs to include the following information:

- Buspirone is given for the management of anxiety.
- It must be taken exactly as directed.
- Although food slows absorption, this drug may be taken with food to decrease gastric irritation. It needs to be taken either consistently with or consistently without food.
- Alcohol and other CNS depressants are not to be concurrently used.
- Client should consult health care provider before taken any over-the-counter drugs.
- Client should notify health care provider if any abnormal movements noticed while on this drug.
- Side effects can include dizziness and drowsiness so client shouldn't drive until he or she knows the medication is not going to cause these side effects.
- Client should keep follow-up appointments to evaluate effectiveness of medication (Spratto and Woods, 2006).

In addition to buspirone, venlafaxine extended release therapy (Effexor XR) has been found to be effective in treating the symptoms of Generalized Anxiety Disorder (Rose, 1998). Imipramine, opirpramol, paroxetine, and trazodone have also been found to improve symptoms over four to eight weeks (Newman, Consoli, and Andres, 1999).

6. **What are some of the interventions, in addition to antianxiety drugs, that are being used with clients who have GAD?** Cognitive Behavioral Therapy is one of a number of treatment modalities used today with patients who have a diagnosis of GAD. Wells (1999) describes a model in which generalized anxiety is an abnormal state of worrying involving worry about worrying. In the therapy, worry is used as a strategy to control worry and put it to work.

   Newman and Consoli (1999) report a palmtop computer program that can be used to increase the efficiency of Cognitive Behavioral Therapy in working with clients with GAD. The program, as they describe it, assists in ongoing unobtrusive gathering of data about treatment adherence and the impact of the therapy techniques. The computer draws the treatment out beyond the hour with the therapists and motivates clients to do homework assignments by "prompting practice of cognitive behavioral strategies."

7. **At one point the daughter says that she thinks Betty is not showing progress. What progress, if any, do you think has been made? What can you tell the daughter?** The client has made some progress in the area of "trust" and developing trusting relationships. Betty confided her feelings and thoughts about the husband loaning money to the daughter. You can tell the daughter that the medication Betty is taking has a slow onset of action: it tends to require at least two weeks to show benefits and longer for maximum benefit. Frisch and Frisch (2006) point out that the effect of buspirone is delayed, often as much as seven weeks, but it can be as effective as benzodiazepines in controlling anxiety/worry without the abuse potential of benzodiazepines.

8. **What do you think about Betty's sister using herbal remedies and rituals for driving out evil spirits in trying to cure Betty? Do herbal remedies work?** Many herbal remedies do produce some beneficial effects, and herbals are used in the development of new medicines; however, the nurse in this case must caution Betty about the possibility of her herbal medication interacting negatively with her prescribed medications, as well as a lack of control on the quality of herbal medicines. The nurse needs to advise her to check with her prescribing health acre provider before taking herbals. Kava has been found to have an effect on vagal cardiac control in Generalized Anxiety Disorder (Watkins et al. 2001). According to Akhondzadeh et al. (2001), Passaflora (passionflower) is an old folk remedy for anxiety. Treatment effectiveness of passaflora was compared to that of oxazepam (Serax) in a double-blind randomized trial. While oxazepam results were

seen quicker, this drug produced impairment of job performance whereas passaflora was found to be effective with a much lower incidence of job performance impairment.

Rituals to drive out evil spirits may help decrease anxiety for some people. If a person believes strongly enough that a ritual will drive out evil spirits, it could possibly stop the worry or reduce the time spent in worrying.

9. **What nursing diagnoses would you write for Betty related to her Generalized Anxiety Disorder?** Possible nursing diagnoses based on the assessment of Betty's generalized anxiety include:

- Anxiety
- Impaired social interaction
- Social isolation
- Altered role performance

References

Akhondzadeh, S. et al. (2001). "Passionflower in the Treatment of Generalized Anxiety: A Pilot Double-blind Randomized Controlled Trial With Oxazepam." *Journal of Clinical Pharmacy and Therapeutics* 26(5): 363–368.

American Psychiatric Association. (2000). *Diagnostic and Statistical Manual of Mental Disorders, 4th Ed.* Text Revision. Washington, DC: American Psychiatric Association.

Frisch, N.C. and L.E. Frisch. (2006). *Psychiatric Mental Health Nursing, 3d ed.* Albany, NY: Thomson Delmar Learning.

Mason, M. and D. Jacobson. (1999). "Don't Worry, Be Happy." *Health* 13(3): 66–71.

Newman, M.G., G. Consoli, and J. Andres. (1999). "A Palmtop Computer Program for the Treatment of Generalized Anxiety Disorder." *Behavior Modification* 23(4): 597–622.

Rose, V. (1998). "Drug Shows Promise in Treatment of Generalized Anxiety Disorder." *American Family Physician* 58(4): 947.

Spratto, G.R. and A.L. Woods. (2006). *PDR Nurse's Drug Handbook.* Clifton Park NY: Thomson Delmar, 183–186.

Watkins, L.L., K.M. Connor, and J. Davidson. (2001). "Effect of Kava Extract on Vagal Cardiac Control in Generalized Anxiety Disorder: Preliminary Findings." *Journal of Psychopharmacology* 15(4): 283–291.

Wells, A. (1999). "A Cognitive Model of Generalized Anxiety Disorder." *Behavior Modification* 23(4): 526–556.

GENDER	DISABILITY
Female	
AGE	SOCIOECONOMIC
19	
SETTING	SPIRITUAL/RELIGIOUS
■ Day treatment program in psychiatric hospital	■ Voodoo
	PHARMACOLOGIC
ETHNICITY	■ Paroxetine (Paxil)
■ White American	PSYCHOSOCIAL
CULTURAL CONSIDERATIONS	
■ Cajun, voodoo beliefs	LEGAL
PREEXISTING CONDITION	ETHICAL
	ALTERNATIVE THERAPY
COEXISTING CONDITION	
■ Agoraphobia	PRIORITIZATION
COMMUNICATION	DELEGATION

PANIC DISORDER WITH AGORAPHOBIA

Level of difficulty: High

Overview: Requires the nurse to develop an understanding of Agoraphobia and Panic Disorder and to use critical thinking to teach the client ways to minimize symptoms of a panic attack and overcome a fear of leaving her house. The nurse must also help a client's peers understand that voodoo beliefs can be cultural practices, not psychosis.

DIFFICULT

Client Profile

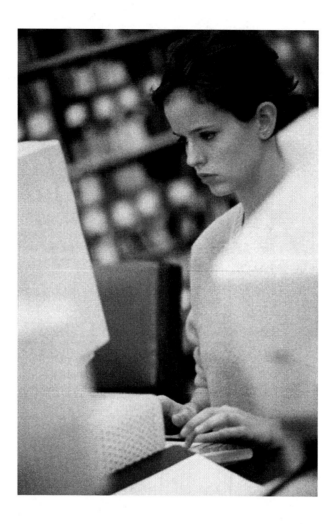

Caroline, a 19-year-old college student from rural Louisiana, is attending a large university in a nearby state. Caroline was doing well at the university until she experienced several unexpected panic attacks. She had a panic attack in the undergraduate library and another one when she went to the gym to work out. The most recent attack occurred about a month ago when she was driving her car. Suddenly and for no reason she could think of, she began feeling short of breath. It "felt like someone was smothering" her, but she was alone in the car. She was afraid she was going to die. Her heart was going very fast; she became dizzy and was feeling numbness and tingling in her hands. She felt a sense of impending danger and wanting to escape. She was so panicked that she had to pull over into a convenience store parking lot and wait until she felt better to call her boyfriend and ask him to come and take her home.

Caroline rode the bus to campus to classes for a while after this panic attack. She parked her car and refused to drive anywhere. She began fearing another panic attack and started skipping classes. A big school football game and party is coming up, and the boyfriend threatens to break up with Caroline if she does not "get a grip."

Case Study

Caroline's mother receives a call from Caroline's roommate telling her of the situation. Her mother takes Caroline to see a psychiatrist who prescribes paroxetine (Paxil) 10 mg/day and suggests an outpatient evening treatment program. Treatment in the evening allows Caroline to go to classes in the daytime. Caroline attends the first two nights of group and individual therapy. Her mother drives Caroline to the evening program on these nights. During group therapy Caroline reveals a fear that she has some life-threatening illness that the doctor has not found on a recent annual physical. Later in group she says she thinks someone has put a voodoo spell on her.

On the third night, Caroline is to take a cab or bus to the evening sessions because her mother has gone back home. It is two hours before the evening program is to begin. Caroline calls the nurse in the outpatient evening treatment program, saying: "I am too afraid to leave the house. I'm sorry. I just can't come tonight. Perhaps I will be able to come tomorrow." The nurse responds, "I want you to take several deep breaths and think about relaxing. Now that you feel very relaxed, I want you to visualize in your mind walking to the door and opening it."

Questions and Suggested Answers:

1. **What is the difference between a panic attack and panic disorder? What symptoms does Caroline have, and do they match the criteria for a diagnosis of Panic Disorder?** A panic attack is one event during a discrete period of time in which the person suddenly experiences intense fear or discomfort, displaying at least four of thirteen cognitive or somatic symptoms. Caroline has at least six of the thirteen symptoms of panic attack.

Thirteen somatic and cognitive symptoms associated with panic attack	Does client Caroline has these symptoms?
Palpitations	Yes
Trembling	
Feeling short of breath or sensation of smothering	Yes
Feeling of choking	Yes
Chest pain or discomfort	
Nausea or abdominal distress	
Sweating	
Dizziness or light headedness	Yes
Derealization or depersonalization	
Fear of losing control or going crazy	
Fear of dying	Yes
Paresthesias	Yes
Chills or hot flushes	

After a sudden onset, a panic attack reaches a peak usually in ten minutes or less; the person may feel a sense of impending doom or danger and wanting to escape. Caroline's last panic attack built to such a peak in ten minutes or less. Panic attacks are divided into three types: unexpected, situationally bound, and situationally predisposed, but only the unexpected type counts in a diagnosis of Panic Disorder (APA, 2000). Caroline's panic attacks seem unexpected because they occurred in a variety of situations. A person must have at least two unexpected panic attacks for a diagnosis of Panic Disorder. In addition, at least one of the attacks has to be followed by a month or more of one or more of the following: persistent worry about more attacks to come, worry about implications of the attack such as dying or going crazy, and/or significant change of behavior related to the attacks (e.g., stopping driving, stopping school attendance, quitting a job).

Physiological causes (e.g., drug abuse, prescription medication, and hyperthyroidism) and other mental disorders have to be ruled out. Provided the health care provider rules out physiological causes for panic attacks, it would appear that Caroline meets the criteria for the disorder.

Note: When a client presents with less than four somatic or cognitive symptoms but meets the rest of the criteria for a panic attack, this is called a limited-symptom attack.

2. **What is the usual onset of panic attacks and Panic Disorder? Is there a gender difference in the prevalence of panic attacks and Panic Disorder?** The age of onset varies but it is usually between late adolescence and the mid-thirties (APA, 2000). The usual onset is in the early twenties (Kwok, Chow, Holt, and Chow, 2003).

   The 2002 National Comorbidity Survey suggests that Panic Disorder is 5.5 times more prevalent in women than in males, with the gender difference increasing with age (Kwok, Chow, Holt and Chow, 2003).

3. **Caroline has Agoraphobia. What is Agoraphobia and what symptoms of this problem does Caroline exhibit?** Agoraphobia can occur with or without Panic Disorder. Anxiety about being in certain places or situations where escape would not be easy or could be embarrassing is an essential feature of Agoraphobia.

   When a person has Panic Disorder, they often have anticipatory fear of the next panic attack and become fearful of being in a place or situation where they cannot get help for their panic attack or cannot escape from the feared situation. Frequently people with Agoraphobia have a zone of safety, such as their own home or their neighborhood. If they get outside this zone, they get anxious. Occasionally a person with Agoraphobia refuses to leave home alone, but will go if a particular person goes with them.

4. **How can Caroline's significant others (e.g., mother, boyfriend, roommate, classmates, and peers in group) best support her in dealing with panic attacks and Agoraphobia?** It will be helpful if Caroline's significant others receive some teaching by the nurse and/or read about Panic Disorder with Agoraphobia in order to better understand what she is experiencing. If people understand that the treatment that is most successful includes medication and specific types of therapy, then they will more likely support her in ways that facilitate attending therapy sessions and taking her medication. Classmates and her roommate may be able to get classroom assignments to her and perhaps taped lecture sessions. They can learn how to get her to take small steps toward going to class.

   The nurse can also help Caroline verbalize what specific support she needs from her significant others.

5. **One of Caroline's group of peers shares with the nurse that he thinks Caroline is psychotic and is paranoid and delusional about somebody putting a spell on her. If you were the nurse, how would you respond?** You can give the peer some positive feedback for coming to you with this concern and for checking it out. You can tell the peer that people of all races and social classes can experience panic attacks and have Panic Disorder and that there do seem to be cultural differences in people's symptoms (APA, 2000; "Understanding Panic Disorder," 2005). You would let him know that people from the Cajun culture can believe in voodoo without being psychotic.

6. **How would you respond if Caroline shares with you that she believes she has a fatal disease that no one has found and that someone is putting a spell on her or choking and putting pins in a voodoo doll that represents her?** You need to respond in a calm voice and let Caroline know that you realize these thoughts must be distressing and that you understand her culture has beliefs about voodoo and spells; however, you think that it is highly likely that the symptoms are only from the Panic Disorder and will decrease then go away when she gets sufficient treatment. You need to explain that it is very common for people experiencing these attacks to believe either that they are in danger or that they might have a fatal illness. You need to do some education about panic disorder and agoraphobia as an early intervention. Keep in mind that, although unlikely, it is possible she has a fatal illness separate from the Panic Disorder.

7. **Why did the nurse respond by encouraging relaxation and visualization when Caroline called to say she would not make it to the evening therapy program?** It is difficult if not impossible to be anxious if you are relaxed enough. It is also easier to hear and to make good decisions if your stress level is not much higher than mild stress. Visualizing the walk to the door and turning the knob is the first step in a series of steps to gradually getting outside the house and moving toward the evening therapy program.

8. **What teaching does the nurse need to do with Caroline in regard to the paroxetine (Paxil) she has begun to take for her Panic Disorder? What problem associated with paroxetine (Paxil) often causes clients, particularly men, to stop taking it, and what can be done about this? What assessments does the nurse need to do because Caroline is on paroxetine (Paxil)?** Special instructions that the nurse would include in patient education regarding Paxil and other selective serotonin reuptake inhibitors (SSRIs) includes the following information:

   - This medication does not begin to work immediately and may take up to eight weeks to reach maximum effect.
   - The dosage is small to begin with and increased gradually to a dose that works best. When you no longer need this medication, you will be tapered off of it. Do not stop it abruptly on your own. Notify the health care provider and/or nurse if you are having problems with the medication. Do not double up on the medication. Take as prescribed.
   - Avoid alcohol and other CNS depressants.
   - Do not drive or do other activities requiring you to be alert for safety if you are experiencing dizziness or drowsiness.
   - Report any side effects to the health care provider and/or nurse. A common side effect is dry mouth, which is often relieved by mouth rinses, sugarless gum, or candy.
   - Wear sunscreen and protective eyewear and clothing, as medication increases photosensitivity.

   The client and nurse need to monitor the client's appetite and the client needs to be weighed weekly as the medication could cause weight gain or loss as a side effect. Since there is some recent concern that SSRIs may increase suicidal risk, the client's mood needs to be assessed and the client needs to be screened frequently for suicidal ideation. Frisch and Frisch (2006) provides a nursing alert saying that clients with Panic Disorder tend to think a lot about death and actually consider or engage in suicidal acts more than clients with depression or other psychiatric conditions. This suggests there may be suicidal ideation with or without the SSRI.

   The nurse must continue to assess the frequency and severity of panic attacks or periods of anxiety. Some, but not all, men and some women complain of symptoms associated with sexual dysfunction while on paroxetine (Paxil) or on some other SSRIs. The nurse can assess for this problem. If a client experiences impotence, particularly a male client, he is likely to stop taking the drug abruptly. If they are forewarned, screened for this problem, and advised that the health care provider needs to know if they experience this problem, the health care provider can change the client to another drug.

9. **What medications have been found to be effective in reducing the number and/or severity of panic attacks?** Many psychiatrists use an SSRI as a first line drug of choice for treatment of Panic Disorder. Some of the SSRIs used in treating panic disorders are fluoxetine (Prozac), fluvoxamine (Luvox), setraline (Zoloft), paroxetine (Paxil), citalopram (Celexa), and venlafaxine (Effexor), which have been found, in various studies, to be more effective in treating Panic Disorder than placebos (Beamish, Granello, and Belcastro, 2002; Sturpe and Weissman, 2002). If a client does not respond to SSRIs, clinicians often switch them to tricyclic antidepressants (TCAs). Some clinicians and researchers suggest monoamine oxydase inhibitors (MAOIs) as a third line of defense. Jefferson (quoted in Beamish, Granello, and Belcastro, 2002) reports many clinicians finding MAOIs the "most potent anti-panic medication," while others such as Kwok, Chow, Holt, and Chow (2003) say MAOIs have no role in the management of Panic Disorders.

   Zamorski and Albucher (2002) state that while SSRIs are the drug of choice for treating Panic Disorder, 30 percent of people placed on these drugs won't be able to tolerate them or will have an unfavorable response and need tricyclic antidepressants. These authors suggest starting SSRIs out at a low dose, aiming for a higher dose and being patient as it may take up to eight weeks to get a maximum therapeutic response.

   Some of the side effects of SSRIs include weight loss, drowsiness, orthostatic hypotension, light-headedness, skin rash, and sexual dysfunctions such as delayed ejaculation or anorgasmia. Kwok and associates (2003) state that 15–30 percent of clients taking SSRIs and 30–40 percent of those taking TCAs reporting an inability to ejaculate or delayed ejaculation or anorgasmia. For males, adding buspirone (BuSpar) was found to help libido (Kwok, Chow, Holt, and Chow, 2003).

One problem with MAOIs is the need for the client to be on a tyramine-free diet for a day or two before starting an MAOI and staying on this diet until two weeks after the drug is discontinued. It takes a good bit of discipline and commitment to stay on this diet. If a client is on an MAOI and is to switch to an SSRI or tricyclic, they need to be off the MAOI for at least two weeks as a potentially fatal interaction (neuroleptic malignant syndrome) can occur when the system is not cleared of the MAOI and the SSRI or tricyclic is started.

10. What therapies other than medication are currently being used to treat Panic Disorder and Agoraphobia?
The most successful treatment of Panic Disorder and Agoraphobia seems to involve more than one methodology. In addition to pharmacological intervention, cognitive-behavioral interventions—such as cognitive restructuring to change thinking errors such as catastrophizing, as well as panic education, guided imagery, breathing retraining, and panic inoculation—have been found to be effective when used in combination. Having the client keep a log or journal is one way that nurses trained in working with clients who have Panic Disorder with or without Agoraphobia can get the client to look at their beliefs and challenge them when necessary. Some treatment programs have clients stop negative thoughts by snapping a rubber band on their wrist or splashing their own face with water. In regard to breathing retraining, it has been found that clients hyperventilate during panic attacks, which possibly accounts for many of the uncomfortable physical symptoms. Clients are encouraged to hyperventilate during a nonpanic attack time and recognize that hyperventilating can cause some of their symptoms. Clients are trained to breathe slow and deep in a controlled way and to breathe using abdominal muscles.

Another therapy used to treat Panic Disorder is interoceptive exposure therapy. In this therapy, physiological symptoms of panic are induced by methods such as short periods of rigorous exercise, spinning, or imagery. The client counselor team works to identify a range of symptoms from least to most fear generated from the various methods of fear inducement. The client begins dealing with the ones that induce low degrees of fear and works up to those creating the most fear. Over a number of sessions, the fear diminishes.

Panic inoculation is a term used for a multimodal treatment approach involving four interventions: education, cognitive restructuring, breathing training, and interoceptive exposure (Beamish, Granello, and Belcastro, 2002).

Another therapy approach was developed at the Applied Technology for Neuro Psychology Lab at the Instituto Auxologico Italian in Verbania, Italy, in collaboration with the University of Milan. An article by Wiederhold and Wiederhold (2003) describes the treatment system as a four zone virtual environment called virtual reality graded exposure therapy (VRGET) with audio and visual images delivered through head-mounted display.

11. What nursing diagnoses would you write for Caroline?

- Anxiety
- Risk for self-directed violence
- Social isolation

12. Discuss some nursing interventions for at least one of the likely nursing diagnoses.

- Anxiety: relaxation tapes, breathing exercises, massage, laughter induced by humorous movies as it is impossible to be stressed while laughing.
- Social isolation: maintaining contact with others through the telephone, having a friend visit in the home, doing short walks with a friend and increasing the distance, writing a letter to a friend, e-mailing to friends.

Frisch and Frisch (2006) discusses some techniques used by Agoraphobics to maintain social functioning. Some of these techniques include carrying something like an umbrella or cane or a folded newspaper under the arm. He further states that Agoraphobics are usually more comfortable out at night or in a dark place such as the theater. People with Agoraphobia also may venture out if accompanied by someone they know or trust or even a dog.

13. Carolyn's boyfriend asks: "What causes Panic Disorder?" How would you answer him? Why might he be concerned? You would tell him that the etiology is uncertain. Some researchers have proposed serotonergic dysfunction and possible genetic defect causing this dysfunction. This proposed etiological theory fits with the fact that many people with Panic Disorder are benefited by taking an SSRI.

In a genome-wide scan of an Icelandic population, looking for "genes conferring susceptibility to anxiety disorders," a connection was found between Panic Disorder and Chromosome 9q. This connection could be for other anxiety disorders also and no final conclusions were drawn in this early genome study (Thorgeirsson et al., 2003).

The boyfriend may be concerned that if Panic Disorder is genetic, this may be a problem for any children that he and Carolyn might have in the future. You need to encourage him to talk about his thoughts and fears in relation to Caroline's diagnosis and if and when appropriate refer them to genetic counseling.

References

American Psychiatric Association. (2000). *Diagnostic and Statistical Manual of Mental Disorders, 4th ed.* Text Revision. Washington, DC: American Psychiatric Association.

Beamish, P.M., D.H. Granello, and A.L. Belcastro. (2002). "Treatment of Panic Disorder: Practical Guidelines." *Journal of Mental Health Counseling* 24(3): 224–247.

Frisch, N.C. and L.E. Frisch. (2006). *Psychiatric Mental Health Nursing, 3d ed.* Albany, NY: Thomson Delmar Learning.

Kwok, M., S.L. Chow, J. Holt, and M.S. Chow. (2003). "Panic Disorder: A Pharmacological Armamentarium." *Formulary* 38(7): 431–439.

Sturpe, D.A. and A.M. Weissman. (2002). "What Are the Effective Treatments for Panic Disorder." *Journal of Family Practice* 51(9): 743.

Thorgeirsson, T.E. et al. (2003). "Anxiety with Panic Disorder Linked to Chromosome 9q in Iceland." *American Journal of Human Genetics* 72(5): 1221–1231.

"Understanding Panic Disorder." (2005). National Institute of Mental Health publication 95-. Available online at http://www.nimh.nih.gov/healthinformation/panicmenu.cfm and through NIMH.

Wiederhold, B.K. and M.D. Wiederhold. (2003). "A New Approach: Using Virtual Reality Psychotherapy in Panic Disorder with Agoraphobia." *Psychiatric Times* 20(7): 31–34.

Zamorski, M.A. and R.C. Albucher. (2002). "What to Do When SSRIs Fail: Eight Strategies for Optimizing Treatment of Panic Disorder." *American Family Physician* 66(8): 1477–1485.

Claudia

GENDER

Female

AGE

25

SETTING

■ General hospital

ETHNICITY

■ Central American

CULTURAL CONSIDERATIONS

■ Colombian

PREEXISTING CONDITION

COEXISTING CONDITION

COMMUNICATION

DISABILITY

SOCIOECONOMIC

SPIRITUAL/RELIGIOUS

PHARMACOLOGIC

■ Trazodone (Desyrl)

PSYCHOSOCIAL

■ Impaired social interaction
■ Situational low self-esteem

LEGAL

■ Confidentiality
■ Consent for release of information

ETHICAL

■ Client's right not to report a crime vs. nurse and health care team members' views

ALTERNATIVE THERAPY

PRIORITIZATION

DELEGATION

DIFFICULT

POST TRAUMATIC STRESS DISORDER (PTSD), ADULT

Level of difficulty: High

Overview: Requires the nurse to select therapeutic communication techniques to use with a client who has signs and symptoms of PTSD. The nurse must decide what action to take when the client reveals being raped in the past and asks the nurse to keep this information confidential. The nurse is challenged to do holistic nursing with this client who has psychological needs and sexual education and support needs as well as medical needs.

Client Profile

Claudia is a single, bright 25-year-old graduate student from a small town in the mountains of Colombia in Central America. She came to the United States to do her graduate work at a large state university. One night she decided to go meet friends at a local bar frequented by college students, locals, and tourists. Her friends did not show up. A nice-looking man bought her a few drinks and then offered to take her home. When she arrived home this man forcibly performed sexual acts and made her perform sexual acts on him. He then forced her to shower to "wash away evidence" and threatened to kill her if she reported the incident. She felt a great deal of fear and helplessness. Claudia thought perhaps this rape was her fault for dressing too sexy or going out unescorted. Almost immediately Claudia began to have a feeling of being numb and detached from everything and seemed to be in a daze, and she seemed to not be able to recall much of the incident at all. She continued her studies and moved in with her boyfriend, but did not tell him about the incident, and she has not told her family in Colombia that she has moved in with her boyfriend. She avoided the bar and the friends that she was supposed to meet. She decided she would move on with her life.

Eventually she started having trouble falling asleep and had nightmares, and her boyfriend recognized she was less interested in intimacy and had begun talking about never getting married or having children. She asked him not to wear a certain aftershave, which she had always complimented him on before.

Case Study

About a year after the rape episode, Claudia is admitted to the general hospital for an appendectomy. The night after surgery Claudia screams in the middle of the night and the night nurse finds her crying. The night nurse decides to sit with Claudia until she relaxes. The nurse offers to sit with Claudia and to listen if she wants to talk and then sits quietly.

Claudia is silent for a while, and then says: "I have had bad dreams almost every night for about a year, and I have bad memories come on me sometimes in the daytime. I have not told anyone about it, and I don't want to talk about it, but I was raped about a year ago and please do not put that in my chart. I am here to have surgery and not talk about the rape. That is in the past. Even my boyfriend does not know about it." The nurse notices that Claudia is hypervigilant, alert to every small noise and is easily startled.

Two days later, the health care provider gives Claudia a tentative diagnosis of Post Traumatic Stress Disorder (PTSD) and asks a psychiatric mental health nurse clinician employed by the hospital to work with the client and the medical team.

Questions and Suggested Answers

1. **What communication techniques did the night nurse use that encouraged the client to reveal that her bad dreams had to do with being raped? Were these recognized therapeutic communication techniques? What other therapeutic communication techniques could the nurse use in response to the client saying she was raped a few months ago?** The approaches the night nurse used were recognized therapeutic communication techniques. The approaches used were offering self and silence. In response to the client saying she was raped a few months ago, there are probably several therapeutic responses, for example: "Talking about it may help. Tell me a little about it." The nurse opens the door for the client to begin talking and is not leading the client in any way, (i.e., suggesting any ideas or set answers).

2. **If you were the night nurse and the client asked you not to tell anyone about the rape, how would you respond, and what would you do with the information?** If the client was a minor and told you she had been sexually or physically abused, you would be obligated by law to report this. The client in this case is an adult and has the right to decide whether to report or not. One of your major concerns as her nurse is getting her

the help she needs to deal with the trauma of rape. You can strongly suggest the client share this information with her health care provider and get a referral for help in dealing with this trauma. Another option would be to talk gently with the client and explain that you would like to call the health care provider so he can prescribe some safe medication for sleep and talk to her in the morning.

As the nurse, you need to consult with your supervisor about this unusual situation. You can tell the client that you need to share the information with your supervisor and hopefully the client will agree. If not, you can talk with the hospital's ethics committee chairman about your legal and ethical responsibilities in a hypothetical case.

3. **The client promises you she will talk with her health care provider in the morning. What could you chart about the client's crying out?** One acceptable option is to chart the date and time and that the client "cried out and was awake at this time. This nurse sat with client for ten minutes during which time she stated: 'I had a bad dream, a dream I have been having for about a year.' Promised to talk with physician in the morning about these dreams and probable cause of the dreams."

4. **If the client were to agree to let you call the health care provider in the middle of the night, what would you say to this provider?** You need to just present the facts and let the health care provider respond. The provider will probably say that he or she will see the client the next day and prescribe something for sleep.

5. **The client is talking about the rape being all her fault for not using better judgment and dressing provocatively. Is this unusual behavior from a rape victim? How do you, as her nurse, respond?** It is not unusual for women to blame themselves for rape, and sometimes others will blame the victim out of lack of knowledge. Latina women are often more likely to take blame due to cultural beliefs that men are not responsible for their own behavior around women or that women are responsible for controlling male sexuality (Hensley, 2002).

In the cultural practices of Colombia and other Central American countries, families do not permit young unmarried women to live alone, live with girlfriends or boyfriends, or go out at night alone. A young unmarried woman still answers to her parents even if she has finished college and has her own salary.

6. **Do you pass on this information about the client saying she had been raped in the report to the next shift?** This is an ethical dilemma. This information could be helpful to the health team in caring for the client, yet this adult client has asked you not to pass this information on. You cannot be sure of the reaction of the staff nurses. Some of the nurses may be agency nurses hired just for the night; student nurses may listen to report in the morning; nurses on your team may seem highly judgmental of clients. Perhaps letting the health care provider and your supervisor make the decision is all you want to do. The client may agree to let you pass this information on to only the primary nurse who will care for her in the morning, especially if you express confidence in the nurse and introduce this oncoming nurse to the client.

7. **Looking at the information in the client profile and the case study, what signs and symptoms has this client had, and perhaps still has, that led the health care provider to a tentative diagnosis of PTSD? If diagnosed with PTSD, would this client likely be diagnosed as having acute, chronic, or delayed onset PTSD?** PTSD is considered acute if the symptom duration is less than three months, and it is said to be chronic if the symptoms last three months or more. Delayed onset refers to symptoms that begin at least six months after the traumatic event. This client will likely be diagnosed with chronic PTSD.

8. **What events can place individuals at risk for PTSD, and which events have the highest risk?** The highest rates of PTSD—about a third to one half—are found in those who survived rape, military combat and captivity, internment for ethnical or political reasons, and genocide (APA, 2000). Stressors with potential to cause PTSD as identified by Khouzam and Donnelly (2001), Birmes et al. (2001), and Russoniello et al. (2002) include: general crime, criminal assault, school shootings, hostage taking, being imprisoned, a natural disaster (flood, hurricane, tornado, fire), military duties, sexual abuse, physical abuse, torture, serious accident (automobile traffic, boating, gunshot), terrorist attack, exodus of refugees during ethnic wars, and vicarious traumatization that can occur when living with someone who has PTSD.

Criterion for PTSD	Client's Signs and Symptoms
Has been in, viewed, or learned about a situation or situations involving death or threatened death or severe injury or some threat to physical integrity or that of others.	Claudia experienced being raped and forced to perform sexual acts and had some physical injuries from this as well.
Responses include great fear, helplessness, or a sense of horror.	Claudia was afraid and felt helpless.
Repeatedly experiences the traumatic event in one or more of five ways: 1. Recurrent and distressing dreams of event, 2. Recurrent intrusive and distressing recall of event with images, thoughts, or perceptions, 3. Acting or feeling the traumatic event like reliving it, and/or hallucinations, dissociative flashbacks even when awake or intoxicated, 4. Intense distress when exposed to cues symbolizing or reminding client of some part of the event, 5. Reacting physiologically to internal or external cues reminding person of event.	Claudia is having recurrent distressing dreams of the rape event. She alludes to daytime flashbacks. This needs further assessment. She has asked her boyfriend to stop using a certain aftershave. This could be a clue that she is having distress when smelling something like the smell of the rapist.
Engaged in three or more of seven ways to avoid stimuli associated with trauma or to numb general responsiveness and this was not present before the trauma: 1. Tries to avoid anyone, any place, or any activity associated with the trauma, 2. Tries to avoid thoughts, feelings, or talks connected with the trauma, 3. Unable to remember an important aspect of the trauma, 4. Greatly decreased interest or engagement in significant activities, 5. Feeling detached or separated from others, 6. Narrow range of affect (e.g., inability to feel love), 7. Unable to see a future (e.g., not seeing a career, marriage, or a normal span of years to life).	Claudia has tried to avoid places and thoughts and feelings associated with the trauma. She has decreased interest in significant activities. She has admitted feeling detached from others, and she has talked about not getting married or having children.

Two or more persistent symptoms of increased arousal (not present before the trauma):
 	
  1. trouble falling or remaining asleep
  2. irritability or outbursts of anger
  3. trouble concentrating
  4. hypervigilance
  5. exaggerated startle response
	Claudia has trouble falling asleep and remaining asleep and appears to be hypervigilant.

Symptoms above must have lasted more than one month.	Claudia's symptoms have lasted almost one year.
Must be clinically significant distress or impairment in an important area of functioning such as social or work (including school) areas caused by the traumatic event.	The rape resulted in impairment in Claudia's school activities and in her intimate relationship with her boyfriend.

Adapted from APA, 2000.

The criterion for the diagnosis, according to the current APA manual of diagnoses, does not change with the type of event. The symptoms are similar and fit those described in the criteria, but they do vary from individual to individual. While most people with PTSD will tend to have the same cluster of nursing diagnoses, the priority of these may vary and the nursing interventions will vary on an individual basis depending on the client's needs, strengths, support system, and other factors.

9. **What nursing diagnoses would you write for this client, given the limited amount of information that you have?** Nursing diagnoses can include but are not limited to:

- Rape Trauma Syndrome
- Risk for self-directed violence

- Powerlessness
- Disturbed sleep pattern
- Ineffective sexuality pattern
- Situational low self-esteem
- Impaired social interaction
- Knowledge deficit (North American Nursing Diagnosis Association, 2005)

10. What are some of the current treatments for PTSD? Treatment of PTSD today usually involves antidepressants and some form of Cognitive Behavioral Therapy in individual and/or group therapy.

Barry Krakow and his colleagues in New Mexico at the Sleep and Human Health Institute studied 168 women, 95 percent of whom had a diagnosis of moderate to severe PTSD. All had been sexually abused at an early age, sexually assaulted in a life-threatening way, or raped. Krakow and his associates used image reversal therapy, a dream- and sleep-oriented therapy to reduce insomnia and change nightmares to better dreams. In the initial therapy session the subject were "encouraged to recognize that nightmares may be both trauma-induced and a learned behavior." The women were then taught and prompted to practice pleasant imagery exercises. In the second session the women were told to write down their nightmare and to change it anyway they wanted and to write down the changed dream. In subsequent sessions the women rehearsed the new dream. Next the women were to rehearse the new dream five to twenty minutes a day while awake. At the end of the study, the women's nightmares were substantially reduced with improved sleep quality and reduction of even the other PTSD symptoms (*Women's Health Weekly*, 2001).

Another therapy that has a long history of use is Exposure Therapy (ET). In this therapy, the client has to do "imaginal reliving" of their trauma on a repeated basis. The idea of reliving the trauma is to confront the belief that anxiety will last forever unless the experience is avoided or that there is some form of escape from the trauma. In the reliving of the trauma in a therapeutic setting, new information is incorporated into the trauma memory to help the client realize that it is not dangerous to remember the traumatic event. The process of "imaginal reliving" is also said to change the meaning of the client's symptoms from personal failure or lack of competence to that of courage and mastery. Reliving in imagination is a chance to modify self-evaluation (Rothbaum and Swartz, 2002).

Some therapists use what is called in vivo exposure and have the client confront places, situations, and objects that remind them of the trauma in order to reduce the strong emotions about these things.

Another treatment being used today is called Virtual Reality Exposure (VRE). The client uses head-mounted display and stereo earphones, which provide some visual and audio clues consistent with the trauma. The therapist must have the skill and knowledge to know how much exposure to the trauma to give the client. While the patient goes at his or her own speed and exposure, the therapist helps the client get through the experience in a therapeutic way (Rothbaum and Schwartz, 2002).

In addition to talk therapies, the client is often prescribed medication to target symptoms of PTSD. The antidepressants most often prescribed for PTSD are SSRIs, which target depression associated with PTSD and other symptoms such as difficulty concentrating, flashbacks, angry outbursts, irritability, hyperarousal, and intrusive thoughts. SSRIs are said to be preferable to tricyclic antidepressants (TCAs) because they have fewer side effects, and overdose of TCAs can cause death. However, about half the patients taking SSRIs have adverse effects, some of which are common to all SSRIs and some of which are more specific to individual SSRIs.

Another antidepressant used for PTSD is trazodone (Desyrl). It has some anxiolytic properties, is believed to inhibit serotonin reuptake, and is quite sedating and helpful in reducing chronic insomnia and the intensity of nightmares. Some clients cannot tolerate adverse effects of SSRIs, TCAs, and trazodone so they are then usually tried on one of the atypical antidepressants, which include: mirtazapine (Remeron), venlafaxine (Effexor), nefazodone hydrochloride (Serzone), and bupropion hydrochloride (Welbutrin).

Bupropion is often prescribed for clients who complain of sexual dysfunction on other antidepressants, as this adverse effect is rare with this drug. It also does not seem to produce weight gain. Bupropion is usually not used in clients with seizure disorders as seizures are a risk with this drug. It is also contraindicated in clients with bulimia and anorexia nervosa. Bupropion is also prescribed as Zyban for smoking cessation.

MAOIs are occasionally used for patients with PTSD. There are not prescribed unless the client can adhere to a strict tyramine-free diet and can abstain from alcohol, as ingestion of tyramine-rich foods can cause a potentially fatal hypertensive crisis and ingestion of alcohol can cause a drug-to-drug interaction.

11. **What teaching would you do about trazodone (Desyrl) with this client?** You would tell this client that trazodone is an antidepressant that has been used in managing symptoms of PTSD and for the treatment of insomnia. It can cause drowsiness and blurred vision so the client needs to avoid driving and using machinery after taking this medication and should avoid changing position rapidly as orthostatic hypotension can occur. Note the nurse needs to take lying and standing blood pressure and pulse at least daily. You would instruct this client to notify health care providers that you are taking this medication before having surgery or medical treatments and to notify your provider before stopping the medication.

12. **How can the primary nurse work with the client in regard to sexuality? How can the primary nurse teach the boyfriend ways to be supportive as well as to deal with his expressed concerns about the client's decreased interest in sexual intimacy?** The nurse will need to do a lot of listening and assessing to find out the boyfriend's perspective and to find out what he sees as his needs, as well as to ascertain the client's needs and goals. The nurse will want to educate the boyfriend about PTSD and its treatment and the importance of Claudia getting professional help in individual therapy and, if her therapist deems it helpful, among a group for survivors of sexual abuse.

   The nurse can also work with the client in terms of good interpersonal communication techniques and also in terms of ways to improve intimacy in general. Sexual intimacy may be improved as the relationship is strengthened and trust is increased and as issues are addressed associated with the rape and perhaps cultural, religious, personal, or family taboos about sex before marriage. Claudia may also feel safer if she is told that some women who are survivors of sexual abuse prefer to initiate the sexual intimacy and play a greater role in controlling the pace and content of the sexual foreplay and sexual acts. The idea is to go slow with lots of patience and build a sense of safety in relations with the boyfriend. While the nurse is not an expert in sex therapy or relationship therapy, sexuality is an important part of life, and in a holistic nursing approach the primary nurse will pay attention to this area of the client's health needs and consult with the psychiatric/mental health nurse clinician and the health care provider on sexual issues.

References

American Psychiatric Association. (2000). *Diagnostic and Statistical Manual of Mental Disorders, 4th ed.* Text Revision. Washington, DC: American Psychiatric Association.

Birmes, P. et al. (2001). "Peritraumatic Dissociation, Acute Stress, and General Posttraumatic Stress Disorder in Victims of General Crime." *Canadian Journal of Psychiatry* 46(7): 649–652.

Hensley, L.G. (2002). "Treatment for Survivors of Rape: Issues and Interventions." *Journal of Mental Health Counseling* 24(4): 331–348.

Khouzam, H. and N.J. Donnelly. (2001). "Posttraumatic Stress Disorder." *Postgraduate Medicine* 110(5): 60–69.

Rothbaum, B.O. and A.C. Schwartz. (2002). "Exposure Therapy for Posttraumatic Stress Disorder." *American Journal of Psychotherapy* 56(1): 59–76.

Russoniello, C.V., et al. (2002). "Childhood Posttraumatic Stress Disorder and Efforts to Cope after Hurricane Floyd." *Behavioral Medicine* 29(2): 61–72.

Women's Health Weekly Editors. (2001). "Image Reversal Therapy Improves Sleep, Reduces Victim's Nightmares." *Women's Health Weekly*, 8/23/01 -8/30/01.

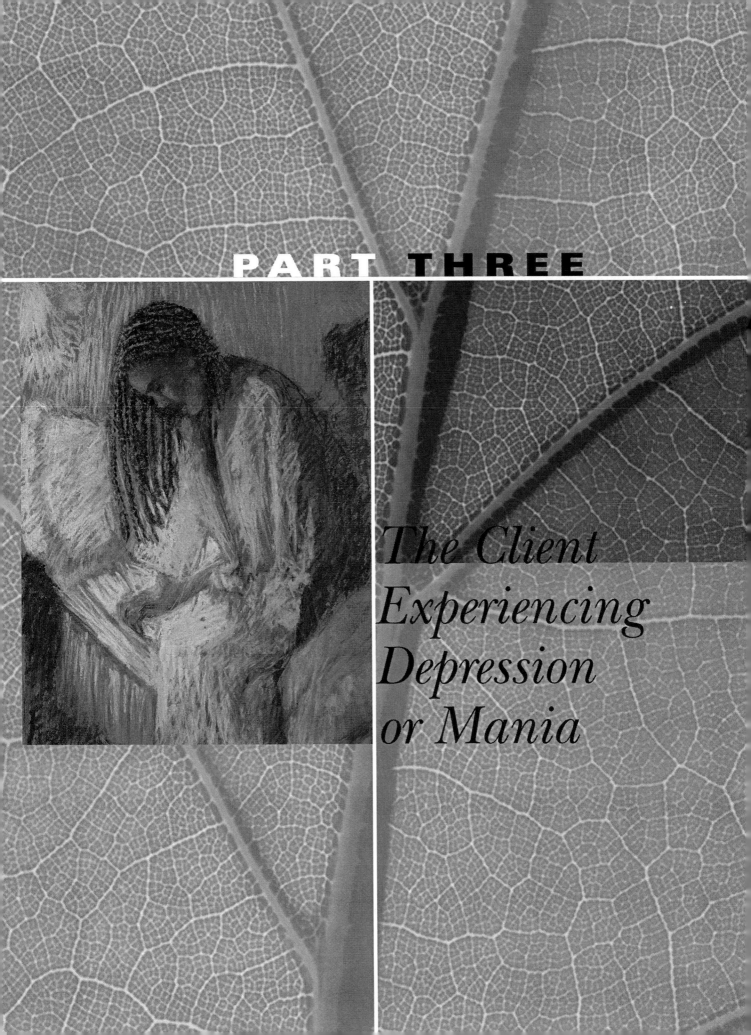

PART THREE

The Client Experiencing Depression or Mania

John

GENDER

Male

AGE

14

SETTING

- Adolescent unit of a psychiatric hospital

ETHNICITY

- Black American

CULTURAL CONSIDERATIONS

PREEXISTING CONDITION

COEXISTING CONDITION

- Obesity Hypoventilation Syndrome

COMMUNICATION

DISABILITY

SOCIOECONOMIC

- Low-income family
- Public assistance
- Housing project

SPIRITUAL/RELIGIOUS

PHARMACOLOGIC

- Vitamins
- Sertraline (Zoloft)

PSYCHOSOCIAL

- Social relationships with peers limited due to obesity/depressed mood
- Low self-esteem

LEGAL

- Obtaining permission for a child or adolescent to take an antidepressant

ETHICAL

ALTERNATIVE THERAPY

PRIORITIZATION

- Addressing physical and psychological conditions while acknowledging self-esteem and identity-building needs

DELEGATION

- Delegation of crisis on unit to another team member

DYSTHYMIA

Level of difficulty: Easy

Overview: Requires the nurse to build a trusting relationship with a young client and his mother. The nurse must determine whether to respond to a unit crisis or delegate that task to a nurse colleague, so a promise to the client and mother can be kept. Challenges for the nurse also include making the mother part of the team identifying treatment goals and interventions. The nurse is called upon to describe current theories of treatment of dysthymia and to demonstrate understanding of a coexisting physical problem: Obesity Hypoventilation Syndrome.

Client Profile

John is a 14-year-old male who lives in urban public housing with his mother. John's father is not in contact. John has had a low level of energy and is described by his mother and teachers as looking sad and being somewhat irritable for the past eighteen months. His major activities outside of school are watching television, using the computer, eating, and attending the native Baptist Church with his mother. Peers in the housing project make fun of John for attending church with his mother, but he likes the church music and the church potluck suppers.

John resists joining activities. He declines peer activity and offers one or more reasons why the activity is not desirable. "I don't care" is a phrase he frequently uses (e.g., if he doesn't do his homework and is given a consequence, he says: "I don't care"). His teachers describe John as "easily distracted" unless he is doing something he is extremely interested in. He is morbidly obese and short of breath after walking a short distance. John is found on a routine school physical to be somewhat depressed and so overweight that it affects his breathing. The health care provider doing the physical refers John to an endocrinologist and a psychiatrist.

Case Study

John is admitted to the adolescent unit of a private psychiatric hospital by his endocrinologist and psychiatrist. The hospital is interested in receiving additional future admissions with similar psychiatric diagnoses and endocrine problems combined, and agrees to accept this case without payment.

On admission, the admitting nurse greets the client and his mother and introduces himself. The nurse interviews John's mother while John is given a tour of the unit. During the interview, a staff member comes and asks the admitting nurse to step out to discuss something urgent. The nurse tells John's mother he will be right back. The staff nurse describes an urgent situation on the unit and indicates the admitting nurse should take care of it; however, the admitting nurse delegates it to someone else and returns quickly to continue the interview. The mother is asked to describe a typical day in the family in chronological sequence and to write down what she and John had eaten at meals the previous day. Later, when the nurse interviews John alone, he asks John: "What do you like to do that you are good at?" John replies: "I can cook, do really cool magic tricks, and play computer games." John tells the nurse that other kids are mean to him and tell him he is too fat to play with them. He says he would like to be able to play football. John is shown a page of faces with various expressions and asked to pick out the way he feels most of the time. He picks out the sad face.

Just before mother leaves, she says to the nurse: "John's birthday is next week; I want to bring a birthday cake for him. Would that be all right if I brought a second cake for the other kids?"

John's tentative diagnoses are early onset Dysthymic Disorder and Obesity Hypoventilation Syndrome. He is admitted for professional help in safely losing weight, to begin medication for dysthymia, and to participate in group, family, and individual therapy. In addition to orders for these therapies, the admission orders include daily vitamins and a strict diet (e.g., protein diet drink to be mixed by the nutritionist and sent to the unit three times a day, one cup of salad, and a four-ounce skinless broiled chicken breast or broiled piece of fish at lunch and dinner). The orders also include nocturnal polysomnography testing in the sleep studies laboratory. Oxygen saturation levels are to be taken four times a day, and John is to wear a pulse oxymeter at night and recordings of the readings are to be made every hour. A $PaCO_2$ level is to be drawn during the day. In the progress notes, the health care provider writes: "Consider Sertraline (Zoloft)."

Questions and Suggested Answers:

1. **Discuss how John's observed behavior may or may not match a diagnosis of Dysthymic Disorder (DD). How do the criteria for a diagnosis of DD differ for adults compared to children and adolescents? What does the psychiatrist mean when he refers to John as having early onset Dysthymic Disorder (EODD)?** The essential

feature of DD is for a child or adolescent to describe a sad or down-in-the-dumps mood and/or display an irritable mood for a minimum of one year. John has appeared sad and been irritable for about eighteen months. From a page with faces depicting various moods, he has picked out both the sad and the irritated face to describe his mood most of the time. The child or adolescent must have at least two more specific symptoms during the period of irritable or sad mood in order to meet the criteria for a diagnosis of Dysthymia: poor appetite or overeating, sleeping too much or not enough, lack of energy or feeling fatigued, low self-esteem, trouble making decisions or poor concentration, and feelings of hopelessness. John overeats, lacks energy, is easily distracted, and likely has low self-esteem as a result of teasing from classmates.

While a child or adolescent can be diagnosed as having Dysthymic Disorder after one year with an irritable mood, the adult must have a depressed mood for at least two years. This means children can get diagnosed sooner than adults, although the mean episode duration in children has been found to be three to four years, according to Nobile, Cataldo, Marino, and Molteni (2003). During the one-year period (two years for adults) the person can be symptom free no longer than two months at any given time. During the required time period the client cannot have a major depressive episode, a manic episode, a mixed episode, or a hypomanic episode and be diagnosed with Dysthymic Disorder. Once the person meets the initial time and other requirements for Dysthymic Disorder without a major depressive disorder, there can be an episode of major depressive disorder superimposed over the Dysthymic Disorder and both diagnoses may be given (APA, 2000).

Additionally, in order to meet the criteria for a diagnosis of Dysthymic Disorder, the client's symptoms must cause significant distress in social, occupational (school for children), or some other area of functioning. A case could be made for John having significant distress in relating to peers who tease him and his inability to enjoy active play.

If the onset of the disorder occurs before age 21, it is referred to as early onset Dysthymic Disorder; if at age 21 or later, it is called late onset (APA, 2000).

2. **What is the risk for a person in a clinical setting with a diagnosis of Dysthymic Disorder to develop a major depressive disorder?** It is thought that up to three-fourths of the persons in clinical settings with a diagnosis of Dysthymic Disorder will have an episode of major depression within five years (APA, 2000).

3. **Is ethnicity a risk factor for Dysthymic Disorder? Are there other risk factors? What gender differences, if any, are there in the occurrence of Dysthymic Disorder in children and in adults?** A recent study of 8,449 subjects with depression or Dysthymia revealed that major depression has a higher incidence in White Americans compared to Black Americans, but this was reversed in Dysthymic Disorder, which has a higher incidence in Black Americans. Other risk factors found for DD include not progressing past middle school and poverty (Riolo, Nguyen, Greden, and King, 2005). A transgenerational factor, which could be heredity and/or learned behavior, has been described by Flory, Vance, Burleson, and Luk (2002). In children, Dysthymic Disorder appears to occur equally in both sexes, but by adulthood, women are two to three times more likely to develop Dysthymic Disorder.

4. **Describe the usual course of Dysthymic Disorder.** Frequently Dysthymic Disorder appears early in childhood, adolescence, or young adulthood and has an insidious and chronic course. There are some reported spontaneous remissions (perhaps 10 percent per year), but the outcome is usually better with active treatment (APA, 2000). According to Nobile, Cataldo, Marino, and Molteni (2003), without treatment DD often has a "worse outcome than observed in major depression" with the long duration of depressive symptoms seen as responsible for "disabling consequences on social skills learning."

5. **Discuss what you know about Obesity Hypoventilation Syndrome from your reading on this subject.** This syndrome was first described by a clinician named Burwell some forty-five or forty-six years ago. He coined the term "Pickwickian Syndrome" to describe clients who had sustained hypoventilation leading to daytime hypercapnia and hypoxemia. This name was chosen because the clients with this syndrome resembled Joe in Charles Dickens's novel *Pickwick Papers*. Pickwickian Syndrome was later renamed Obesity Hypoventilation Syndrome (Teichtahl, 2001).

Obesity can have a detrimental effect on respiratory function. In some clients, obesity leads to chronic hypoventilation, which explains the name Obesity Hypoventilation Syndrome (OHS). Some obese persons with chronic hypoventilation also have sleep apnea. The term Sleep Hypoventilation Syndrome (SHVS) is also now in use, as is Obesity Sleep Apnea Syndrome (OSAS). Researchers debate how many syndromes are associated with obesity and hypoventilation, what signs and symptoms fit with each, and what to call them.

There have been several studies involving clients who have obesity and hypoventilation. One study, reported in the publication *Chest* (August 2001), found that of thirty-four such clients, twenty-three out of twenty-six subjects who had sleep studies demonstrated sleep apnea. The researchers in this study also concluded that their subjects without sleep apnea demonstrated that obesity per se could lead to chronic hypoventilation.

Clients with OHS tend to have daytime elevated $PaCO_2$ and may have low O_2 saturation levels. Some patients' daytime $PaCO_2$ levels reportedly normalize with use of a CPAP machine at night while others require noninvasive mechanical ventilation. Some clients have had a tracheotomy performed when the client could not tolerate the nasal or facemask of CPAP and or if the trachea is being compressed by increased neck fat. Some researchers suggest that there may be multiple pathophysiologic mechanisms leading to OHS.

6. **When the staff member called the nurse out of the interview with John's mother, why do you suppose he delegated whatever needed doing and went right back into the interview?** The nurse was cognizant of his statement to the mother that he would be right back. The nurse was trying to build a trusting relationship with the mother and wanted to keep his word about any promises, as this fosters trust. A nurse must be very careful about promises he or she makes to a client, family member, or others. If the nurse is unsure about how long he or she will be before returning, the nurse could say: "If I am going to be longer than five minutes, I will send someone to tell you and to give you something to do or read."

7. **The nurse asked John what he likes to do and what he is good at. What can the nurse and the treatment team use this information for?** The nurse and the treatment team can help the client to build his self-esteem by encouraging him to do activities he is good at and can feel a sense of pride in doing. Peer appreciation of his talent is also helpful in building self-esteem. For example, a client who likes to do magic tricks could be encouraged to perform a magic trick for first one other person and then a small group of peers as the person gains confidence. Also, doing things he likes to do or is good at doing will tend to improve the mood as the client focuses on a positive activity rather than negative thoughts. The nurses can use the client's talents to keep his mind on activities and away from thoughts of food.

8. **Describe the possible reasons for John to go to individual, group, and family therapy sessions.** In individual and group therapy, the therapist leader can help John try out relating to peers in different ways in a safe environment. John can begin to identify and work on issues that may be contributing to his depressed mood and weight gain. Some peers may have had similar issues and be willing to share how they dealt with these issues. He can get realistic feedback as well as support and encouragement from peers. Through Cognitive Behavioral Therapy, he can learn to avoid thinking errors that tend to reinforce depressed mood.

In family therapy with his mother, John can learn to communicate with his mother and let her know what his needs are, as well as to negotiate with her on things that are negotiable. His mother can learn how to be consistent in applying rules, set appropriate limits, and give logical and reasonable consequences. In therapy his mother and John can work through how they will deal with situations in which they tend to eat too much (e.g., at church potlucks), with stressful emotions, and with using food as rewards or to show love.

9. **If you were the admitting nurse and John's mother asked you if she could bring him a birthday cake the following week, what would your response be?** You could start by asking mother what type of cake she has provided for John in the past, what kind of cake she would like to provide this time, and how much cake he has eaten at one sitting in the past. This is an opportunity to help John's mother to look at the kind of cake and amount of cake she has allowed or encouraged in the past. John's mother has given him a whole

cake to eat by himself and expects to do so again. You can help her look at the calories in the type and amount of cake she plans to give John. You must listen respectfully and make sure your nonverbals as well as verbals are not disapproving in nature. Are you crossing your arms and frowning or do you lean forward and listen attentively? After you and mother talk about the calories in the cake she plans, you might say to her something like: "John is going to be on a very strict diet to improve his health; however, it is going to be his birthday and since I understand you want to do something special, we may be able to negotiate some special treat with the rest of the health care team. You are on our team, and we want you working with us as we figure out what to prepare for John." You could suggest that one possibility is a slice of angel food cake without icing, but that the team must be in agreement to allow this. Hopefully his mother will see that John can thoroughly enjoy just one piece of angel food cake without icing.

10. **From the limited information you have been given, what nursing diagnoses are most likely for this client?** Possible nursing diagnoses include:

   - Ineffective coping related to depression (as evidenced by statements reflecting discouragement such as "I don't care")
   - Imbalanced nutrition: More than body requirements
   - Activity intolerance
   - Ineffective breathing pattern
   - Disturbed body image
   - Chronic low self-esteem related to being teased about weight

11. **Describe some interventions you would use for at least one of these nursing diagnoses.** Activity intolerance and low self-esteem can both be addressed by slowing the peers to the client's pace. The group leader could tell the group on outings that since the staff is old, the group has to go slow. Another idea is to suggest a "slow contest" to see who can go somewhere the slowest. These interventions take the focus off the obese child's need to go slow and decrease teasing by peers and the peers' tendency to leave him behind. Being part of the group and staying with the activity will help him decrease his focus on food.

   To combat ineffective coping, the treatment team is challenged to get the client to care and be able to elevate his own mood without looking to food for the answer. One useful intervention in this area is a behavioral reward chart with a sticker or point awarded for each participation in planned activities. A certain number of stars or stickers could be designated as the amount needed to shop in the unit store if the unit has one, while other designated amounts could be tied to the opportunity to choose an activity on the unit or to do some chore that is considered fun, such as feeding the fish for a day.

12. **What is the health care provider likely considering before starting sertraline (Zoloft)? What assessments need to be done prior to the client being started on sertraline, and what teaching needs to be done with the client and the client's mother? Who needs to sign permission for the client to take sertraline?** Selective serotonin reuptake inhibitors (SSRIs) have received a fair amount of publicity in regard to possibly increasing suicidal risk in adolescents. While being regarded as first line medications, SSRIs are sometimes not prescribed until the health care provider determines if the client will show sufficient improvement on other nonmedication therapies alone.

   In the case of the minor child, the parents need to sign permission for the child to take sertraline. If one parent has custody and the other does not, the custodial parent signs. If John's parents are still married and the father returns and objects to the medication, he may have legal grounds to stop the medication. The nurse must check this with the nursing supervisor who may check with the hospital legal department. In this case the mother being the only available parent will be given instruction about the medication benefits and side effects including the possible increased risk of suicide, and she will then be given the opportunity to sign permission for John to be given the medication. John can also be given information about the medication benefits and side effects and asked to sign the permission for the medication unless the hospital practice is not to ask minors to sign. While not legally necessary, having John sign gives him a sense of control and increases chances of compliance.

References

American Psychiatric Association. (2000). *Diagnostic and Statistical Manual of Mental Disorders, 4th ed.* Text Revision. Washington, DC: American Psychiatric Association.

Flory, V., A. Vance, P. Burleson, and E. Luk. (2002). "Early Onset Dysthymic Disorder in Children and Adolescents: Clinical Implications and Future Directions." *Child and Adolescent Mental Health* 7(2): 79–85.

Nobile, M., G.M. Cataldo, C. Marino, and M. Molteni. (2003). "Diagnosis and Treatment of Dysthymia in Children and Adolescents." *CNS Drugs* 17(13): 927–947.

Riolo, S.A., T. Nguyen, J.F. Greden, and C.A. King. (2005). "Prevalence of Depression by Race/Ethnicity: Findings from the National Health and Nutrition Examination Survey III." *American Journal of Public Health* 95(6): 998–1000.

Teichtahl, H. (2001). "The Obesity-Hypoventilation Syndrome Revisited." *Chest.* 120(2): 369–377.

GENDER

Female

AGE

35

SETTING

- Inpatient hospital psychiatric unit

ETHNICITY

- Central American

CULTURAL CONSIDERATIONS

- Hispanic culture, rural Nicaraguan

PREEXISTING CONDITION

COEXISTING CONDITION

COMMUNICATION

- Speaks little English; Spanish preferred language

DISABILITY

SOCIOECONOMIC

- Raised by poor parents; now upper middle class

SPIRITUAL/RELIGIOUS

- Catholic

PHARMACOLOGIC

- Birth control
- Lithium carbonate (Eskalith)
- Olanzapine (Zyprexa)

PSYCHOSOCIAL

LEGAL

- Confidentiality
- Right to refuse medication

ETHICAL

- Birth control vs. Catholic teachings

ALTERNATIVE THERAPY

PRIORITIZATION

DELEGATION

- collaborating treatment planning with team
- collaborating management of lithium levels with team

MODERATE

BIPOLAR I MANIC EPISODE

Level of difficulty: Moderate

Overview: Requires critical thinking to therapeutically deal with the client's lack of judgment in areas such as spending, sexuality, and dress. Requires the nurse to consider how a client's culture and religion can affect treatment. The client's high levels of energy, activity, and distractibility require the nurse to develop strategies to get the client to eat, sleep, and attend to hygiene tasks. Requires management of the client's medication at a therapeutic level and to delegate this aspect of care at discharge.

Client Profile

Maria is a 35-year-old married female born and raised in a small village in Nicaragua, Central America. Her parents are poor. Her husband is a university professor who was serving as a Peace Corps worker when they met. She has been in the United States for two years and speaks a little English but requires Spanish for clear understanding. They have a 4-year-old daughter. Maria has been diagnosed with Bipolar I and takes lithium carbonate. Recently she stopped taking her lithium and has been staying up all night and eating very little. She is dressing and behaving in a sexually provocative manner and going on spending sprees buying things she does not need and cannot afford (e.g., a motorcycle that she does not know how to ride and a drum set that she does not know how to play). Her husband decides she is out of control and calls Maria's psychiatrist who suggests admission to the psychiatric unit of the hospital.

Case Study

During the admission process, the nurse observes that Maria is dressed in a short and tight-fitting dress. Her speech is clear but sprinkled with profanity as she moves rapidly from topic to topic. At the nurse's request, Maria sits down, then jumps up and moves about the room.

Maria's husband says that Maria has stopped taking her lithium and has not been sleeping or eating enough. He describes her extravagant purchases, some of which were returned or given away to strangers (e.g., Maria gave part of a drum set to a man she met in a bar). The husband explains that Maria has put the family in serious debt and states she is unfit to care for their child. With her husband translating for her, Maria objects to being admitted to the hospital, but then agrees to admission. The husband expresses concern about her sexually provocative behavior and states he fears that she will get sexually involved with other clients.

At the first meal after admission, Maria is in the dining room with the other clients. Instead of eating, Maria carries napkins to, and talks to, all the other clients and ignores the food. Staff members have told Maria several times to sit down and eat, and she has not complied.

The nurse asks the dietitian to prepare a sandwich and a banana for Maria. After the clients are finished with lunch, the nurse suggests Maria go to her room to wash her face and hands.

The psychiatrist-ordered pregnancy test comes back negative. The psychiatrist orders Lithium carbonate (Eskalith), olanzapine (Zyprexa), and birth control pills.

At medication time, the nurse gives Maria her medications and then examines Maria's mouth. The nurse does some teaching about the medications with Maria, who becomes upset when she learns she has been prescribed birth control and says she will not take it as it is not allowed in her religion.

The nurse notices that Maria is irritable and verbally hostile at times as well as inappropriate during her first days on the unit. During one encounter with Maria, the nurse senses great hostile energy coming from Maria, who says, "You think you so smart! You don't know nothing!" Sometimes Maria is demanding or threatening. For example, she demands that the nurse send someone to the store to pick up items for her and take her credit card to pay for them. Maria continues to dress and talk in a sexually provocative manner. She asks the male nurse, who passes medications in the early morning, to perform some sexual acts with her. At one point Maria is intrusive with another client in the day room and the client is threatening to harm Maria. The nurse observes that both clients are loud and their behavior is escalating.

After one month, during a meeting of the psychiatric health team, the psychiatrist discusses Maria's past psychiatric history, which includes two episodes of depression and one of mania. He offers a diagnosis of Bipolar I, Manic Episode for Maria. He orders that blood be drawn for a lithium level. The lithium level comes back at 1.5.

Questions and Suggested Answers

1. What criteria is essential for a diagnosis of Bipolar I? What would need to be different for Maria to have a diagnosis of Bipolar II Disorder? Which of Maria's behaviors are consistent with the criteria for a manic

episode? A Bipolar I diagnosis requires a clinical course characterized by one or more manic episodes. The person may have had depressive episodes in the past but is not required to have had them to be diagnosed with Bipolar I.

To have a Bipolar II diagnosis Maria would need to have at least one major depressive episodes accompanied by at least one hypomanic episode. If she has a manic or mixed episode in the course of Bipolar II, the diagnosis is changed to Bipolar I.

Criteria for a manic episode includes having a specific period in which the client's mood is elevated above normal consistently or is expansive or irritable for at least a week. If hospitalization is needed, any length of time where there are mood changes as described is sufficient. During the mood disturbance the client must have at least three of seven symptoms (four symptoms are required if the mood is only irritable). Maria has at least five of the symptoms, which include: inflated self-esteem or grandiosity, decreased need for sleep, more talkative than usual, distractibility, and excessive involvement in pleasurable activities, such as buying sprees and sexual indiscretions, which have a high potential for painful consequences. Another criteria is that the mood disturbance must cause marked impairment in some area of functioning or necessitate hospitalization to avoid harm to self or others, or psychotic features must be present (APA, 2000). Maria meets at least the marked impairment in functioning and the need for hospitalization.

2. **What would it feel like to be manic, and why would someone who is manic stop taking medication to bring their mood down to "normal"?** In the book entitled *An Unquiet Mind: A Memoir of Moods and Madness*, Kay Redfield Jamison (1997) describes what it is like to be manic as well as seriously depressed: "My body is uninhabitable. It is raging and weeping and full of destruction and wild energy gone amok." She discusses at length her reluctance to take lithium in the early period of treatment, as she, like many other manics, feared losing the "intoxicating poetic exhilarations of pure mania." Manics can clean the entire house in a short time in the middle of the night and can be very creative when the manic energy is high.

3. **If you were Maria's nurse, what needs would you assess in relation to her culture and communication? What accommodations would you most likely try to make for her?** You will want to find out about any customs that are important to Maria. You will need to arrange for a Spanish-English translator for teaching sessions, therapy sessions, and any other sessions where understanding is critical. If you don't speak Spanish, it would be helpful to learn a few phrases. You will want to find out if Maria is using any alternative medicines and/or healing. It is important to learn Maria's beliefs about mental illness. Habel (2004) states that many Hispanics and some in other cultures have a "magicoreligious health belief system" believing that supernatural forces "influence health and illness." They "have aspects of magic (as well as religion) in their health belief practices"; it is fairly common for poor rural Hispanics of Nicaragua to view someone with mental illness as being possessed by the devil and to offer herbal remedies and prayer for a "cure."

Many Catholics in Central America view the Church as a central part of life, so you will need to arrange for Maria to attend Mass if she wants Mass or, if this is not possible, accommodate insofar as possible a request to have a priest visit.

You need to assess Maria's usual diet. The poor of Nicaragua eat a diet consisting mainly of beans, rice, and tortillas and, when they have it, some small amount of chicken and/or eggs. In some areas of Nicaragua fish are available and part of the diet. When ill, Maria may prefer the diet of her childhood.

While you may have some general ideas about the Hispanic culture or the rural Nicaraguan culture, it is important to assess Maria as an individual because, as Kavanaugh and Gardiner (2003) point out, "every culture has incredible diversity and subcultures."

4. **Why did the nurse ask the dietitian to prepare a sandwich and a banana for Maria, and why did the nurse take Maria to her room?** Finger foods are easier for a manic person to eat when they are restless and moving about. The foods ordered are finger foods and soft foods, which are less likely to cause choking if the client does not take time to chew well. The nurse probably took Maria to her room so she would have fewer distractions during the time she has to eat.

5. **What is the most likely reason for the psychiatrist ordering a pregnancy test on admission? Why did he order birth control pills? The client has refused the birth control pills. How do you feel about this, and what action**

would you take if you were the nurse in this case? Lithium is toxic to the embryo in the first three months of pregnancy. The physician wants assurance that Maria is not pregnant before giving her lithium. Female clients of childbearing years must have a negative pregnancy test before being started on lithium and neuroleptics. The psychiatrist ordered birth control pills for this female client as he wants to insure that she does not become pregnant while on lithium and olanzapine (Zyprexa) in a hypersexual state. Regardless of how you feel about birth control in general or the doctor ordering birth control, in this specific case, the client has refused the pills and she has the right to do so as a voluntary admission to the hospital.

6. **What reason did the nurse have for inspecting Maria's mouth after giving her the medication?** The nurse needed to make certain that Maria was not "cheeking" the medication. The health care provider will order these checks if he or she suspects the client of holding the medication in the cheeks and spitting it out when and where the staff will not discover it or saving it up to take all at once. A prudent nurse will do these checks routinely with or without an order by the physician.

7. **What teaching did the nurse need to do about lithium for Maria? What is the significance of the lithium level, and what action(s) does the nurse need to take, if any?** When taking lithium, a person needs to keep fluid and salt intake stable with a normal moderate salt intake and a fluid intake of 2,000 to 3,000 ml of water a day. The client can be taught to increase the sodium some if they are perspiring a lot. The client is taught to limit intake of coffee, tea, and cola due to the diuretic effect of those drinks. Taking lithium with meals reduces nausea. Some side effects, such as thirst, nausea, dry mouth, thirst mild hand tremors, weight gain, bloated feeling, insomnia, will lessen with time. The client needs to be taught which symptoms to report immediately, such as the symptoms of mild to moderate toxicity: vomiting, diarrhea, tremors, overall muscle weakness, vertigo, lack of coordination, and feeling very sedated, as well as the symptoms associated with major toxicity, which are ringing in the ears, blurred vision, dilute urine, and a sense of giddiness (Spratto and Woods, 2006).

 The therapeutic range for serum lithium levels is 0.6 to 1.2 mEq/L. A serum lithium level of 1.5 falls into the mild to moderately toxic range. The nurse needs to immediately hold any lithium doses and notify the client's health care provider of the lab results. In addition, the nurse needs to assess for signs of lithium toxicity described above. The nurse needs to collaborate with the rest of the team in looking for causes of lithium toxicity, which could be too high a dose of lithium, not drinking enough water, eating a salt poor diet (lithium competes with salt for reabsorption in the renal tubules), diarrhea, and/or fever.

8. **What is olanzapine (Zyprexa), and what is the likely reason that Maria is being prescribed olanzapine?** Olanzapine is an atypical antipsychotic agent. Atypical antipsychotic medications, including olanzapine, have been shown in studies to be "effective for acute manic episodes associated with bipolar disorder. Some atypical antipsychotics have been demonstrated to have mood-stabilizing properties while at the same time less side effects are reported" (Tugrol, 2004). The Federal Drug Administration (FDA) approved olanzapine for the short-term management of acute mania in bipolar disorder, and in 2004 the FDA approved it for maintenance therapy in long-term treatment of bipolar disorder. The American Psychiatric Association (APA) Practice Guidelines for Bipolar Disorder recommend that antipsychotic drugs be used in conjunction with mood stabilizers (e.g., lithium).

9. **What would you do or say if you were the nurse standing in front of Maria when she says: "You think you so smart. You don't know nothing"?** One theory is that when clients are hostile they are afraid of others and the behavior is a protective mechanism to keep others at a distance. Nurses may need to excuse themselves and not try to approach the client for a while. Another staff member may be able to approach without difficulty when necessary.

10. **What strategies could a nurse use when Maria is demanding that a staff member be sent to shop for her using her credit card? Do strategies differ depending on whether the client has supportive family and/or friends, or not?** The nurse could offer to help Maria determine what things her husband, family, and/or friends could bring to her. In this case Maria has a husband who will probably shop for her. In some cases the

family has abandoned the client due to their behavior and ongoing needs. In these cases, the nurse needs to set some limits such as telling the client that no one can use his credit card and go over his shopping list to determine which things are allowed on the unit and are priorities at this time and to keep the list within the client's amount of money. The nurse need to advise staff that it is unethical to spend any of the client's money on themselves or to borrow it or use it for any purpose other than to purchase items the client has asked for.

11. **What might you say or do in response to the husband's expressed fear that his wife will become involved sexually with a peer on the unit?** You will want to acknowledge that you hear and understand his concerns and take them seriously. Tell him that you and the staff will do your best to keep his wife safe. You need to instruct the staff to be vigilant in preventing inappropriate contact between client and peers. The client must not go off the unit unescorted. Many facilities have the capacity for the clients' bedrooms to be locked from the outside to prevent peers from entering, but with egress from the inside to allow the clients to leave the room. The halls must be monitored. Routine checks to determine the clients' whereabouts need to be carried out at least every half hour.

12. **How would you feel and what would you say or do if you were the male nurse passing medications and Maria was talking seductively and using profanity?** Responses to this situation vary from person to person. Some people might feel repulsed at this language and behavior while others might be fascinated with it. As the nurse, you need to stay professional and therapeutic. You can tell the client that the language and behavior is inappropriate and that you are not going to listen to her unless she stops the profanity. If she does not stop, you can walk away in some situations. When passing medications, you cannot leave your medicine cart or station and walk away, but you can do some other ignoring behaviors such as not giving eye contact or not responding verbally.

13. **When the nurse finds Maria has been intrusive with another client and that both clients are escalating and threatening, what is the best response by the nurse?** The nurse needs to immediately summon additional staff and not work with the two clients single-handedly as this is not safe. The clients need to be separated with Maria taken to a quiet place.

14. **What are some potential nursing diagnoses that you could likely write for this client?** Some nursing diagnoses likely to be appropriate for this client after further assessment include:

   • Noncompliance (medication regimen)
   • Knowledge deficit related to medications
   • Thought processes altered
   • Risk for violence directed to others
   • Nutrition less than body requirements

15. **What developmental stage is Maria in, and what behaviors, if any, does she have to match the tasks of this stage?** Maria is entering her middle adult years (35 to 64) and Erickson's stage of generativity vs. stagnation. A person who is mastering generativity engages in caring for and guiding children as a parent, mentor, community leader, or volunteer. There is little evidence that Maria is focused on guiding the next generation. The nurse will continue to assess her behaviors, and as Maria becomes better, the nurse can guide Maria to work on the tasks of generativity. Earlier stages of development may also need work as Maria may not have mastered the tasks of those stages (Frisch and Frisch, 2006).

References

American Psychiatric Association. (2000). *Diagnostic and Statistical Manual of Mental Disorders, 4th ed.* Text Revision. Washington, DC: American Psychiatric Association.

Frisch, N. C. and L. E. Frisch. (2006). *Psychiatric Mental Health Nursing, 3rd ed.* Albany, NY: Thomson Delmar Learning.

Habel, M. (2004). "Caring for People of Many Cultures." *Nurse Week.* January 2, 2004.

Jamison, K.R. (1997). *An Unquiet Mind: A Memoir of Moods and Madness.* New York: Knopf Publishing.

Kavanaugh, K.M. and S.D. Gardiner. (2003). "Culturally Sensitive Care." *Advance for Nurses* 1(3): 28–30.

Spratto, G.R. and A.L. Woods. (2006). *PDR Nurse's Drug Handbook.* Clifton Park, NY: Thomson Delmar Learning.

Turgol, K.C. (2004). "Evolving Role of Antipsychotic Therapy in the Management of Bipolar Disorder." *Advanced Studies in Nursing* 2(11): 24–32.

Candice

GENDER

Female

AGE

13

SETTING

- Adolescent unit of private psychiatric hospital

ETHNICITY

- White American

CULTURAL CONSIDERATIONS

PREEXISTING CONDITION

COEXISTING CONDITION

- Marijuana use

COMMUNICATION

DISABILITY

SOCIOECONOMIC

- Upper class; has trust fund

SPIRITUAL/RELIGIOUS

PHARMACOLOGIC

PSYCHOSOCIAL

LEGAL

ETHICAL

ALTERNATIVE THERAPY

PRIORITIZATION

- Prioritizing urgent vs. important tasks

DELEGATION

- Delegating to mental health technician

MODERATE

MOOD DISORDER IN A CHILD, BIPOLAR EPISODE

Level of difficulty: Moderate

Overview: Requires critical thinking to determine least restrictive yet effective interventions with an adolescent who has a family history of Bipolar Disorder (BPD) and symptoms of a Manic Episode. Requires therapeutic communication skills as well as empathy to help the client's parents understand treatment approaches and feel they are an essential part of the treatment team. Requires an understanding of the basic principles involved in seclusion and restraint.

Client Profile

Candice is a 13-year-old female whose grandfather made a fortune in the oil business and left her a trust fund when he died. Her grandfather was known to have required little sleep and to have a phenomenal amount of energy at times. He was said to have had a number of mistresses, sometimes gone on spending sprees, and given extravagant tips to waitresses even when he only ordered a cup of coffee. Once when he was in a private psychiatric hospital, he ordered two hundred steak dinners and called a taxi to pick them up and deliver them to the hospital for all the patients and staff. He called a jeweler and ordered a diamond ring for one of the nurses he had just met and then threatened to get five lawyers to come to the hospital when she refused to marry him. Grandfather eventually committed suicide, but not before he was diagnosed as manic-depressive (term used before Bipolar Disorder came into use) and put on lithium, which he refused to take.

Candice recently has been having a somewhat elated mood (e.g., giggling about things that others don't find funny and taking about the exquisite beauty in mundane things such as a light bulb). The speed of her speech has increased, and she jumps rapidly from topic to topic. She has been staying up all night drawing original cartoons and/or rearranging her room and the family living room. At school, Candice has recently been going to the principal's office or catching her in the hall to tell her how to run the school better. She also tells the teacher how to make the classroom better. At school Candice was caught kissing a boy in the boy's restroom and the teacher intercepted a note that Candice wrote to another boy suggesting they engage in sex. Candice's father discovered that she was e-mailing a 27-year-old man that she had never met and planned to run away with him. She denied drug use but admitted that she had started smoking cigarettes and occasionally smoked marijuana, which she had gotten from her father's desk. Candice's father had her evaluated by a child-adolescent psychiatrist, and she was admitted to the adolescent unit of a private psychiatric hospital for evaluation and treatment. Candice's parents were worried that they could not keep Candice from running away and getting into trouble so they agreed to pay whatever it cost.

Case Study

Candice has been admitted to the adolescent unit. The nurse notices that Candice is pacing rapidly in the day room and goes to talk to her. Candice talks rapidly, moving from topic to topic. One of her themes is getting out of the hospital to meet her "friend." As the nurse walks away, she hears one of Candice's peers on the unit tell her: "Back off; get out of my face." The nurse then sees Candice scratching and hitting the peer. When a male mental health technician tries to pull Candice away from the peer, Candice scratches him deeply with her long fingernails and kicks him. Other staff members, including the nurse, take Candice to the seclusion room. The nurse calls the psychiatrist for an order to seclude Candice, who is in the seclusion room scratching herself superficially with her nails and smearing blood on the walls. The mental health worker reports later that Candice is asleep in the seclusion room. When she awakes the nurse talks with her and decides to let her out of seclusion but not before cutting Candice's fingernails. When Candice's parents come to visit, they are very angry about her long nails being cut and about her being put in seclusion. They express concern about the possibility of sexual activity with boys on the unit and whether or not Candice is stopping her seemingly constant motion long enough to eat.

Questions and Suggested Answers

1. **Should you, if you were the nurse in this case, have gotten an order from the physician before secluding the client? When secluding a client, is it ever correct to delegate all communication with the client to another team member such as a mental health technician?** Frequently there is not time to call the health care provider for an order before secluding the client because the client exhibits rapidly escalating behavior and would benefit from immediate seclusion as a protection from harming themselves or others. You need to

call the health care provider for an order to seclude the client before secluding whenever circumstances permit this, but when this is not possible for safety reasons, you can make the call as soon as possible after the seclusion has occurred.

It is common practice and policy, in some facilities, to have one designated trained person to communicate with the client during seclusion. Hearing and responding to one staff member is less confusing to the client than hearing a variety of things from various team members. The selected person is usually the scheduled designated seclusion team leader or has the best relationship with the client being secluded. Team members have signals for communicating without words to each other.

2. **Discuss safety precautions and tasks required of the staff when a child or adolescent is secluded. What needs to be documented? How would you decide when to release the client from seclusion?** Seclusion rooms are designed so that the person in seclusion can be seen in a mirror in the corner of the room, no matter where he or she is located in the room. A staff member is required to visually check the client every fifteen minutes and document the activity of the client at the time of the check. It is the nurse's responsibility to make certain that the safety checks are done every fifteen minutes and that needed as well as required care is given. State rules and regulations and facility policies and procedures require that food and water and toileting are offered at certain intervals. This care, the fifteen-minute checks, the reason for and time of secluding the client, the behavior justifying the seclusion, and the time of release and the behavior justifying release must all be documented.

Occasionally secluded clients have hurt themselves or killed themselves between fifteen-minute checks. A client might bang on the walls or door so hard they break a bone, might bite off a finger and lie bleeding with their hand hidden under their body, or might hang himself or herself if there is a doorknob inside the seclusion room or any object strong enough to hold their weight. An article on the Child and Adolescent Bipolar Organization Web page (www.bpkids.org, 2005) states, "Bipolar Disorder is a life-threatening medial condition with a mortality rate of over 10% from suicide."

A staff member can be assigned to the client in seclusion to help the client feel safe and to relax instead of using the more restrictive option of restraint. Use of restraints requires a staff member to be present at arm's length to protect the restrained client from harm. If a client in seclusion needs restraint, the nurse will have to obtain a specific order for a time-limited restraint and read and follow the facility's seclusion and restraint policies and procedures.

At the time they are secluded, clients must be told the reason for their seclusion and the behavior that is required for release from seclusion. All states have regulations and facilities have rules and policies about when a client must be released from seclusion. A common requirement is to release a client who has fallen asleep or who has been quiet for a specified time and agreed to control their behavior. Seclusion orders are time limited. If the order is to seclude for up to four hours, the client must be released on or before the four hours are up; if not ready for release another order must be obtained. Each seclusion must have its own order.

3. **Just as you pick up the phone to call the health care provider for orders for secluding Candice, another adolescent client comes running up to you and says: "I need to talk with you right now about something very important." Do you stop what you are doing and listen, get the orders first then listen, send this child to another staff member, or come up with another solution?** You need to talk with the health care provider and get the order for seclusion without much delay; however, this can wait a few minutes. You need to try to quickly get an idea from the child as to how much of an emergency the situation is. If the situation cannot be handled quickly or wait for you, then delegate this child's situation to another nurse. You must be careful that the child, wanting to talk with you, does not overhear your telephone conversation with the health care provider about the seclusion order. Some children or adult clients stay near the nurses' station hoping to pick up some interesting information about peers or themselves, while others do it accidentally and then may become focused on the peer's issues rather than working on their own. As a matter of confidentiality, you must be very careful about who hears your conversations in the nurses' station/staff office, at home, and elsewhere.

4. **After the client is out of seclusion, you sit in on a debriefing with the seclusion team. Do you think that the situation in the day room that led to seclusion was handled well, or could seclusion have been avoided?**

Could the injuries have been avoided? What would you say or do in the briefing? Clients are to be in the least restrictive environment based on their behavior and response to interventions. Before secluding a client, staff are to try less restrictive options like talking with the client, redirecting the client, or taking the client to a quiet place that is not secluded. Medication can be considered a medical restraint in some circumstances, but it is less restrictive than seclusion. Once Candice started attacking a peer, the mental health technician had limited options. Getting Candice into a safe and approved hold and secluding her was one option. Mental health technicians are trained in approved holds and releases as well as ways to manage aggressive behavior by getting the client to talk and listening to the client and negotiating with them. The staff member and/or the nurse did need to call for help. If several staff would have been made visible to the client, this "show of force" may have brought the client to a state of compliance.

As the nurse you must think about whether or not you need to get an order for restraint for this client when she is scratching herself and smearing the wall with blood. If this behavior goes on for any length of time, Candice needs to be restrained and observed on a 1:1 staff to client basis.

You can ask each team member to think about anything that could have been handled in a way that would have resulted in a less restrictive means of calming the client. You can ask each member about what they think they did well during this seclusion and what they think could be improved upon in secluding the next client. You will want to stress the idea of preventing seclusion whenever possible and discuss ideas such as careful observation of clients for clues they may need to be calmed down by going to a quiet place or talking or getting into some activity. You will also want to stress using less restrictive options and get the staff to talk about these. You may decide to request additional training in management of aggressive behavior for the staff and/or additional practice sessions.

5. **What behaviors do children and adolescents who are diagnosed with a Bipolar Disorder exhibit? What diagnostic criteria would Candice, or other children and/or adolescents, have to meet to be diagnosed as having a Bipolar Episode or Bipolar Disorder? Does her behavior match any of these criteria?** One behavior of children and adolescents with Bipolar Disorder comes out of the grandiosity associated with these disorders and involves the child or adolescent telling the teacher what to teach or telling the principal or vice principal to fire a teacher or what to do to make the school better. Other behaviors seen in children with Bipolar Disorder include: giggling inappropriately at things they should be concerned about such as grades falling, moving rapidly and illogically from topic to topic, and sleeping very little. Some children and adolescents as well as adults tend to stay up all night when in a manic phase and may be very creative and/or clean or rearrange a room or the house in a record amount of time. Children and adolescents may have trouble paying attention. They may be hyperactive, irritable, euphoric, grandiose, and have pressured speech, which are symptoms also seen in adults. Similar to adults, some adolescents in a manic episode may be hypersexual compared to peers. These children and adolescents may carry out daredevil acts or have a lot of anger that comes and goes. Some children and adolescents with Bipolar Disorder describe feeling out of control, not feeling right with the world, and not having friends (Wilens et al., 2001).

Bipolar diagnoses vary depending on the types of episodes experienced. *The Diagnostic and Statistical Manual of Mental Disorders IV-TR* (APA, 2000) divides Bipolar into Bipolar I and II, with the diagnostic criteria being the same for children and adolescents as for adults. A Bipolar I diagnosis requires at least one Manic Episode or a Mixed Manic and Major Depressive Episode. A diagnosis of Bipolar II requires one or more Major Depressive Episodes plus at least one Hypomanic Episode. Candice's behavior would appear more manic than hypomanic. Criteria for a Manic Episode include:

1. A mood that "is abnormally and persistently elevated, expansive, or irritable" and lasts one week or more or any amount of time if the person is hospitalized.

2. At least three of the following seven symptoms (four symptoms if mood only irritable) that are persistent during the time of the mood disturbance:

- Self-esteem inflated or grandiosity
- Need for sleep is less than usual (may feel rested with three hours of sleep)

MOOD LOG

Name: _____

Month: _____ Year: _____

Rate mood

0 ——— 50 ——— 100
Dep   Normal   Mania

Days of Month →	1	2	3	4	5	6	7	8	9	10	11	12	13	14	15	16	17	18	19	20	21	22	23	24	25	26	27	28	29	30	31
Mania																															
Depression																															
Anxiety (1–10)																															

Medication

_____

_____

_____

_____

_____

_____

	1	2	3	4	5	6	7	8	9	10	11	12	13	14	15	16	17	18	19	20	21	22	23	24	25	26	27	28	29	30	31
Menses																															
Sleep																															

A mood log can be used to document periods of mania and depression.

- Hypertalkative or pressured speech
- Feeling as if thoughts are racing or having flight of ideas
- Distractibility (responds easily to unimportant or irrelevant external stimuli)
- Increased psychomotor agitation or goal-directed activities
- Overinvolvement in activities that are viewed as pleasurable but that have high risk for painful consequences, such as going on buying sprees, having sexual indiscretions, or engaging in foolish business investments
- The symptoms do not meet criteria for mixed episode (depression and mania)
- Mood disturbance is severe enough to cause marked impairment in some important area of functioning such as in relationships or social activities, or to require hospitalization to prevent harm to self or others, or to cause psychotic features
- Symptoms not due to a medicine, a general medical condition, or use of addictive substances.

Candice has at least three or four listed symptoms that have caused impairment in her social life, her family life, and perhaps life at school. In your assessments and those of other professionals on the team, you will be trying to get a good history of any previous episodes, any depressive periods or mixed periods of depression and mania or hypomania, and you will be documenting the behaviors that you see and what the client says as this documentation provides clues to the client's moods during your shift. Eventually a mental health professional qualified to diagnose and having sufficient information about Candice's moods and other behaviors could diagnose her as having either Bipolar I or II.

6. **Describe why clinicians have difficulty diagnosing mood disorders in children and adolescents and why parents and clinicians confuse it with other disorders.** Bipolar Disorders and some other disorders have the same or similar symptoms (e.g., mania and ADHD share the symptoms of hyperactivity, irritability, and distractibility); however, only the child or adolescent with Bipolar Disorder has elated mood exhibited in such behaviors as giggling and grandiosity exemplified in such behaviors as telling the teacher what to teach (Wilens et al., 2001). The symptoms of alcohol abuse and abuse of other substances include depressed as well as manic or hypomanic behavior, which can make it difficult to discern if the behaviors are due to drugs or to a mood disorder or to both.

Gracious, Youngstrom, Findling, and Calabrese (2002) point out that not only is it difficult to differentiate Bipolar Disorder from ADHD, but it is difficult to differentiate it from Conduct Disorder and Schizophrenia. Ramasamy, Ambrosini, and Coffey (2003) point out that "although young patients may present with classic symptomatology consistent with adult mania (e.g. elevated mood, grandiosity, and flight of ideas), younger patients may also present with less florid though no less challenging symptoms (e.g. unrelenting irritability, aggressive dyscontrol, and mixed states)."

7. **What do you think causes Bipolar Disorder? Does genetics play a role in the cause of Bipolar Disorder? What is the age of onset and the usual course of Bipolar Disorder? Is the course the same in children compared to adults?** Most theorists/scientists think there is no single cause for Bipolar Disorder, though most scientists today think genetics plays some role in causing Bipolar Disorder. You will note that Candice's grandfather was diagnosed with Manic-Depressive Disorder (an older term for Bipolar Disorder). Having a biological family member with a Bipolar Disorder makes the diagnosis somewhat more plausible for Candice.

Scientists are trying to identify the genes that play a role in development of the disorder and what that role is. Identical twin studies have shown that genetics alone cannot explain Bipolar Disorder. The second identical twin is more likely to develop Bipolar Disorder than a nontwin sibling, but does not necessarily develop the diagnosis. Scientists lean toward a multifactorial cause including not only genetics but environment as well. One theory is that genetics provide a predisposition to Bipolar Disorder and a client's strengths hold off the development of the disorder until environmental and internal stressors and genetics are too much for the client's strengths to overcome.

Scientists are using MRI and PET scans to study the brains of people with Bipolar Disorder and those without the disorder to see if there are differences in structure or functioning (www.nimh.nih.gov/publicat/bipolar.cfm, 2005).

According to Geller, (Wilens et al., 2001) the principal investigator in a study of ninety-three children with Bipolar Illness conducted at Washington University, adults will typically have episodes of either depression or mania lasting a few months with apparently normal functioning between episodes. Children do not have this pattern. Geller has found many children to be both manic and depressed at the same time and often staying ill for years without the well periods that adults demonstrate.

Bhangoo et al. (2003) did a study involving children with BPD classified as either having chronic or episodic symptoms. These researchers stated that their preliminary data indicate that "among children being treated for BPD in the community, those with discrete episodes of mania may be more likely to have a lifetime history of psychosis and a parental history of BPD."

Looking at onset of Bipolar Disorder, Geller and other researchers at Washington University found children as young as age 7 with Bipolar Illness resembling the severest form in adults. In the Washington University study the average age of participants was 10, with 43 percent of the subjects between 7 and 10 years of age.

Other studies have reported a later age of onset. Aarkrog (1999) reported on a study by Olsen who looked at twenty-eight patients with manic-depressive illness whose first episode came before age 19. The average age of onset of first manic episode for females was age 16 and for males the first Manic Episode was at 15 years.

APA (2000) reported 20 years old as the mean age of onset for the first Manic Episode, with some cases starting in adolescence and some after age 50.

Some theorists have speculated that the use of newer antidepressants in children and adolescents who have exhibited symptoms of major depression or some form of depression will cause the children who would eventually exhibit symptoms of mania to exhibit the mania much younger.

8. **What is your response to the parents' anger about Candice being in seclusion and having her nails cut? How would you answer the parents in regard to their concerns about their daughter's possible sexual activity while in the facility?** You must avoid being defensive. You need to stay calm and try to use a caring voice to convey the idea that you care about Candice's well-being and that you really felt badly about having to seclude her and cut her beautiful nails but needed to do so for safety. Try to work closely with the parents, conveying the idea that they are part of the team and that the staff will work with them to help Candice and try to prevent having to seclude her in the future.

You can describe the equipment or staff practices that keep the male and female adolescent groups separated. A number of child and adolescent units in private psychiatric treatment facilities have motion detector systems operating when clients are in bed at night or assigned to be in their rooms. Some units have closed-circuit TV monitors on the hall. It is somewhat reassuring to parents to know that such equipment is in place and being monitored by staff. Units without such equipment may house the boys on one half of the hall and the girls on the other half with a colored tape on the floor to mark the line each gender cannot cross. There are consequences for crossing the line and rewards for following the rules.

Facilities also have periodic routine room checks. In some facilities the nurse can delegate bed checks every half hour to nurses' aides or mental health workers, but must do a certain number herself or himself. Know your facility policy on room checks. Whether the facility requires it or not, you as the nurse need to do some checks yourself. You can get input from the team about how to insure that Candice does not engage in sexual activity with peers.

You cannot absolutely guarantee to the parents that their child or adolescent will be safe from sexual contact with another child, but you can do your best to prevent such contact and can discuss the safety measures with the parents.

9. **What nursing diagnoses are you likely to write for this client given what information you have? What are some tentative goals that you might develop with input from the client/family/colleagues on the unit? What**

interventions do you think would be necessary and/or helpful? Some possible nursing diagnoses for Candice include:

- Violence, self-directed
- Violence, other-directed
- Noncompliance
- Knowledge deficit
- At risk for imbalanced nutrition

Tentative goals could include:

- Will have no incidences of harm to self or others
- Will maintain weight

Or:

- Will eat 75 percent or more of meals served
- Will keep a social distance from peers on unit
- Will comply with treatment regimen
- Will attend 100 percent of education classes and groups assigned

Observe for clues of suicidal ideation on an ongoing basis. Have the client sign a No Harm/No Suicide contract (an agreement to contact the nurse immediately if the client is having thoughts of hurting or killing himself). Serve small-sized finger foods and food easy to eat without choking and easy to carry, such as sandwiches or chicken fingers. People who are in a manic episode often won't stop to eat. They also tend to be busy looking after other people (e.g., getting everyone napkins). They don't have time to chew and will try to swallow large pieces and start to choke if not watched closely. Clients need close observation by staff at mealtimes and anytime food is served.

Close observation by a staff member may also be a necessary intervention to keep Candice from inappropriate touching with peers. Assign tokens or points or some reward system for complying with a "no touch" rule and consequences for inappropriate touch. Peers can be taught to tell Candice to stop if she is touching them inappropriately or making inappropriate sexual remarks.

You could provide some education about the risks of nicotine and marijuana use/abuse and plan some interventions to get her to commit to stopping the use of these substances. The issue of her getting the marijuana from her father's desk could be addressed with the father individually. The nurse could use therapeutic communication techniques and enlist his support in being a good role model for the client. This issue could perhaps be addressed in family therapy sessions.

Parents will need to be educated about the serious risk of suicide. In Letters to the Editor in the *Journal of the American Academy of Child and Adolescent Psychiatry* (Wilens et al. 2003), Martha Hellander, the Executive Director of the Child and Adolescent Bipolar Foundation, describes preschool children who have made suicidal attempts or threats. She describes parents reporting such things as their preschoolers deliberately laying down under the wheels of cars, tying ropes around their necks, and cutting themselves with various instruments and much later being diagnosed with Bipolar Disorder. Hellander points out that professionals can make the mistake of assuming such acts are only active imagination and harmless when they can be serious attempts and/or diagnostic clues.

10. **What medications and treatments are being used today for children and adolescents who are exhibiting signs of mood disorders, particularly signs of Bipolar Disorder?** Antidepressants, especially SSRIs, have been prescribed for children and adolescents as well as adults with depression. Some children who present with symptoms of Major Depressive Disorder will later have a Manic Episode and be diagnosed with some type of bipolar illness. According to Ascribe Newswire, Health (Wilens et al. 2004), the Child and Adolescent Bipolar Foundation asked the Food and Drug Administration (FDA) to require that drug companies warn parents and physicians that antidepressants have the potential to worsen or trigger suicidality and can make

mania and rapid cycling Bipolar Disorder worse in some children. Antidepressants may precipitate mania according to Cicero, Mallakh, Holman, and Robertson (2003), who also noted that antidepressants have been increasingly used in children and adolescents and that Bipolar Disorder is increasingly being diagnosed in children and adolescents. In a study by these researchers they claimed that "although far from conclusive, [their] data [is] consistent with the hypothesis that antidepressant treatment is associated with a Manic Episode earlier than might occur spontaneously."

Ramasamy, Ambrosini, and Coffey (2003) stated, "There is some evidence to suggest that lithium (Eskalith, Lithobid), valproic acid or divalproex sodium (Valproate, Depakote) and carbamazepine (Tegretol, Tegretal XR) may be effective in treating mania in youth." These authors did caution that compliance is a significant issue in a client with Bipolar Disorder who is on medicine. People who are Bipolar often hate to give up their highs and the creativity that comes with these highs.

There is some relatively recent evidence reported by Delbello (as cited by Ramasamy, Ambrosini, and Coffey, 2003) suggesting that olanzapine (Zyprexa), risperodone (Risperdol), and quetiapine (Seroquel) along with divalproex sodium have antimanic effects.

Findling et al. (2003) did a study using a combination of lithium and divalproex sodium with ninety subjects aged 5 to 17 with a diagnosis of Bipolar Disorder. These researchers concluded that this combination of medication could safely and effectively be used in the treatment of mania and depression in juvenile Bipolar Disorder.

In addition to medication, treatment includes such modalities as individual, group, and family therapy. Many communities have family support groups for the families of clients with Bipolar Disorder. Since many clients with Bipolar Disorder resist treatment, it is especially important to educate the family about the disorder and ways to help the client be more compliant with treatment regimens.

11. *Note: The following two studies are examples of research being conducted in Bipolar Disorder in children and adolescents.* **What research has been done, or is currently being carried out, with children and adolescents who have a diagnosis of Bipolar Disorder?** Wilens et al. (2000) conducted research with 31 adolescents from a group of 128 boys with Attention Deficit Hyperactivity Disorder who were also diagnosed with Bipolar Disorder and a group of 109 subjects with neither ADHD or Bipolar Disorder. These researchers found that "the developmental onset of BPD in adolescence (ages 13–18 years) conferred a greater risk for cigarette smoking compared to those youths with the onset of their BPD prepubertally (less than 12 years) even after controlling for conduct disorder and other confounds." The rate of cigarette smoking in youths with BPD was significantly higher than in non-BPD youths after controlling for ADHD confounds. In addition to the higher risk of smoking with later adolescent onset of BPD, there was a significantly greater incidence of cigarette smoking in adolescents with BPD compared to those without this diagnosis after controlling for ADHD.

Gracious, Youngstrom, Findling, and Calabrese (2002) examined the usefulness of a parent report version of the Young Mania Rating Scale developed by Young and colleagues in 1978. The subject group included parents and 117 youths aged 5 to 17 years old. These researchers concluded "this rating scale (Parent Version of the Young Mania Rating Scale) may be used to derive clinically meaningful information about mood disorders in youths."

References

Aarkrog, T. (1999). "Psychotic Adolescents 20–25 Years Later." *Nord Journal of Psychiatry* 53(Supplement 42): 1–38.

American Psychiatric Association. (2000). *Diagnostic and Statistical Manual of Mental Disorders, 4th ed.* Text Revision. Washington, DC: American Psychiatric Association.

Bhangoo, R.K. et al. (2003). "Clinical Correlates of Episodicity in Juvenile Mania." *Journal of Child and Adolescent Psychopharmacology* 13(4): 507–514.

Cicero, D., R.F. Mallakh, J. Holman, and J. Robertson. (2003). "Antidepressant Exposure in Bipolar Children." *Psychiatry* 66(4): 317–318.

Findling, R.L. et al. (2003). "Combination Lithium and Divalproex Sodium in Pediatric Bipolarity." *Journal of the American Academy of Child Adolescent Psychiatry* 42(8): 895–901.

Gracious, B.L., E.A. Youngstrom, R.L. Findling, and J.R. Calabrese. (2002). "Discriminative Validity of a Parent Version of the Young Mania Rating Scale." *Journal of the American Academy of Child Adolescent Psychiatry* 41(11): 1350–1360.

Ramasamy, D., P. Ambrosini, and B. Coffey (2003). "Clinical Case Presentation: Therapeutic Challenges in Adolescent-Onset Bipolar Disorder." *Journal of Child and Adolescent Psychopharmacology* 13(4): 425–430.

Wilens, T.E. et al. (2000). "Is Bipolar Disorder a Risk for Cigarette Smoking in ADHD Youth?" *American Journal on Addictions* 9(3): 187–186.

———. (2001). "Bipolar Disorder in Children Appears More Severe Than in Most Adults Say Washington University Researchers." Ascribe Newswire, Health, June 14, 4–6.

———. (2003). Letters to the Editor, "Depression and Suicidality in Preschoolers." *Journal of the American Academy of Child Adolescent Psychiatry* 42(10): 1141.

———. (2004). "Parents of Bipolar Children Praise FDA Warning on Antidepressants, Suicidality." Ascribe Newswire, Health, March 22, 9–11. Available online at www.bpkids.org.

www.bpkids.org. Accessed January 2, 2005.

www.nimh.nih.gov/publicat/bipolar.cfm. Accessed January 2, 2005.

GENDER	**SPIRITUAL/RELIGIOUS**
Female	
AGE	**PHARMACOLOGIC**
41	■ Citalopram hydrochloride (Celexa)
SETTING	**PSYCHOSOCIAL**
■ Psychiatric unit of a general hospital	■ Isolating
ETHNICITY	**LEGAL**
■ German	■ Confidentiality
	■ Client right to refuse treatment
CULTURAL CONSIDERATIONS	**ETHICAL**
■ German	■ Respect for confidentiality vs. informing
■ Military	neighbor to ensure client safely
PREEXISTING CONDITION	**ALTERNATIVE THERAPY**
COEXISTING CONDITION	**PRIORITIZATION**
	■ Safety issues
COMMUNICATION	**DELEGATION**
DISABILITY	
SOCIOECONOMIC	

MAJOR DEPRESSIVE DISORDER

Level of difficulty: High

Overview: Requires the nurse to identify symptoms of major depression, look at factors contributing to depression, and identify strategies to prevent suicide.

DIFFICULT

Client Profile

Elke, a 41-year-old female, came to the United States five years ago, shortly after marrying a career U.S. military soldier. Elke has two children: a 10-year-old from a previous marriage and a 6-year-old from the current marriage. Elke has been a meticulous housekeeper and has managed the family finances. Since arriving in the United States, she has not been back to Germany to see her parents and siblings. Although she would very much like to visit her family, she can't afford to do so.

Case Study

Elke is admitted to the psychiatric unit of the city's general hospital. Her husband had noticed that she was so depressed she no longer laughed or smiled. She had admitted to him that she had been having thoughts of killing herself. She was not eating or drinking enough, had lost fifteen pounds in three weeks, and was not attending to her hygiene. Elke seemed to have little or no interest in anything except sleeping or sitting in a chair. The client's husband accompanies her on admission and shares with the staff that he is afraid Elke will kill herself and he is unable to watch her around the clock. He says that he believes if she does not kill herself by some means such as hoarding pills and overdosing that she will deteriorate by not eating or drinking enough.

On admission the psychiatric nurse asks Elke about any prior episodes of depression. The client admits to having had a deep depression about a year prior. The nurse assesses Elke for suicide ideation and finds her describing feeling like she is in a deep dark hole with no way out and her life is hopeless. The nurse first assesses the client alone and then talks with the husband and client. At one point the nurse asks Elke to tell her what it means when someone says: "Don't cry over spilled milk." Elke says: "Don't cry when milk is spilled because you can buy some more at the store."

The nurse takes Elke's vital signs, weight, and height. Her vital signs are normal: height is 5 foot 5 inches and weight is 100 pounds.

The psychiatrist puts Elke on citalopram hydrochloride (Celexa), an SSRI. The nurse who admits Elke, and who continues to be assigned to her, notices that Elke isolates, verbalizes very little, and does little except when she is prompted and rewarded with points. Elke refuses to play volleyball or go to the movies with peers and staff. About five weeks after admission, Elke seems to be doing better. Her affect is brighter. She begins to play the piano in the dayroom. She asks the doctor for a pass to go home briefly to pay some bills and check on things there. Her children are now at her mother-in-law's home and her husband is away on military duty, and she has to take care of paying the bills.

Questions and Suggested Answers

1. **Which signs and symptoms does Elke have that are consistent with those of a major depressive episode?**
   The "key symptoms of a Major Depressive Episode are depressed mood; significant change in sleep pattern; significant change in appetite; psychomotor agitation or retardation; loss of energy; loss of interest in pleasurable activities; feelings of guilt or worthlessness; difficulty with memory, attention span, or concentration; and suicide ideation" (Breen and McCormac, 2002, 28). A diagnosis of a major depressive episode can be made if a person presents with depressed mood or anhedonia and any other four symptoms listed above. Elke is not eating or drinking, a significant change in appetite. She has had a significant change in sleep pattern as she sleeps or sits in a chair most of the time. Her lack of activity and slow movements are indicative of psychomotor retardation and also suggest a loss of energy. Her refusal to attend the movies, play volleyball, or do much of anything on the unit indicate a lack of interest in pleasurable activities, also known as anhedonia. She has admitted to suicide ideation.

2. **What factor(s) do you think could have contributed to Elke's depression?** It is possible that there is a hereditary factor and that others in Elke's family have depression or had depression. Other possible factors contributing to Elke's depression could be guilt at not attending to her family in another country, the stress of being in a culture different than her culture of origin, some situation or incident that is troubling to her or guilt producing for her, or hormonal changes at her stage of life. A significant percentage of women with depression report symptoms of depression worsening just before menses (APA, 2000). Having a military husband who is gone and turns the control of the house over to her, then returns and wants to resume control, may cause the client to feel out of control.

3. **Why is the nurse interested in whether Elke has had prior episodes of major depression?** If a person presents with no evidence of prior episodes of major depression, the diagnosis will be Major Depressive Episode. If there is a history of one or more prior major depressive episodes, the diagnosis is Major Depressive Disorder. Elke has had a prior Major Depressive Episode and qualifies for a diagnosis of Major Depressive Disorder.

4. **The nurse makes an observation that Elke has had an episode of depression one year ago. What does the nurse need to learn from Elke and/or her husband, and what significance could it possibly have if Elke were depressed every year at the same time?** The nurse needs to discover what was going on in the client's life one year ago. The anniversary of the death of a loved one or the anniversary of some traumatic event could be triggering a Major Depressive Episode. It could be the anniversary of leaving her home country.

5. **Why does the nurse ask Elke to interpret what is meant by "Don't cry over spilled milk"? What does the nurse learn from Elke's response?** The nurse is going to learn from the client's response whether she is capable of abstract thinking or if she is a concrete thinker. The client who can abstract will answer the nurse with something like: "Don't worry over things already done because worrying does not help." A concrete thinker

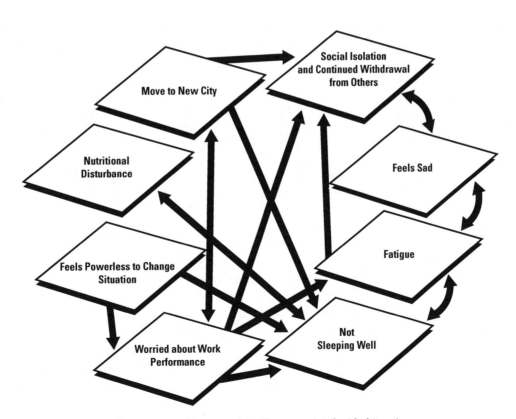

Concept map of issues and problems associated with depression.

will say something like: "If you spill milk on the floor, don't cry; just wipe it up." Knowing that a client is a concrete thinker tells the nurse that the client will take whatever she says quite literally and she must keep this in mind when determining what to say to the client.

6. **What percentage of people with Major Depressive Disorder kill themselves? What could the nurse do to help keep Elke from killing herself?** Morris (2003) states that "up to 15% of deaths of people with major mood disorders occurs from suicide."

All clients who have symptoms of major depression need to be assessed on an ongoing basis for suicide ideation, access to means to kill themselves, amount of energy, and degree of intent to carry out the ideation. All threats of suicide must be taken seriously. Hospitals and other facilities admitting clients with psychiatric diagnoses will have policies about what items the client is permitted to have. The nurse must be familiar with these policies, and whether the policy states it or not, the client who has suicidal ideation, or is at risk of developing such thoughts, must not be allowed to have sharp items or items he or she might use to hang himself or herself. For example, the client should not have soda tabs, belts, ties, or shoelaces. The nurse can develop a no-suicide contract with this client and others who are at risk of self-harm. The contract essentially says that when the client thinks about killing herself, she will talk with the nurse on duty about these thoughts rather than acting on them. The nurse will work to develop a trusting nurse-client relationship in which the client can talk about her feelings, learn about medication and other treatment modalities, begin to move out of social isolation, develop treatment goals, and work toward going home.

7. **How would you feel if you were Elke, and what would you need if you were Elke? What would it be like to be Elke's spouse or to be the spouse of any person with Major Depressive Disorder?** If you have ever been down in mood and felt like escaping through sleep or just couldn't get motivated to do anything or just felt like doom was impending and things were not only beyond your control but hopeless, you can probably magnify this feeling and imagine it lasting most of the day nearly every day for two weeks or more. If you were to put yourself in Elke's place, you would feel perhaps like you could not get out of your bed or your chair and as if you didn't care about anything or anyone because you are not worthy and they don't care about you. You still want someone to care about you and to care for you until you can do it yourself. You need someone to put food in front of you and tell you it is time to eat, to prompt you to make your bed or to get into it when it is time to sleep, to prompt you to do your hygiene chores. You need someone to stay with you and wait until you are ready to talk and then to listen.

Being the spouse or significant other of someone who is depressed can be trying. You might suggest an activity or something to cook, and his or her response is "no" or "I don't care." He or she perhaps refuses to talk with you, eat with you, or go anywhere with you, or perhaps to even acknowledge your presence. The depressed person may refuse treatment or stop taking medication.

8. **What interventions would you most likely initiate if you were writing a care plan for someone like Elke?** Interventions would include ongoing and periodic assessment for suicide ideation and intent, perhaps one on one staff to client if suicide intent is evident, and a gradual building of client's interactions with others to decrease social isolation. This might start with the nurse-client relationship; communication classes; playing the piano for one person and building up to playing it for a group (building on client's strengths); medication classes; leisure activities class; group, family, and individual therapy; and cognitive therapy.

"No-suicide contracts," also called "no-harm contracts," have been utilized by many nurses in all types of psychiatric care facilities. Frisch and Frisch (2006) state, "Most therapists agree that when clients readily agree to not harm themselves during a prescribed period, risk is decreased. Often such contracts are written and signed and the client is assured he has someone to call if he can not bear to be alone." The "no-suicide" or "no-harm" contract is used in combination with other interventions. Some institutions have stopped using no-suicide/no-harm contracts based on the premise that this technique is not scientifically proven to be effective while other institutions continue to use it on the premise that it is a useful technique in combination with other techniques.

9. **When Elke's mood seems to improve greatly and she wants to get a pass to go home and take care of some urgent business, would you support her having a pass? Why or why not?** Depressed patients who suddenly brighten in mood may have just reached the point where the medication has improved their energy levels enough for them to kill themselves. The thought of relief at not having to deal with feeling hopeless and helpless and/or extreme guilt after death may be behind the brightening of mood. Note: SSRIs tend to take effect in four to six weeks. This client is four to five weeks into treatment with an SSRI.

10. **The health care provider signs the pass allowing Elke to go home for four hours, provided an adult accompanies her, and she gets her neighbor to drive her home and back. What would you do if you were Elke's nurse?** If you were Elke's nurse under these circumstances, you would need to assess her for suicide ideation at this time. The hospital may have a formal suicide assessment tool you can use. You can ask Elke: "Are you thinking of killing yourself while you are home?" Clients most often tell the truth when asked this question. If the client says "yes," you will obviously not sign the client out and you will alert the health care provider and your supervisor. If the client says "no" or the health care provider and supervisor permit the client to go on pass, you will discuss with the neighbor the importance of not leaving the client alone by herself. Explain that the health care provider has written an order that the client can go home if accompanied by a responsible adult. Explain that this means the client must be accompanied at all times when out of the hospital on this pass. You should worry about confidentiality and choose your words carefully, but realize that if the client goes home and kills herself, you will then have to worry about being named as contributing to her death in any lawsuit that is filed.

11. **What is a token economy or a point system, and how is this used to change behavior?** A token economy or a point system economy in a treatment setting provides the client with a set number of tokens or points for complying with expectations on the unit. For example, a client might get a token or a certain number of points for attending class and a token or a certain number of points for participating in class. Often the unit milieu has a store that trades goods and/or privileges, such as cigarettes or a private room, for a certain number of tokens or points. Levels, in some economies, may be determined not only by points but by a vote of treatment team members.

12. **Is ECT used today for clients with depression? How do you feel about this?** ECT is used currently in some facilities and not in others. Clients who have been found to respond better to ECT are those with psychotic depression, melancholic depression, medication refractory depression, chronic/recurrent depression, suicidal depression, Schizophrenia with catatonic features, and depression in geriatric patients and those with Bipolar Depression. It is not usually used for clients who respond to SSRIs or other antidepressants. ECT has changed drastically in recent years. A qualified and experienced health care provider gives clients receiving ECT a planned and closely monitored amount of current. Student nurses sometimes have the opportunity to observe a client or clients receiving ECT. These student observers must watch closely to see even the slightest movement of a toe or an eyelid. There is no great jerking of muscles as seen in classic movies in which psychiatric patients received ECT (Rassmussen, 2003).

References

American Psychiatric Association. (2000). *Diagnostic and Statistical Manual of Mental Disorders, 4th ed.* Text Revision. Washington, DC: American Psychiatric Association.

Breen, R. and R.J. McCormac IV. (2002). "Fresh Look at Management of Depression." *Nursing* 112(3): 28–35.

Frisch, N.C. and Frisch, L.E. (2006). *Psychiatric Mental Health Nursing, 3rd ed.* Albany, NY: Thomson Delmar Learning. Morris?

Rassmussen, K.G. (2003). "Clinical Applications of Recent Research on Electroconvulsive Therapy." *Bulletin of the Menninger Clinic* 67(1): 18–32.

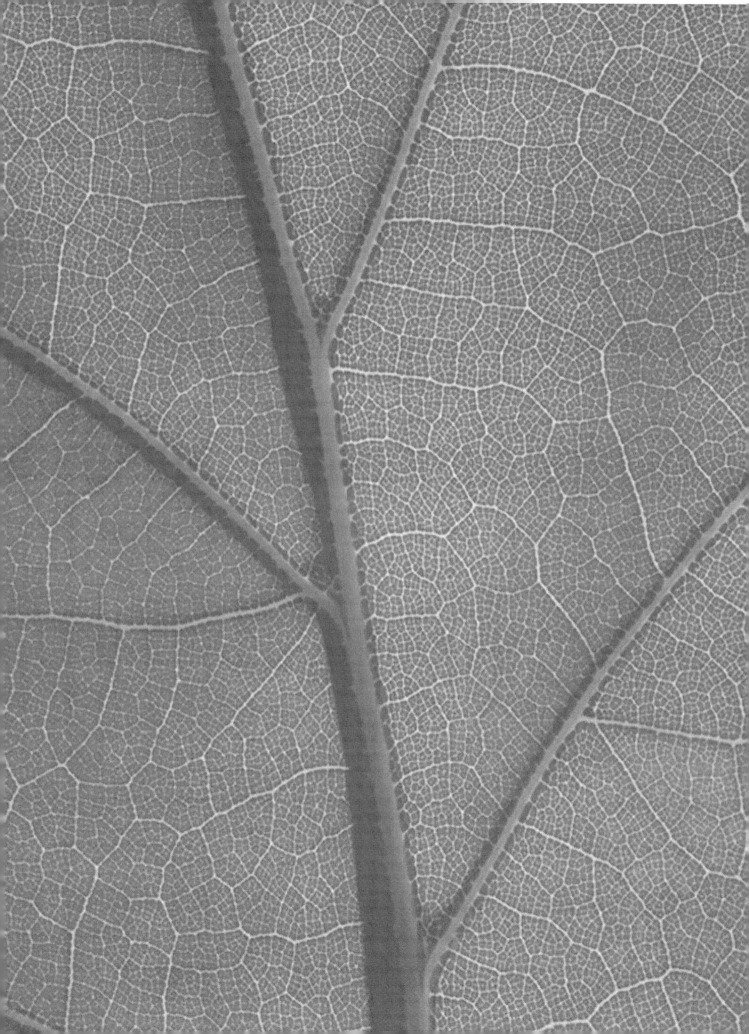

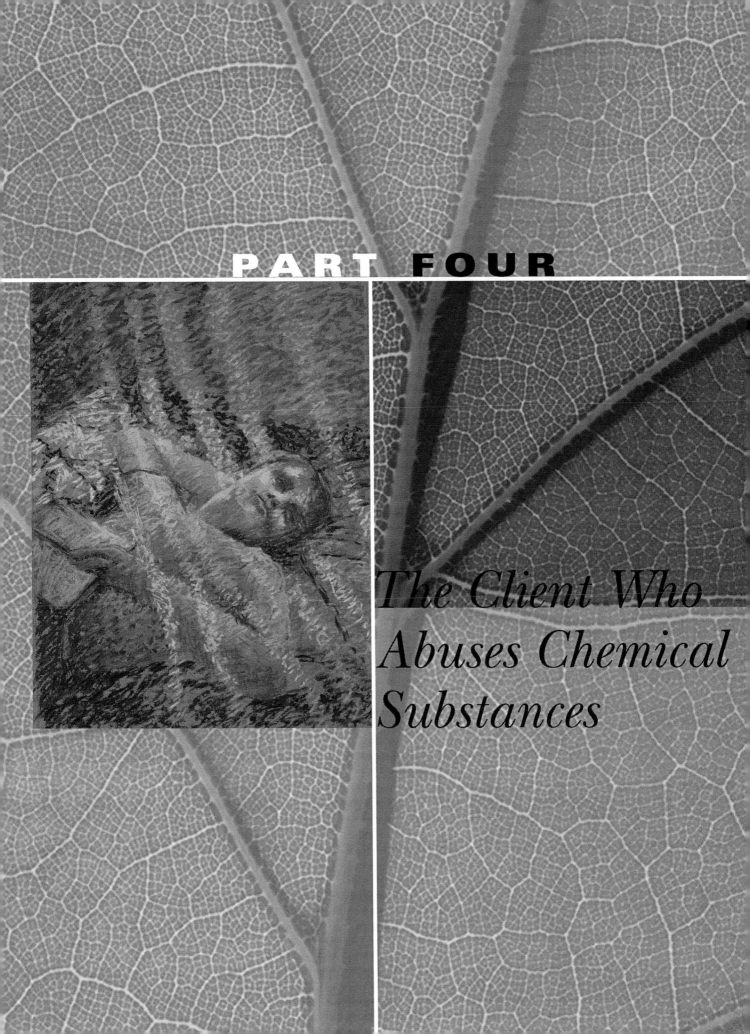

PART FOUR

The Client Who Abuses Chemical Substances

Ron

GENDER

Male

AGE

42

SETTING

■ Hospital

ETHNICITY

■ White American

CULTURAL CONSIDERATIONS

■ "Hippie" culture

PREEXISTING CONDITION

COEXISTING CONDITION

COMMUNICATION

DISABILITY

SOCIOECONOMIC

■ Middle class

SPIRITUAL/RELIGIOUS

■ Buddhist

PHARMACOLOGIC

PSYCHOSOCIAL

LEGAL

■ Illegal drug possession and use
■ Charting must be factual
■ Possibility of nurse involvement in court proceedings

ETHICAL

■ Care based on client lifestyle

ALTERNATIVE THERAPY

■ Acupuncture

PRIORITIZATION

DELEGATION

MODERATE

CANNABIS ABUSE

Level of difficulty: Moderate

Overview: This case involves treating an illegal drug user with additional health concerns.

Client Profile

Ron is a 42-year-old high school teacher who smokes marijuana (Cannabis sativa) occasionally. He has been using marijuana with varying intensity since junior high school. His drug use prolonged his college education, but he did eventually earn a bachelor's degree and teaching certificate for high-school-level history, English, and science. The drug use also contributed to the dissolution of his first marriage. Since then he has become fascinated with Buddhist teachings and studies them often.

Ron continues to smoke marijuana "to relax," although it makes him anxious, paranoid, and impacts his short-term memory. He has to be particularly careful that none of his students or their parents see him, so he only smokes at his home or the homes of close friends, and never within several hours of teaching. The school has a zero tolerance policy on drug use.

After an argument, Ron's girlfriend, Patsy, hid some marijuana in his briefcase and then anonymously notified the principal of his school once Ron had gone to work. Due to the tip, the principal inspected Ron's briefcase, found the marijuana, and notified the police. Ron was suspended from his job, but after Patsy admitted to planting the marijuana, the school board agreed to give Ron another chance if he would complete a twenty-eight-day (two weeks inpatient and two weeks outpatient) treatment program and agree to abstain from marijuana or other illegal substance use following treatment. Ron consented to save his job. He has a court date in a month for a charge of marijuana possession.

Case Study

Ron decides to smoke a little marijuana to control his nerves and mellow himself out before going to be admitted to the drug treatment program. He also reasons that he should smoke the remainder of his marijuana rather than flush it down the toilet. On the way to the program he is in an automobile accident, is injured, and ends up being admitted to the orthopedic unit of a large medical-surgical hospital. Patsy arrives just as Ron is admitted and blurts out: "He was on his way to the outpatient treatment program to be treated for marijuana abuse when he had this accident. He is going to lose his job if he doesn't go for treatment. This is awful."

Questions and Suggested Answers

1. **Why do you think Ron smoked the last of his marijuana before going to the first night of inpatient treatment for drug abuse? How did Ron's behavior demonstrate the difference between insight and judgment?** Ron's thinking and behavior was typical of the thinking and actions of many drug abusers—to use up drugs instead of wasting them or to have one last drug use before going into treatment to prepare them to deal with the treatment.

    Insight involves awareness of a situation and possible consequences of actions you might take, for example, knowing that it may be dangerous to go home with a stranger after a party. Judgment is what you decide to do about a situation (i.e., this invitation). Ron seems to have had good insight in the past about when he can smoke marijuana and when he cannot in order to preserve his job and to avoid driving while under the influence of the drug. His insight was probably not the problem. It was his judgment that was poor. Ron had a lapse of judgment in smoking the marijuana and then driving himself rather than taking a taxi or calling a friend.

2. **How would you respond if you were the nurse listening to the girlfriend comment about the client using marijuana before his accident and his need to complete the drug abuse treatment program in order to save his job as a teacher?** It is important to keep an open mind as the girlfriend's statements are hearsay and the girlfriend may or may not be a reliable source of information. You should clarify whether she was with Ron when he allegedly smoked the marijuana before the accident. You should share the possibility that Ron smoked marijuana or used other substances, which may be in his system, with the rest of the health care team, especially with the health care provider who is prescribing for Ron and anyone providing care to

him. The information you choose to include in your chart requires thought and careful attention to facts and avoidance of hearsay and speculation. Because there was an accident and an allegation of drug abuse, this could become a court case, particularly if anyone was hurt in the accident. You could be subpoenaed to testify, and you will have only your recall, which could be distorted by time, and your charting notes to use in your testimony. You may decide to chart what Patsy said in an exact quote and her response to whether she was actually with the client when she alleges he smoked the marijuana.

3. **How would you feel if you were assigned to work with this client who has been abusing cannabis (marijuana) and teaching high school students and is now in need of medical care, possibly due to using cannabis then driving?** You will probably have both negative and positive feelings and attitudes toward this client. You may feel compassion for this client for a variety of reasons, for example, you could believe that he has an inherited genetic predisposition to drug abuse. You may view working with this client as a professional challenge that you enjoy because you look forward to putting your therapeutic communication skills to work.

Possible negative feelings about working with this client include being angry with Ron because you think he put his life and other people's lives in danger by being under the influence of an illegal substance. You could think he is stupid for abusing drugs and taking the risk of losing his job.

Some nurses have friends or family members who abuse drugs and because of this might feel emotions associated with them. Whatever your feelings, it is important that you recognize and understand them and then make sure you are providing the best care you can, regardless of your personal feelings and background. Two studies (McLaughlin and Long, 1996; and Happell and Taylor, 2001) found that a majority of nurses and other health professionals hold negative stereotypical perceptions of illicit drug users. They concluded that these negative perceptions become prejudicial, hence "blocking the professional from carrying out effective and human nursing care to this client group." You will want to be aware of this risk and avoid bias.

4. **What are the criteria for cannabis abuse, and does this client appear to meet any of those criteria? What is the difference between someone who abuses marijuana and someone who is dependent on it?** Cannabis abuse is substance use in a maladaptive pattern that leads to clinically significant impairment or distress as demonstrated by at least one of the following, happening within a one-year period:

   1. Repeated substance use with a failure to carry out major role obligations at home, work, or school as exemplified by such behaviors as repeated work or school absences, suspensions, or expulsions and/or neglect of household duties or children.
   2. Repeated substance use in ways that are physically hazardous such as driving a motor vehicle or operating machinery while impaired by substance use.
   3. Repeated legal problems related to substance use (for example, arrests for disorderly conduct related to substance use).
   4. Ongoing use of substance even when having persistent or repeated social or interpersonal problems due to or made worse by effects of the substance (for example, fights with spouse about consequences of substance use, having marijuana in the house or around children). The client must never have met the criteria for cannabis dependence in order to have cannabis abuse (APA, 2000, 199).

   In the past twelve months, Ron has had trouble at work related to substances, has had one accident that we know of related to substance use, and has an impending court case to address his drug use. Therefore, Ron meets the criteria for cannabis abuse.

   When a person has "psychological or physical problems associated with cannabis in the context of compulsive use," a diagnosis of cannabis dependence instead of abuse is considered. Clients with cannabis dependence will persist in using even though they have physical problems such as chronic cough associated with smoking or psychological effects such as heavy sedation and reduction of goal-oriented activities from continued high doses. This person may spend a lot of time each day obtaining and using cannabis, and it frequently causes problems in the family, work, recreation, and school (APA, 2000).

5. **Would you expect this client to have withdrawal symptoms if he does not have marijuana to smoke? How would withdrawal manifest?** The client who abuses cannabis may have some psychological cravings triggered

by situations or people that he normally uses marijuana in or with, but the client with cannabis dependence will suffer from withdrawal. Part of the difficulty in stopping the use of cannabis is likely found in the withdrawal symptoms experienced, according to Budney, Moore, Vandrey, and Hughes (2003), who found in a study that cannabis withdrawal patterns include "aggression, anger, anxiety, decreased appetite, decreased body weight, irritability, shakiness, sleep problems, and stomach pains" (393).

Ron will be in the inpatient program for two weeks, which will probably clear his urine of cannabis, and the next two weeks he can be randomly checked for cannabinoids in his urine after going home or daily. The difficulty with outpatient treatment is that the client can go home part of the day or evening and can use during that time. His first two weeks in the inpatient treatment program hopefully will fortify him to resist temptations to smoke marijuana when he progresses to outpatient work.

6. **What is/are the current treatment(s) for cannabis abuse?** There is very little written in the current literature about treatments used today for cannabis abuse. Many cannabis abusers do not seek treatment. Of those who do end up in treatment programs, most are treated in an inpatient or outpatient treatment program for alcohol and other drug abuse so they are on a unit socializing and engaging in educational classes, individual therapy, family therapy, and therapy groups with peers who abuse not only cannabis but alcohol, cocaine, heroin, amphetamines, and other illegal drugs as well as prescription drugs. There are usually few clients in the treatment mix who use/abuse only cannabis. The client may be asked to do the twelve-step work of Alcoholics Anonymous and to attend Narcotics Anonymous (NA) meetings. One concern with this is that the person who is abusing only cannabis may learn about the use of other drugs and where to obtain these drugs. Not all clients abusing cannabis will go on to abuse other drugs, according to Stenbacka, Allebeck, and Romelsjo (1992), who wrote, "Several studies show cannabis is usually the first illicit drug that people use" and "a minority of abusers seem to continue with other drugs and intravenous drug abuse."

The person in treatment for abusing cannabis may be provided with ways to relax, such as acupuncture, deep breathing exercises, music, or guided imagery. Dr. Long (2005) stated treatment can include antianxiety medications to treat cannabis-induced anxiety or panic; an antipsychotic if cannabis induced psychosis; antidepressants if the cannabis is being used to deal with depressed mood or if the client is depressed for any reason; lifestyle changes such as staying away from people, places, and things related to cannabis use; and teaching ways to manage anxiety such as assertiveness training and self-esteem building.

7. **You are to instruct Ron about harmful effects of cannabis, but he is skeptical and thinks there are no harmful effects. Has cannabis been shown to adversely affect the health of someone who abuses it?** Cannabis has had many supporters who claim it is not harmful, and many more who claim it is not as harmful to the body as is alcohol. Walling (2004) called cannabis the most commonly used illicit substance, especially among young people, and yet the "consequences of cannabis use remain unclear and highly controversial." Walling explains that even though marijuana "has been associated with psychological problems, decreased educational achievement, antisocial behavior, and a range of psychosocial conditions," there are those who believe cannabis does not cause these problems but instead that the problems predispose the person to drug use. It is the underlying adverse circumstances that need to be addressed.

The harmful effects of cannabis appear to be overall either less damaging to the body or less researched and documented, compared to the effects of alcohol. However, the harmful effects of cannabis appear to include increased risk of motor vehicle accidents while driving under the influence, harmful effects on lungs and air passages (Kalant, 2005), a possible but unclear link with Schizophrenia, depression, and other psychiatric disorders (Trosini, Pasini, Saracco, and Spalletta, 1998), increased risk of suicide in chronic users (Beutrais, Joyce, and Mulder, 1999), cognitive impairments including impact on memory (Herning, Better, Tate, and Cadet, 2005; Walling, 2004), and decreased overall quality of life for some clients (Walling, 2004).

8. **Are there medical uses for cannabis, and is there a medical source of cannabis?** Cannabis has been found to be effective in treating loss of appetite, wasting syndrome, and nausea and vomiting associated with cancer and HIV/AIDS.

While cannabis is a schedule I drug just as LSD and heroin are, Marinol (dronabinol) is a synthetic version of THC (delta 9-tetrahydrocannabinol) schedule II oral capsule, which comes in 2.5, 5, and 10 mg capsules, and is FDA-approved to treat nausea and vomiting in cancer patients who fail to respond to conventional treatments. The most often reported side effects are drowsiness, thinking abnormally, exaggerated happiness, and paranoid reaction (www.marinol.com). Medical uses described on the Southern Illinois University website (www.siuedu~ebl/leaflets/hemp.htm) also include the treatment of anxiety, high blood pressure, and intraocular pressure in glaucoma.

However, clients with medical symptoms are "most often disappointed with Marinol compared to marijuana" (Walling, 2004), because smoking will provide relief in minutes but the oral Marinol may take four hours or more to provide relief with a goodly amount of the swallowed substance metabolized into other compounds in the liver. The psychoactive effects of oral THC can be intense, and the cost of enough Marinol for a month runs $500 to $900 (Arkansas Alliance for Medical Marijuana Smoking).

9. **Is marijuana use for medical purposes permitted in your state? If not, are there nearby states where it is?** Nine states have passed initiatives for medical marijuana: Alaska, Arizona, California, Colorado, Maine, Montana, Nevada, Oregon, and Washington. The state legislatures in Hawaii and Vermont passed bills protecting users of marijuana for medical purposes. You should be aware of the laws in your state because they may impact your responsibilities regarding reporting drug use.

10. **Would you feel better caring for this client if he had a medical prescription for marijuana or if smoking marijuana for personal use were legal? If so, under what circumstances should a client smoke marijuana for personal use?** You would probably feel better about working with a client who is not engaged in an illegal behavior and is taking a medicine for symptoms such as pain and nausea that have not responded to other conventional pain therapies. You have been trained and educated to comply with the law. You may also feel it is unethical to support or encourage or ignore a client smoking marijuana when it is illegal.

You may have a variety of feelings or attitudes about whether people should smoke marijuana for personal use and whether it should be legalized or not. It would be good to discuss your thoughts on this in class or informally with your peers. Being aware of your feelings and attitudes will help you provide the best care for your clients.

11. **How does this client's belief in Buddhism impact or affect your care?** If you are unaware of the teachings of Buddhism, the most therapeutic and professional approach would be to encourage the client to talk about his religious preference and try to understand his perception of it. You might read about Buddhism and try to understand its major ideas. You can then not only help the client meet his spiritual needs but help the client to see that the teachings of Buddha may have direction for change in his behavior and lifestyle. For example, the Gautama Buddha (Siddhartha) taught that human beings need to seek truth and reality as they are. This concept could be useful in working with this client. Keep in mind that Buddhism varies from country to country and that the most important thing is to assess the client's perception and utilize teachings he believes in for planning and implementation, as appropriate.

12. **The client's mother comes to visit and you talk to her about the importance of support and compassion. She asks you to explain the difference between support and compassion and enabling. She tells you that she was told in the past not to enable Ron's abuse of marijuana.** Support involves not giving up on a person's ability to change or to give up drugs and stay in recovery. Support can be concrete, such as driving the person to the treatment program, saying encouraging things, and attending family night at the treatment program. Support is based on the idea that people can change even if they have tried before and been unsuccessful.

Compassion involves seeing the good in the person who is using/abusing drugs and believing that the person is engaging in this behavior for a reason and not because they are just a bad person. Student nurses learn in their nursing program that all behavior has meaning and purpose to the individual. The compassionate person uses empathy—trying to feel and understand what the client is going through—to gain insight into the client's struggles and pain and treats the client as they would want to be treated or they would want someone they love to be treated. Being compassionate does not mean that you give the client everything they ask for. Often the compassionate nurse must set limits and say "no" if this is what she believes is in the best interest of the client to get him to change his behavior. Setting limits needs to be a well-thought-out response planned on an individualized basis. It would be helpful for nurses to have discussions with peers about what enabling, support, and compassion mean.

Enabling a person's use/abuse of illegal substances would include such things as buying their drugs or giving them money for drugs. It would include calling in sick for them when they are unable or unwilling to go to work because of the drug use. Lying for a person to cover their drug use/abuse is also enabling.

13. **If you were to write a care plan for this client, what assessment data would you like to have?** You would want to assess the client's physical and mental status. You not only have to assess this client for physical and mental problems associated from injuries in his accident but problems associated with his recent and chronic cannabis abuse. Clients who have recently used cannabis (marijuana) may present with red eyes, dry mouth, an increased pulse and lowered blood pressure, and problems concentrating. Cannabis stimulates appetite, hence the statement from some users that they have the "munchies." If the client received a high dose of THC, he may be edgy or have brief periods of panic-like behavior. You would want to assess mood and affect.

You would need to assess the client's strengths and limitations as well as leisure skills and interests. An assessment of stressors that trigger marijuana use would be helpful in your planning phase. Also the client's usual methods, other than marijuana, for dealing with stressors need to be assessed. The client's sources of support need to be assessed as well as the family dynamics. The client's problem-solving skills need to be assessed. You would assess the client's perception of the benefits and harmful consequences of smoking marijuana. He smokes it because he feels it benefits him in some way. You need to assess his reasons for smoking marijuana as well as to get him to look at the harmful and possible harmful effects.

You will want to assess his motivational level for quitting the use of marijuana and whether he has a plan that he thinks will work or is open to working with the health care team to develop a plan. It would be helpful to assess his knowledge of Buddhism, his perception of the teachings of Buddha, and the degree of importance it holds in guiding him in his day-to-day life.

14. **What nursing diagnoses would you write for this client? What goals are likely for this client?**

- Altered role performance related to hospitalization, injuries, and cannabis abuse
- Knowledge deficit related to harmful consequences of smoking cannabis
- Low self-esteem (either situationally or chronically)
- Possibly anxiety or depressed mood
- Powerlessness related to having to adhere to hospital schedule and routine and being in a treatment program.

Possible and likely goals for this client would include:

- Client will describe four harmful consequences of smoking cannabis.
- Client will remain free of cannabis or other substance of abuse.
- Client will agree to attend individual and family therapy sessions, education classes, and other classes or activities as scheduled 100 percent of the time as soon as he can be taken to the hospital drug and alcohol treatment unit or as soon as he can be discharged from the hospital and admitted to the drug treatment program he was scheduled to attend.

15. **What interventions would you likely write for this client?** You will have interventions pertaining to the injuries of the client, but you can also intervene in problems associated with cannabis abuse. Have the client write two columns of information about the consequences of smoking cannabis. One column would be for the benefits as he sees them and the other column would be for harmful effects. It is important to recognize and acknowledge that the client sees some benefits in smoking marijuana. If you indicate that you are hearing what he is saying and listening to him, he will be more willing to listen to you talk about the harmful consequences of smoking cannabis.

Provide teaching about harmful and possible harmful effects of smoking marijuana in a language and way that he can understand. Encourage the client to attend individual and family therapy sessions if they are scheduled while he is on the general hospital unit. Give positive reinforcement for any efforts to work on goals. Provide opportunities for the client to engage in leisure activities and model participation in such activities for him. The nurse spending a few minutes demonstrating how to play a computer game or a card game of solitaire or working a puzzle with a client may appear to some to be neglecting work, but in reality modeling engagement in acceptable leisure activities is important.

Encourage the client to discuss his Buddhist religious beliefs and how they impact his daily life and how he sees them impacting his behavior in the future. Provide the opportunity to read about Buddhism and to practice if the client desires. Provide supplies and encouragement for journaling. Provide opportunities for the client to have control when possible, for example, give the client a choice of activities. Ask for his ideas and suggestions. Show respect for the client. Ask the client by what name he prefers to be called and within reason call him by that name. You may indicate his behavior needs to be changed and what behavior you don't like, but you want to convey that the client has worth and is valued and respected.

References

American Psychiatric Association. (2000). *Diagnostic and Statistical Manual of Mental Disorders, 4th ed.* Text Revision. Washington, DC: American Psychiatric Association.

Arkansas Alliance for Medical Marijuana. Synthetic THC/Marinol www.ardpark.org/reference/marinol.htm. Accessed June 3, 2006.

Beautrais, A., P. R. Joyce, and R. T. Mulder. (1999). "Cannabis Abuse and Serious Suicide Attempts." *Addiction* 94(8): 1155–1165.

Budney, A.J., B.A. Moore, R.G. Vandrey, and J.R. Hughes. (2003). "The Time, Course, and Significance of Cannabis Withdrawal." *Journal of Abnormal Psychology* 112(3): 393–402.

Happell, B. and C. Taylor. (2001). "Negative Attitudes toward Clients with Drug and Alcohol Related Problems: Finding the Elusive Solution." *Australian and New England Journal of Mental Health Nursing* 10:87–96.

Herning, R.I., W.E. Better, K. Tate, and J.L. Cadet. (2005). "Cerebrovascular Perfusion in Marijuana Users During a Month of Abstinence." *Neurology* 64: 488–493.

Kalant, H. (2005). "Regular Heavy Use of Cannabis Adversely Affects Health." *Women's Health Weekly*, January 13, 90–91.

Long, P. (2005). "Cannabis Abuse Treatment." Available at www.mentalhealth.com/rx/p23-sb03.html.

McLaughlin, D. and A. Long. (1996). "An Extended Literature Review of Health Professionals' Perception of Illicit Drugs and Their Clients Who Use Them." *Journal of Psychiatric Mental Health Nursing* 3(5): 283–288.

Reinarman, C., P. Cohen, and H.L. Kaal. (2004). "The Limited Relevance of Drug Policy: Cannabis in Amsterdam and San Francisco." *American Journal of Public Health* 94(5): 836–843.

Stenbacka, M., P. Allebeck, and A. Romelsjo. (1992). "Do Cannabis Drug Abusers Differ from Intravenous Drug Abusers? The Role of Social and Behavioral Risk Factors." *British Journal of Addiction* 87(2): 259.

Trosini, A., A. Pasini, M. Saracco, and G. Spalletta. (1998). "Psychiatric Symptoms in Male Cannabis Users Not Using Other Illicit Drugs." *Addiction* 93(4): 487–492.

Walling, A.D. (2004). "Marijuana Research." *Scientific American* 291(6): 8.

www.marinol.com. Accessed April 21, 2005.

www.siuedu/~ebl/leaflets/hemp.htm. Accessed April 24, 2005.

Margaret

GENDER

Female

AGE

51

SETTING

- Home/visiting nurse

ETHNICITY

- White American

CULTURAL CONSIDERATIONS

- Appalachian/Northern European descent

PREEXISTING CONDITION

- Possible Alpha-1 Antitrypsin deficiency

COEXISTING CONDITION

- Chronic Obstructive Pulmonary Disease (COPD) related to Chronic Emphysema

COMMUNICATION

DISABILITY

- Disabled due to Emphysema and COPD

SOCIOECONOMIC

- Husband on social security; client receives social security disability payments; subsidized housing

SPIRITUAL/RELIGIOUS

- Used to attend church but now too tiring to attend

PHARMACOLOGIC

- Nicotine spray
- Bupropion (Zyban)
- Ipratropium bromide (Atrovent)

PSYCHOSOCIAL

- Decreased social life due to tiring easily because of COPD and Emphysema
- External locus of control

LEGAL

- Confidentiality

ETHICAL

- Should people have the right to smoke when it harms their health and that of others in their environment?

ALTERNATIVE THERAPY

- Hypnosis
- Acupuncture
- Guided imagery

PRIORITIZATION

DELEGATION

NICOTINE DEPENDENCE

Level of difficulty: Moderate

Overview: Requires critical thinking to come up with strategies to motivate a client, who is disabled due to Emphysema, to give up smoking. The nurse must get the client to move beyond her external locus of control thinking. The nurse must explore her own thinking about, and issues regarding, smoking in order to be effective with the client.

Client Profile

Margaret is a 51-year-old woman who smokes a package of cigarettes a day even though she has Chronic Obstructive Pulmonary Disease (COPD) from Chronic Emphysema. She has severe shortness of breath at times during the day. She cannot walk from the car to the house or carry her own groceries without tiring. Margaret's husband, John, smokes too, but just a cigar each day in the evening along with a glass of beer. Margaret has a "little glass of beer" with him. Margaret's daughter won't let her children go to Margaret's home because of the secondhand smoke and Margaret does not have the energy to climb the stairs to her daughter's home, so she has not seen her grandchildren for over a year. John does all the cooking, and the daughter takes Margaret's list and does the shopping. Margaret doesn't go to the church she has attended since she was a child because she does not want her many friends there to see her so short of breath and easily exhausted.

Sometimes Margaret cuts back on the groceries she puts on her list so she can have enough money for cigarettes and beer. Her daughter won't buy the cigarettes when she does the shopping, so Margaret calls the liquor store to deliver them along with a case of beer.

Margaret developed pneumonia recently and was hospitalized for treatment. The doctor mentioned to her on discharge that it would be a good idea for her to stop smoking and that he was sending the visiting nurse to work with her to quit smoking.

Case Study

The visiting nurse calls Margaret and tells her that the doctor has asked her to stop by for a visit. Margaret says she is doing OK and doesn't think she needs to see the nurse. The nurse replies: "I'd like to see you even though you are doing fine. Would you like me to come on Tuesday at 10 AM or Thursday at 4 PM?" Margaret agrees to the Tuesday visit. When the nurse arrives at Margaret and John's home, she visits a few minutes with Margaret and John and then checks Margaret's vital signs, listens to her lungs and heart sounds, does oxygen saturation, and draws some blood to send to the lab for CBC. She checks the capillary refill and then asks Margaret if they could have a cup of tea and just visit.

The nurse has brought some "special" tea bags. The nurse makes the tea and begins to discuss smoking with Margaret. The nurse asks Margaret how long she has been smoking, and the answer is: "Since I was 18 years old." The nurse asks her if she has ever thought about quitting, and she says: "No, I need it to calm my nerves." The nurse replies: "Perhaps the doctor can prescribe something to help you calm your nerves. While there are pros to smoking like increased alertness and relaxation, there are some cons to smoking like it increases the risk of serious illness and it makes your Emphysema worse." Margaret tells the nurse that she has known lots of people who smoked and none of them got Emphysema or pulmonary disease or cancer or lung problems: "It is just bad luck that I got this Emphysema, and I have hospital insurance and cancer insurance." Margaret tells the nurse that her father raised tobacco and tobacco is a good plant. She describes how she used to help her father by cutting the blooms out of the tobacco to keep them from sucking energy from the plant. Then Margaret asks: "Do you smoke or did you ever smoke, nurse?"

Before the visit ends, the nurse asks Margaret about her ancestry. Margaret says her father's parents came from Denmark and her mother's great-grandparents came from Finland. When the nurse reports back to Margaret's doctor, she tells him that it will be difficult to get Margaret to quit smoking but that she has some ideas, and she asks him about the possibility of Alpha-1 Antitrypsin (AT) deficiency.

Questions and Suggested Answers

1. **Why do you think the health care provider wants Margaret to give up smoking? What would be some common feelings of nurses assigned to work with a client like Margaret?** The health care provider, no doubt, hopes that smoking cessation will slow or stop the progression of Margaret's Emphysema and COPD. Smoking

cigarettes is the main cause of COPD, and smoking cessation is the "most effective means of stopping the progression of Chronic Obstructive Pulmonary Disease" (Marlow and Stoller, 2003, 172). These authors point out that one benefit of quitting smoking is that it will result in a "slowing of the accelerated rate of lung function decline that occurs in susceptible smokers."

Some nurses would be excited about the challenge of helping a client give up smoking and full of patience and plans for helping a client like Margaret. Other nurses might feel that clients have the right to smoke if they want to, regardless of the consequences. A number of nurses would be angry with clients like Margaret, or critical of them, for smoking when they have health problems.

Clients who smoke but want to or need to quit smoking are more likely to be successful if the nurse is supportive and patient. Swartz (1992) pointed out that many people can quit, but "staying off requires maintenance, support, and additional techniques such as relapse prevention." Quit rates can be improved if clinicians provide "counseling support rather than simple advice and warnings." Ask yourself if you only want to work with clients who are able to make healthy choices and do healthy things or if you want to work with people who need more help from the nurse to change their unhealthy patterns.

2. **If you were the nurse, how would you respond when the client asks if you smoke or ever smoked? Do you think a nurse who smokes can help a client successfully give up smoking?** One option is to tell Margaret honestly whether you smoke or not. If you do smoke, what will it mean to Margaret that you want her to give up smoking, but you won't do likewise? If you don't smoke, Margaret may feel that you could not possibly understand how hard this is for her or what smoking means to her. Another option is to tell Margaret that the smoking is not about you, but about her and you want to help her quit smoking. Deciding how to respond involves two questions: "Is it truthful?" and "Is it therapeutic for the client?"

Patkar, Hill, Batra, Vergore, and Leone (2003) compared smoking habits of over eleven hundred medical and nursing students and said: "The approach and credibility of future doctors and nurses as treatment providers for smoking and tobacco related diseases may be influenced by their smoking habits." These researchers found significantly fewer medical students who smoked compared to nursing students (3.3 percent compared to 13.5 percent). The authors concluded smoking among medical students in the United States has declined, but there needs to be increased education and intervention among nursing students. It is possible that a nurse who smokes could help a client give up smoking, but it is also possible the client would smell smoke on the hair, skin, and clothing of the nurse, which would make it more difficult for the client. It is conceivable that the nurse's own acceptance of smoking would come through in the nurse's approach to the client. Do note that a smoke smell does not necessarily mean a nurse smokes as the smoke smell can come from being around people who smoke or from a fireplace or wood-burning stove.

3. **Margaret's family asks: "What is Emphysema and what causes it?" How would you answer? What do you know about Alpha-1 AT deficiency, and what clues point to the possibility Margaret could have this deficiency?** Emphysema is a progressive, long-term lung disease with shortness of breath as the primary symptom. Emphysema is included in a group of diseases referred to as Chronic Obstructive Pulmonary Disease or COPD. In Emphysema, the alveoli in the lungs overexpand and lose their elasticity. COPD is a long-term airway obstruction occurring with chronic Emphysema, bronchitis, or both (Smith, 2005). The client has trouble exhaling air due to the lack of elasticity in the alveoli.

Cigarette smoking is considered to be the most common and most preventable cause of Emphysema. In addition to smoking, risk factors include air pollution and repeated infections, as well as genetic factors such as a hereditary deficiency of Alpha-1 Antitrypsin. Anyone with this deficiency is at risk for developing Emphysema because the destructive effects of neutrophil elastase are unopposed. The normal range for Alpha-1 AT levels is from 104 mg/dl to 276 mg/dl with levels greater than 57 mg/dl believed to provide adequate protection from Emphysema. Alpha-1 Antitrypsin deficiency is an autosomal recessive genetic condition resulting from mutations in the Alpha-1 AT. Both parents are involved in passing this disorder on to their children (Scharnweber, 1999). A deficiency of Alpha-1 AT is mainly (95 percent) found in Caucasian persons of Northern European descent (Murray et al., 2000; Scharnweber, 1999). In Denmark, this genetic deficiency is said to affect about 50 percent of the population (Scharnweber 1999). Alpha-1 AT deficiency affects as many as seventy thousand to one hundred thousand people in the United States, although most people with this disorder are misdiagnosed or undiagnosed (Banasik, 2001). John Walsh, President and CEO of the Alpha-1 Foundation, said to be the "leading research education and consumer organization for ATT deficiency," is quoted as saying: "ATT deficiency is as prevalent as cystic fibrosis and it is widely misdiagnosed or under diagnosed." Estimates say twenty-five million people in the United States are unrecognized carriers of the gene causing the deficiency (*Heart Disease Weekly*, 2004).

When a person does not have sufficient levels of Alpha-1 Antitrypsin, it will, over time, result in early onset Emphysema in the third to fifth decade of life (Scharnweber, 1999).

A simple blood test as well as a buccal swab test is available for checking the level of Alpha-1 AT. Alpha-1 Antitrypsin deficiency has been described as "the most common modifiable genetic factor leading to COPD, the fourth leading cause of death in the United States (*Heart Disease Weekly*, 2004).

Major clues to the possibility that Margaret has Alpha-1 AT deficiency are her northern European ancestry (both parents' families) and especially her Danish ancestry, as well as her early age of onset for Emphysema.

4. **Why would this client, or any client, refuse to have testing for alpha-1 AT deficiency? Why would a client want to have the testing? What are the current treatments for alpha-1 AT deficiency and for Emphysema?** Margaret might refuse if there were no definitive treatment for this deficiency other than quitting smoking, which she will be asked to do regardless of testing. Other reasons clients refuse to be screened include concern about future insurance coverage and prejudice from supervisors and employers (Banasik, 2001). Clients might want to have this testing to know if they might pass on the gene for this disorder to their children. If both parents have this gene, testing of family members would be the next step.

The current treatment for alpha-1 AT deficiency includes getting the client to give up smoking if they smoke and to avoid secondary smoke as well as air pollution. These clients are usually immunized for hepatitis A and B and given the pneumococcal vaccine. Alpha-1 AT replacement therapy is controversial. The client is asked to avoid alcohol and to take measures to avoid infection or treat infection promptly (Banasik, 2001). Some clients may receive replacement alpha proteinase inhibitor made from pooled plasma concentrate. The FDA approved this replacement therapy in 1988. It is made from several thousand liters of plasma from donors without the Alpha-1 Antitrypsin deficiency (Scharnweber, 1999).

If patients with Emphysema have shortness of breath at rest, the health care provider may prescribe albuterol by metered dose inhaler at regularly scheduled times or by nebulizers when the inhaler is no longer adequate. Ipratropium bromide (Atrovent), another bronchodilator, which lasts longer than albuterol and often provides greater relief, may be prescribed. Theophylline (Theo-Durr) oral tablets are prescribed to keep air passages open; however, with theophylline the health care provider has to monitor the blood levels as the client can receive an overdose if too much or won't get relief is the dosing is too little. The health care provider may prescribe steroid medications to decrease inflammation in the lungs, but not everyone responds to steroids. The provider may also prescribe antibiotics even if there are no signs and symptoms of infection as people treated with antibiotics may have shortened episodes of shortness of breath. Some clients have home-based oxygen tanks and portable units.

Lung reduction surgery is sometimes done for advanced Emphysema. Some of the wasted or dead space of the lungs is removed to increase ability to breathe. Transplantation of either or both lungs can provide great relief (i.e. near cure) but not without risks. There is not a sufficient supply of available organs for all who need this transplantation. According to Scharnweber (1999), about 12 percent of the lung transplant candidates have Alpha-1 Antitrypsin deficiency.

5. **What are the criteria for a diagnosis of nicotine dependence, and does Margaret appear to meet these criteria? Is there a measuring tool that measures the degree of nicotine dependency of clients?** The criteria for nicotine dependence are the same as for substance dependence, although according to APA (2000, 264), "Some of the generic criteria for dependence don't seem to apply to nicotine while other criteria require more explanation." The criteria for nicotine dependence using the substance dependence criteria of APA (2000) would include a maladaptive pattern of the use of nicotine resulting in clinically significant

impairment or distress as manifested by three or more of the following seven criteria met and happening any time but within the same twelve-month period:

1. Tolerance. Nicotine tolerance is shown by an increased intensity of effect of nicotine the first time it is used in the day and the lack of nausea and dizziness with repeated smoking in spite of regular use of substantial amounts.

2. Withdrawal. People with nicotine dependence often take nicotine to relieve or avoid symptoms of withdrawal when they first wake up in the morning or after being denied nicotine, as after a flight or at work.

3. Substance often taken in larger amounts or over more time than was the intent.

4. Persistent desire for nicotine or unsuccessful efforts to cut down on smoking or to control use.

5. Much time is spent in activities to obtain nicotine (e.g., chain smoking) or recovering from its effects.

6. Important activities such as social, occupational, or recreational activities are given up or cut back because of nicotine use.

7. The nicotine use continues despite knowing of a persistent or recurrent physical or psychological problem that is likely a result of the nicotine use or is exacerbated by the nicotine use (Adapted from APA, 2000).

Margaret meets criteria 6 and 7 above as she has given up her church activities and her homemaking activities, and she has continued to use nicotine in spite of having emphysema. She also meets criterion 4 as she continues to want nicotine on a persistent basis. She may meet other criteria as well.

There is a tool that measures the degree of nicotine dependency of clients. The Fagerstrom Test for Nicotine Dependency (FTND) is frequently mentioned in the literature on nicotine dependency and smoking cessation. It rates addiction on a scale of 1–10. A major part of the test and the one with the most emphasis for determining addiction to nicotine is the amount of time from awakening to the first cigarette smoked. The person who is highly addicted must reach for a cigarette quickly after awakening, whereas less addicted people may wait an hour or much longer. Patkar, Hill, Batra, Vergore, and Leone (2003) provide a modified version of the FTND. Questions include: 1. How soon after you wake up do you smoke your first cigarette? (less than 5 minutes = score of 3 points, 6–30 minutes = 2 points, 31–60 minutes = 1 point, and more than 60 minutes = 0 points); 2. Do you have difficulty refraining from smoking in places where it is forbidden? (yes = 1 point and no = 0 points); 3. Which cigarette would you hate most to give up? (first in A.M. = 1 point and any other = 0 points); 4. How many cigarettes per day do you smoke? (Less than 10 = 0 points, 11–20 = 1 point, 21–30 = 2 points, and more than 30 = 3 points); 5. Do you smoke more frequently during the first hours after awakening than the rest of the day? (yes = 1 point and no = 0 points); and 6. Do you smoke if you are so ill that you are in bed most of the day? (yes = 1 point and no = 0 points). A score of greater than 6 is said by Patkar, Hill, Batra Vergore, and Leone to suggest a high level of dependency. You may want to observe the behavior of some of your assigned clients who smoke to see how long it is in the morning after awakening when they reach for their first cigarette and whether this cigarette would be harder to give up than others later in the day. If you smoke, you may want to look at your own behavior surrounding the first cigarette of the morning.

6. **What are the current theories on causation of nicotine dependence?** The craving for nicotine may be genetic. Secko (2005) states that "nicotine interacts with nicotinic acetylcholine receptors (nAChRs) in the brain, although how this interaction leads to a chemical dependency remains unclear." Secko goes on to point out that recent research has found a specific area of one nAChR as a "prime target in the development of nicotine dependence." What he is referring to is a mutation in the α4nAChR subunit, which Tapper and colleagues (2004), reporting in *Science*, say lowers the threshold for nicotine addiction in mice. Scientists have been aware that the brain is affected both positively and negatively by nicotine, which not only acts to increase addiction, but also increases mental alertness. Both of these effects have been linked to nAChRs present on the CNS neurons. The nAChRs "form a family of ion channels normally activated by the neurotransmitter acetylcholine" although these receptors also bind nicotine. "Each receptor channel is made up of 5 components assembled from a pool of 12 known subunits and these combinations produce a variety of receptor subtypes each with distinctive properties."

7. **What are the current treatments for nicotine dependence? Would it be easy or difficult to get someone who is nicotine dependent to give up smoking, and what would help a person who doesn't want to give up smoking?** Until recently, the FDA approved only the use of nicotine replacement therapy as first-line treatment for nicotine dependency. In the last few years bupropion (bupropion SR) became the first nonnicotine replacement pharmaceutical recommended for first-line treatment in the updated United States Clinical Practice Guidelines (Jorenby, 2002).

Nicotine replacement therapy is available in various forms: nicotine generic or Nicoderm patches (7 mg, 14 mg, and 21 mg); nicotine gum in generic or the brand product Nicorette and Nicorette mint (2 mg and 4 mg) available over the counter; nicotine nasal spray available in 0.5/spray with the usual usage being one spray per nostril for a total of 1 mg; nicotine inhaler with each cartridge providing 10 mg of nicotine. If delivered with the head tilted a little, this method provides the most rapid nicotine delivery of all the nicotine replacement therapies with a peak effect in five to ten minutes. There also is a nicotine lozenge (Polacrilex, Commit) available in 2 and 4 mg doses. Nicotine lozenges give a client 25 percent more nicotine than the doses in the gum.

The health care provider may prescribe bupropion (Welbutrin, Welbutrin SR, Zyban). The therapeutic effects of this medicine include decreased depression and decreased craving for cigarettes. The usual dosage is 150 mg for three days then 300 mg per day. Bupropion has an added benefit of blunting weight gain often associated with smoking cessation.

A second-line smoking cessation drug is clonidine (Catapress), an antihypertensive medication that can be taken orally or transdermally and has been used to decrease smoking craving. Naltrexone combined with nicotine replacement therapy and psychosocial therapy may enhance smoking cessation rates in women, according to a study by Byars, Frost-Pineda, Jacobs, and Gold (2005).

A number of researchers and clinicians indicate that it is not easy to get people who are nicotine dependent to give up smoking. Most nurses have encountered relatives as well as clients who have tried many times to give up smoking unsuccessfully, who say they want to give up smoking but don't, or who adamantly refuse to give up smoking. Swartz (1992) described smoking cessation treatment in three phases: preparation, intervention, and maintenance. Preparation involves increasing motivation to quit and increasing confidence in a client that success is possible. The nurse can provide smoking cessation information or kits from public or volunteer agencies, books, and tapes; encourage participation in campaigns like the Great American Smoke Out program; and direct the client to counseling and clinics and nicotine replacement. Maintenance involves giving support, teaching coping strategies, and helping the client find substitute behaviors.

Marlow and Stoller (2003) suggested that health care providers use a five-step system of ask, advise, assess, assist, and arrange to help clients give up smoking. These authors stated that to be successful, a cessation program has to be individualized and account for the reasons the client smokes, environment in which the person smokes, available resources for quitting, and individual preferences for how to quit. They stressed patience and persistence in "developing, implementing and adjusting each [client's] smoking cessation program."

8. **Is smoking more common among lower socioeconomic groups or other groups? What general characteristics of individuals from Appalachia have been identified that might be helpful to keep in mind in designing interventions to help the client stop smoking?** Smoking is more common among lower socioeconomic groups and in those with less education, according to Marlow and Stoller (2003). It is possible that as people become more educated, they are better able to see connections between what they put into their bodies, and do with and to their bodies, and their health condition; however, there are educated people who still smoke. It may be that a genetic predisposition to nicotine addiction makes it much more difficult for a person to quit. It may be that worries and anxieties associated with not having sufficient finances cause a person to smoke or smoke more.

Macnee and McCabe (2004) studied smokers in Southern Appalachia and got 659 smokers or former smokers to agree to participate in filling out a questionnaire consisting of six scales that measure constructs from a transtheoretical model of behavior change. These authors found that the culture of Appalachia includes a" strong value of independence and self-sufficiency as well as a strong commitment to traditional values including family, land, religious belief and social equality." The nurse may be able to get the client to commit to lifestyle changes that increase independence and self-sufficiency and encourage family and religious experiences. Macnee and McCabe found that some of the subjects from Appalachia have personally participated in raising tobacco and have experience working in tobacco-related jobs or, like our client Margaret, have relatives who raise or have raised tobacco.

9. **What will you do to help this client maintain a nonsmoking status if she agrees to stop smoking? How will you feel and what attitude will you adopt if she relapses again?** You want to maintain close contact with the client or have her establish close contact with a counselor or therapist whom she can call when she is considering smoking. One counselor told the client to promise if she did smoke to only smoke as much of the cigarette as tasted wonderful and then to put it out and call him. Oftentimes cigarettes do not taste good to the client and he or she will smoke very little and then go back to abstinence. Silver acetate, an aversive therapy that makes a bad taste in the client's mouth if they smoke, has been given along with the nicotine patch, but was found in some studies to be less effective than mecamylamine, a nicotine agonist, combined with the nicotine patch (Marlow and Stoller, 2003). You may want to do a review of the most recent literature to see what is reported as working best with highly nicotine dependent persons, then determine what will work for your individual client. The more you know about Margaret and the more you open your mind to new and creative ways to help her based on your ongoing assessments, the more likely it is that you will think of a way to motivate her to stop smoking and to stay smoke free.

You will no doubt want to be sure that the client has lots of positive reinforcement for every day that she is smoke free and that her husband has the same reinforcement if he is smoke free. If he does not give up his cigar, maybe you can talk him into smoking it while outside or away from the client so it does not trigger smoking on the part of the client. She is used to smoking cigarettes when he smokes a cigar. Seeing him smoking a cigar could well stimulate the client to want to light up and smoke a cigarette.

One idea is to have the client set up a reward system for herself if she gives up smoking for a week, a month, and a year. She could put the money saved each day or week into a bank or envelope and buy herself something special with the money she saves.

Another idea is to find pictures of the lungs of smokers and pictures of lungs of former smokers showing improvement. The client needs to have a clear idea that smoking will improve her lung condition. You might also have her daughter put a picture of the granddaughter on the refrigerator with a message saying something like: "Smoke free equals time with your granddaughter." If the client relapses again, you could think of it as being one step closer to success. Some clients relapse several times before success. Every try at smoking cessation is a practice for success. The inclination is usually to be discouraged and perhaps even upset with the client, or to blame oneself for not planning better or doing something differently or better, or blaming family members for the failure. There is hope that the client will be successful in smoking cessation at some point. Relapse calls for an evaluation and reassessment.

10. **What are the withdrawal symptoms this client will probably have?** The symptoms of nicotine withdrawal can extend for up to several weeks and include physical symptoms such as anxiety, irritability, depressed mood, trouble concentrating, impatience, and restlessness. The intensity of the withdrawal signs and symptoms seems to be related to the degree of nicotine dependency.

11. **What data do you want to gather on this client? What nursing diagnoses, goals, and interventions would you likely write if you were writing a care plan for this client?** You need to do a physical assessment, taking vital signs, listening to heart and lung sounds, assessing breathing pattern(s), and paying particular attention to signs and symptoms associated with the respiratory system, but also doing a complete physical assessment to see if the client has other health problems. You will want to look at lifestyle changes due to Emphysema and how this has affected the client and whether the client might be motivated to stop smoking and make other changes to get some of her former lifestyle back. You can get the client to talk about pros and cons of smoking and see which of these might motivate her to quit smoking. Perhaps not being able to have her granddaughter in her home is a strong motivator.

What is the client's thinking and feeling about not attending her church anymore when it was her social life in the past? What is possible in regard to attending church activities in person or having someone from church visit her?

You will want to assess the family dynamics and the client's coping methods. You will look at the environment and its contribution to smoking. Would the husband giving up cigar smoking increase the client's motivation to stop smoking and stay smoke free? Will the daughter continue to insist the mother give up smoking to have the granddaughter in the house? Will the daughter support the mother in smoking cessation efforts and be patient if she relapses and help her try again?

Some possible nursing diagnoses depending on findings from the assessment would likely include some or all of the following nursing diagnoses:

- Impaired gas exchange RT inadequate alveolar function
- Self-care deficit
- Altered role performance
- Knowledge deficit
- Anxiety
- Altered nutrition: less than body requirements due to energy required to eat, or Altered nutrition: more than body requirements due to insufficient exercise and activity.

Some possible goals to write for this client would be:

- Will identify four pros and four cons for smoking
- Will state a willingness to give up smoking within one month
- Will contact her church and reconnect with the church in some manner
- Will develop a plan for smoking cessation
- Will decrease number of cigarettes smoked per day and gradually stop smoking at a chosen time
- Will agree to seek support when she needs it and to identify sources of support.

Nursing interventions could include:

- Build a therapeutic trusting relationship
- Offer planned support and follow up over time
- Educate family about ways to be supportive in any smoking cessation efforts and ways to encourage client to try again if a relapse occurs
- Prepare family members about relapse and what to do and say should it occur
- Do teaching about Emphysema and its relationship to smoking
- Do client education about smoking cessation
- Teach client ways to prevent infection and to monitor for infection
- Teach clients about medication
- Teach client ways to exercise within their tolerance level
- Teach the client ways to organize simple activities and to schedule them to maximize use of available energy
- Teach relaxation techniques to reduce stress and oxygen demand
- Teach client to control breathing
- Encourage client to eat a diet high in calories and protein to provide energy without having to consume large amounts of low-calorie foods

References

American Psychiatric Association. (2000). *Diagnostic and Statistical Manual of Mental Disorders, 4th ed.* Text Revision. Washington, DC: American Psychiatric Association.

Banasik, J. (2001). "Diagnosing Alpha-1 Antitrypsin Deficiency." *Nurse Practitioner* 26(1): 58–62.

Byars, J.A., K. Frost-Pineda, W.S. Jacobs, and M.S. Gold. (2005). "Naltrexone Augments the Effects of Nicotine Replacement Therapy in Female Smokers." *Journal of Addictive Disease* 24(2): 49–60.

Jorenby, D. (2002). "Clinical Efficacy of Bupropion in the Management of Smoking Cessation." *Drugs* 62(Supplement 2): 25–35.

Macnee, C.L. and S. McCabe. (2004). "The Transtheoretical Model of Behavior Change and Smokers in Southern Appalachia." *Nursing Research* 53(4): 243–250.

Marlow, S.P. and J.K. Stoller. (2003). "Smoking Cessation." *Respiratory Care* 48(12): 1238–1254.

Murray, J.F., J.A. Nadel, R.J. Mason, and H.A. Boushey Jr., eds. (2000). *Textbook of Respiratory Medicine, 3rd ed.* Philadelphia: W. B. Saunders.

"New Noninvasive Swab Test for ATT Deficiency Offered." (2005). *Heart Disease Weekly*, June 20, 32–34.

Patkar, A.A., K. Hill, V. Batra, M.J. Vergore, and F.T. Leone. (2003). "A Comparison of Smoking Habits Among Medical and Nursing Students." *Chest* 124(4): 1415–1421.

Scharnweber, K. (1999). "Alpha 1-Antitrypsin Deficiency and the Impact of Nursing Interventions and Treatment." *Journal of IV Nursing* 22(5): 258–264.

Secko, D. (2005). "Craving Nicotine: It's in the Genes." *Canadian Medical Association Journal* 175(2): 175–177.

Smith, B. (2005). "The Nursing of a Patient Following Lung Reduction Surgery." *Nursing Times* 101(6): 61–63.

Swartz, J.L. (1992). "Methods of Smoking Cessation." *Medical Clinics of North America* 76(2): 451–476.

Tapper, A.R. et al. (2004). "Nicotine Activation of $\alpha4$ Receptors: Sufficient for Reward, Tolerance, and Sensitization." *Science* 396(5689): 1029–1032.

GENDER

Male

AGE

19

SETTING

■ Workplace, office of industrial nurse

ETHNICITY

■ White American

CULTURAL CONSIDERATIONS

■ American "Rave" culture

PREEXISTING CONDITION

COEXISTING CONDITION

COMMUNICATION

DISABILITY

SOCIOECONOMIC

■ Middle class

SPIRITUAL/RELIGIOUS

PHARMACOLOGIC

PSYCHOSOCIAL

LEGAL

■ Illegal drug use

ETHICAL

■ Professional vs. personal relationship with client

ALTERNATIVE THERAPY

PRIORITIZATION

DELEGATION

DIFFICULT

HALLUCINOGEN ABUSE

Level of difficulty: High

Overview: Requires the nurse to accept a young adult whose behavior is risky to his health and who is using the illegal stimulant/hallucinogen MDMA (Ecstasy) and has a lifestyle totally different from that of the nurse. The nurse must maintain professional behavior and help the client develop a trusting relationship before attempting to motivate a change in behavior in the client.

Client Profile

Bennie is a 19-year-old adopted male, who has worn leather and chains at times in the past couple of years. His hair has occasionally been spiked up the middle of his head and colored green. His behavior has attracted attention in his parents' conservative upper-middle-class neighborhood. In addition to his hairstyle he has stood in the middle of the street and cursed his adoptive parents, talked to neighbors about smoking "weed," and played his drums loudly. The parents have been concerned about his effect on a younger brother who is their natural child and involved in sports and not at all like their adopted son. Just before graduation from high school, the parents suggested Bennie move out. Bennie moved to an apartment with one of his friends, got a job designing computer games, and started going to raves. His passions are: raves, the drug MDMA (Ecstasy), Macintosh computers, computer games, and cars. His parents have asked him not to come home.

Case Study

Bennie comes to the nurse's office in the company where he works. His chief complaints are insomnia, feeling anxious and nauseated, and experiencing blurred vision. He wants his blood pressure checked to see if something is wrong. As the nurse takes his vital signs, the nurse finds Bennie has a rapid pulse of 124 and tremors in his hands. The nurse notices that his muscles are tense and he is sweating. His mood appears a little depressed, and he thinks people in his department are sabotaging his work.

Bennie tells the nurse he thinks she is cute and asks her to go out with him. The nurse's response is: "When you go out, Bennie, where do you like to go?" The client reveals he likes to go to raves and invites the nurse to go with him to a rave.

Questions and Suggested Answers

1. **If you were the female nurse in this case, would it be acceptable for you to go out socially with this client? Why or why not? What developmental stage, according to Erickson, is this client in and how does that relate to the client's behavior? Could the nurse have professional reason(s) for asking Bennie what he really likes to do in his time away from work?** It is not a good idea to date a client. You need to maintain a therapeutic and professional role with the clients. Psychologists and professional counselors as well as marriage and family counselors are, in most states if not all, prohibited by law from having a dual relationship. These professions consider it unethical to be in a professional role with the client and a personal role as well. Nurse practice acts may or may not list having a dual role with a client as unprofessional conduct, but in some facilities the nurse can lose his or her job for dating a client. This is especially true for nurses working in psychiatric facilities. The client is considered vulnerable and the nurse is in a power position. In this case the client may not be particularly vulnerable and there may not be a company rule against employees dating, but it does change the professional relationship if the nurse has a personal relationship with the client.

   One possible explanation for the client asking the nurse to socialize with him is that the client is in the intimacy versus isolation stage of development. In this stage a person looks for a life mate and life work. When a young adult client asks a nurse if they are married or not, or asks a nurse to go out on a date, the client is actually behaving consistently with the Ericksonian task that they are to fulfill and the life stage that they are in. It is the nurse's responsibility to respond in a therapeutic professional manner.

   There could be a number of professional reasons for the nurse asking Bennie questions about where he likes to go and what he likes to do. It is an unobtrusive way to find out if the client likes to go places where there is apt to be alcohol and/or drugs. In this case it opens the door to finding out about the use of drugs, which might account for the client's symptoms.

   A nurse might use a similar approach to a client who has high blood pressure. Sometimes a client will reveal they like to drink a particular alcoholic drink. This opens the door for the nurse to talk about the effect of alcohol on blood pressure and the importance of avoiding or minimizing the use of alcohol. The answer to the nurse's question also gives the nurse insight into the client's interests, which can be helpful in developing a care plan.

2. **What does the client mean by a "rave"?** Raves started as underground dance parties in Europe in the 1980s. The location of events were usually kept secret until the evening of the party in order to keep the public and law enforcement away. The raves moved secretly from place to place by word of mouth. Now raves are found all over the United States and the world and have moved into small towns as well as cities. These raves are found in permanent dance clubs as well as in temporary locations such as open fields and empty buildings or warehouses. They are usually highly organized and often charge high entrance fees. The raves are seldom formally advertised. Flyers and Internet announcements of a rave may direct people to a location where they are given the location of the actual rave. Rave music DJs or bands are highly skilled performers in mixing extremely fast-paced, pounding beat music with choreographed laser programs. Increasingly, club owners or rave managers seem to promote drug use at raves, especially use of MDMA. Some managers or owners provide bottled water and electrolyte sports drinks to prevent hyperthermia and dehydration as well as pacifiers to prevent involuntary teeth clinching ("Information Bulletin from the U.S. Department of Justice: Raves," April 2001; Weir, 2000). A history of raves and the rave culture can be found at http://en.wikipedia. org/wiki/Rave_party.

3. **What is the most common drug used at raves and why? What other drugs are commonly found at raves? Is there drug paraphernalia associated with MDMA (Ecstasy)? Is the typical way of dressing at raves leather and chains, and if not, what is it?** Weir ("Information Bulletin from the U.S Department of Justice: Raves," 2000) stated that marijuana is the most popular drug at raves, while other sources such as a U.S. Department of Justice Bulletin suggest MDMA (Ecstasy) is the most common drug used at raves. Ecstasy is a stimulant as well as a hallucinogen and is "known for its empathogenic, euphoric, and stimulant effects" ("Information Bulletin from the U.S Department of Justice: Raves," April 2001). The "speeding up" by the drug heightens the fast music experience, and the hallucinogenic experience heightens the senses so the person is more aware of sound and colors. Neon glow sticks also are sold or provided to enhance the effects of MDMA.

Other drugs found at raves and considered an integral part of the events are: Ketamine, GMB (gamma-hydroxybutyrate), Rohypnol, and LSD. Some attendees use alcohol and marijuana as well as other drugs in combination with MDMA.

MDMA users often wear pacifiers on bead necklaces that they use to prevent the involuntary teeth clenching associated with MDMA use. Bead bracelets are common and sometimes attendees at raves have strung MDMA tablets along with candy or beads on the bracelets.

Leather would probably be considered too hot to wear at a rave. Lightweight loose clothing in layers is typically worn. This enables the wearer to remove clothing, as they feel increasingly hotter while dancing for long periods. The dress often includes "baseball hats, T-shirts emblazoned with logos, baggy pants, running shoes, knapsacks, barrettes, infant toys, plastic chains and infant soothers" according to Weir (2000), who points out the "the clothing suggests 'ravers' pride themselves on their lack of pretension and their open acceptance of themselves and their community."

4. **What drugs are considered hallucinogens? How are hallucinogens usually taken, and how is MDMA (Ecstasy) taken? Have there been or are there currently any medical uses for hallucinogens?** According to the American Psychiatric Association (2000), hallucinogens are a diverse group of substances. Hallucinogens include ergot and related compounds such as lysergic acid diethylamide (LSD) and morning glory seeds; phenylalkylamines such as mescaline; MDMA 3.4 methylenedioxymethamphetamine, which is commonly called Ecstasy; and indole alkaloids such as psilocybin, DMT, and various other compounds. PCP and cannabis are excluded from the hallucinogens although they can produce hallucinogenic effects. Hallucinogens, including Ecstasy, are almost always taken orally.

There have been, and are currently, some medical uses for hallucinogens. MDMA was used by some psychotherapists in therapy with their clients up until 1988 when it was declared a schedule 1 drug under the Controlled Substance Act. Ketamine is currently used in anesthesia of humans and in veterinary medicine.

Most of the Ketamine sold in the street is diverted from the offices of veterinarians. Dextromethorphan is an ingredient in cough and cold medications sold over the counter (www.whitedeerrun.com/hallucinogens.asp).

5. **What effect does MDMA have on the person taking it? Is the strength of the drug MDMA consistent, and what is the danger of receiving PMA (paramethoxyamphetamine) as a substitute for MDMA?** Initially the user of Ecstasy experiences feelings of peacefulness, empathy, and acceptance (Yacoubran and Peters, 2005); however, the area of the brain that is critical to thought and memory is damaged by MDMA. This drug causes the release of serotonin, dopamine, and norepinephrine from their storage sites and increases their circulating levels, which increases energy and speeds up the body temporarily. The heart rate and blood pressure are increased. The client can dance for hours. The brain ends up with a depletion of these neurotransmitters, and it takes a long time to rebuild them for important brain functions. MDMA, like other hallucinogens, can cause distortion or transformation of shapes and movements.

In addition to increasing energy, in high doses Ecstasy also increases sexual arousal and suppresses appetite and thirst and sleep needs, while in therapeutic doses it is hypothesized that it will reduce stress and increase feelings of empathy without sedative and other problems ("Ecstasy Under Scrutiny for California Patients", 2005).

Adverse physical effects include the involuntary teeth clenching mentioned before, muscle tension, nausea, blurred vision, tremors, rapid eye movement, sweating, chills, and feeling faint. The user of MDMA is at risk for dehydration, hyperthermia, and heart or kidney failure. According to an article on the effects of Ecstasy in *Pain and Central Nervous System Week* ("The Effects of Ecstasy," 2005), "Ecstasy, Ice, and Speed are variations of amphetamines originally developed as appetite suppressants. The psychedelic effects are reported to last four to six hours. The psychiatric effects can last for weeks and these include: anxiety, depression, insomnia, memory loss, and paranoia."

Overdose symptoms can be mild to severe, "e.g. frank apnea interspersed with periods of violent combativeness" or coma and respiratory depression. With no antidote, there is only nonspecific supportive care, which could include a ventilator and atropine for bradycardia (Weir, 2000).

The strength of MDMA is not consistent. Members of private drug education and drug testing organizations referred to as "harm reduction organizations" have periodically gone to Raves in the last decade to test illegal drugs and inform Rave attendees of the purity level to order to decrease harm ("Information Bulletin from the U.S Department of Justice: Raves," April 2001). The danger of taking PMA and thinking it is MDMA is that the user often believes he has gotten a weak dose of MDMA because the PMA takes longer to take effect. If the user decides to take a second dose of drugs, this can lead to overdose as the drugs stack up.

6. **Does admitting attendance at raves affirm that the client does hallucinogenic drugs? The client admits taking MDMA. What action(s) do you take? What is your top priority with this client?** The nurse must not jump to the conclusion that attendance at a rave means that the client uses hallucinogenic drugs. It is possible for someone to attend a rave and not use drugs.

If the client admits to using hallucinogenic drugs, you need to talk with your supervisor about any policies or rules of the company about employees and illegal drugs; however, since your priority is safety of the client, you need to get this client to see a health care provider. Perhaps the company has a health care provider or one to whom referrals are made. It would be prudent to have the client seen soon. You will have to make a judgment call about whether the client needs to be taken to the emergency room or if he can call someone to take him to the health care provider's office. If you decide the client can be seen in the provider's office, you should call the provider and describe the situation and ask if the client can be seen right away. If you suspect hallucinogen intoxication or overdose, whether the client admits it or not, you will want him to get medical attention.

7. **What are the criteria for Hallucinogen Intoxication? Does this client appear to meet those criteria?** The criteria for Hallucinogen Intoxication are:

   1. Using a hallucinogen recently

2. Obvious maladaptive behavior or psychological changes—such as anxiety or depression, thoughts of losing one's mind, paranoid ideas, using poor judgment, or impaired social or occupational functioning—developing during or not long after hallucinogen use

3. Being fully awake and alert yet having perceptual changes such as "subjective intensification of perceptions, depersonalization, derealization, illusions, hallucinations, synesthesias" occurring soon after taking a hallucinogen

4. Soon after taking a hallucinogen, demonstrating at least two of the following signs and/or symptoms:

    a. Dilation of pupils
    b. Rapid heart rate
    c. Sweating
    d. Palpitations
    e. Blurring of vision
    f. Tremors
    g. Impaired coordination

Note: the signs and symptoms must not be due to a medical condition or another mental disorder (APA, 2000).

From the description of the client and his chief complaints, it would appear that the client demonstrates more than two of the signs and symptoms and has some paranoia and anxiety as well as depressed mood. It is likely that someone qualified to make a diagnosis of Hallucinogen Intoxication could make the diagnosis if their assessment did not reveal other causes for the signs and symptoms.

8. **What are the criteria for Hallucinogen Abuse, and does this client seem to meet the criteria for Hallucinogen Abuse? What diagnoses are associated with hallucinogens that are not associated with some other addictions such as alcohol, and what significance does this have for the nurse?** The criteria for Hallucinogen Abuse are the same criteria for abuse of any substance. It involves a maladaptive pattern of use, which had led to significant impairment or distress, and the meeting of one or more of four criteria: 1. Failing to meet major role obligations at school, home, or work due to recurrent substance use; 2. The substance is repeatedly used in situations that are physically hazardous; 3. The client has repeated substance-related legal problems; and 4. The person continues substance use in spite of having ongoing or reoccurring social or interpersonal problems caused or made worse by effects of the substance (e.g. arguments with significant others). In addition, to have a diagnosis of Hallucinogen Abuse, the client must not be able to meet the criteria for Hallucinogen Dependence and has never been able to meet the dependence criteria. It is possible that this client could meet these criteria if he has indeed been using MDMA or other hallucinogens on a recurrent basis and if this use is the reason for his difficulties in meeting major role obligations in the family and at school.

One diagnosis that is unique to the hallucinogens in terms of addiction diagnoses is "Hallucinogen Persisting Perception Disorder (Flashbacks)," and it refers to periodic brief reoccurrences of disturbances in perception reminiscent of those experienced during earlier hallucinogen intoxications. To meet this diagnosis the client must, during a time when they are not using hallucinogens, re-experience one or more perceptual distortions that they experienced in the past while intoxicated with the drug (e.g., intensified color or halos around objects), and these symptoms must cause significant distress or impairment in functioning in one or more areas of the client's life.

The nurse must assess for any flashbacks the client may have experienced and be aware of the possibility that this client and other clients using hallucinogens may experience flashbacks.

9. **Has the use of Ecstasy increased or decreased in recent years? How is the prevalence of hallucinogen use, particularly that of Ecstasy, estimated?** The use of Ecstasy has been reported consistently, in the literature, to have increased in recent years. Surveys of populations for self-report of use, emergency room admissions of persons having used hallucinogens, and drug seizures by official agencies are sources of estimations of prevalence. The number of new MDMA users was said to be 168,000 in 1993 and 1.8 million in 2001. The National Survey on Drug Use and Health (Information Bulletin from the U.S. Department of Justice: Raves, 2001)

found 15.1 percent of young people ages 18 to 25 had used MDMA at least one time, and in 2002 there were 676,000 reporting use of MDMA in the month they were surveyed.

A 2002 study reported by Yacoubran and Peters (2005) surveying 2,258 high school seniors reported 10 percent lifetime Ecstasy use with only 3 percent in the past thirty days. It is apparent that the figures on Ecstasy use vary, but it still remains a problem. Yacoubran and Peters found it to be mainly a problem of Caucasian rave attendees and suggested targeting this population for help.

Looking at seizure figures, the DEA reportedly seized 196 tablets of Ecstasy in 1993 and more than 5.5 million in 2001. The U.S. Customs and Border Patrol reported a large increase in seized tablets from 1999 to 2000, with 3.5 million seized in 1999 and 9.3 million in 2000.

10. **What treatments are currently being used for clients who use or abuse Ecstasy?** While there may be a program somewhere especially dedicated to treatment of Ecstasy users/abusers or treatments specifically for this type of client, it is not readily apparent from a review of the literature. Clients who need treatment for Ecstasy intoxication may receive help in the hospital emergency room. Clients who need help with Ecstasy abuse or dependence are usually treated in an inpatient or outpatient clinic or program for treatment with clients who abuse or are dependent on other drugs. Treatment often includes a twelve-step program, individual and group therapy, and family therapy and cognitive therapy using such techniques as teaching about thinking errors, reframing, letter writing, and stoppage of negative self-talk.

11. **What data would you like to have if you were the nurse writing a nursing care plan for this client? What nursing diagnoses and goals would you likely write for this client? What interventions could you write for this client?** You would want to have vital signs, a review of body systems, a psychosocial assessment, and a mental status examination. You would gather data on the client's strengths and limitations. The client's knowledge of the effects of MDMA needs to be assessed as well as the client's motivation to continue using hallucinogenic drugs or to stop using them.

Possible nursing diagnoses include but are not limited to:

- Thought processes altered due to MDMA and marijuana
- Knowledge deficit related to MDMA and marijuana
- Ineffective coping
- Family processes altered
- Sleep pattern altered
- Self-esteem chronically low
- Risk for injury to self

There are many appropriate goals you could write, including but not limited to:

- Abstinence from mood altering drugs
- Will describe adverse effects of using MDMA
- Will list five reasons to give up MDMA
- Will identify triggers for relapse
- Will write a recovery plan
- Will state two positive self-affirmations daily
- Will identify appropriate ways of coping such as problem solving
- Will identify appropriate role within family
- Will identify appropriate interactions with brother

There are many appropriate interventions you could write, including but not limited to:

- Monitor vital signs
- Do teaching on MDMA based on client need for information
- Model and teach problem solving
- Role play with client appropriate dialogue with brother and parents

- Encourage and provide positive reinforcement for compliance with treatment
- Have client write a behavioral contract
- Use empathetic and appropriate confrontation
- Set and maintain limits consistently
- Teach client to use reframing
- Teach and encourage use of appropriate leisure activities

12. **What research is being conducted with hallucinogens?** There are several studies that are approved and under way to look at the effects of hallucinogens on such things as late stage cancer anxiety, Obsessive Compulsive Disorder, and Post Traumatic Stress Disorder. UCLA has a study looking at psilocybin and therapy as a treatment for late stage cancer anxiety. The University of South Carolina is looking at MDMA as a treatment for Post-Traumatic Stress Disorder triggered by sexual abuse (Kotler, 2005). The Lahey Clinic, Medical Center Boston, received FDA approval for a four-month study involving twelve clients to see if Ecstasy can lessen client's fears and suicidal thoughts as well as improve relationships with significant others ("Ecstasy Under Scrutiny," 2005).

LSD research in the 1940s and 1950s lead to the discovery of the neurotransmitter serotonin, and this "jump started the brain chemistry revolution" (Kotler, 2005).

References

American Psychiatric Association. (2000). *Diagnostic and Statistical Manual of Mental Disorders, 4th ed.* Text Revision. Washington, DC: American Psychiatric Association. http://en.wikipedia.org/wiki/ Rave_party. Accessed January 22, 2006.

"Ecstasy Under Scrutiny for California Patients." (2005). *Nursing* 35(3): 30.

"Information Bulletin from the U.S Department of Justice: Raves." (April 2001). Document ID: 2001-L0424-004. Available at www.usdoj.gov/ndic/pubs/656. Accessed May 2005.

Kotler, S. (2005). "Drugs in Rehabilitation." *Psychology Today* 38(2): 28–30.

"The Effects of Ecstasy: It Takes Two to Tango in the Cell." (2005). *Pain and Central Nervous System Week*, March 14.

Weir, E. (2000). "Raves: A Review of the Culture, the Drugs and the Prevention of Harm." *Canadian Medical Association Journal* 162(13): 1843–1848.

www.erowid.org/chemicals/mdma/mdma.shtml. Accessed May 2005.

www.whitedeerrun.com/hallucinogens.asp. Accessed January 21, 2006.

Yacoubran, G.S., Jr. and R.J. Peters. (2005). "Identifying the Prevalence and Correlates of Ecstasy Use Among High School Seniors." *Journal of Alcohol and Drug Education* 49(1): 55–73.

CASE STUDY 4

Pena

GENDER

Female

AGE

13

SETTING

- School nurse called to the girl's restroom

ETHNICITY

- White American

CULTURAL CONSIDERATIONS

PREEXISTING CONDITION

- Neglect; physical, sexual, and psychological abuse

COEXISTING CONDITION

COMMUNICATION

DISABILITY

SOCIOECONOMIC

- Lower socioeconomic group; living below poverty line

SPIRITUAL/RELIGIOUS

PHARMACOLOGIC

PSYCHOSOCIAL

LEGAL

- Laws requiring reporting suspected child abuse
- Legal issues when child is truant

ETHICAL

- Question of when it is all right to plant an idea in the client's mind and when it is not

ALTERNATIVE THERAPY

PRIORITIZATION

- Nurse has several students needing care

DELEGATION

- Question of what to delegate to nonnursing personnel

DIFFICULT

INHALANT ABUSE

Level of difficulty: High

Overview: Requires perseverance and patience to work with a teenager who has been "huffing" gasoline and inhaling spray paint fumes. The nurse must use therapeutic communication skills, observational skills, and other means to discover what is going on with the client. The nurse is required to prioritize and delegate some tasks to others as there are other students seeking services at the same time this client is experiencing problems.

Client Profile

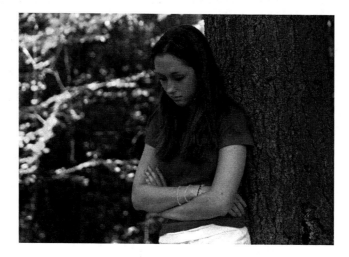

Pena is a 13-year-old girl whose parents are alcoholics. The family is below the poverty level in income and lives on social security disability and the food stamp program. They often sell or trade food they get with food stamps or from the WIC program to get alcohol and cigarettes, since food stamps are not accepted in payment for these items. The father tells Pena that she will never amount to anything and frequently tells her she is "stupid." Her parents don't like to ruin a good alcoholic "buzz" by eating, and they rarely prepare a meal for Pena. She eats whatever she can find in the refrigerator or cupboard. Her mother slaps Pena and yells at her. Her father sexually abuses her. Pena has learned to be as invisible as possible at home and school. She has begun to realize that some of her classmates make fun of her because she doesn't have clothes and shoes like they do and she always looks forlorn. Pena sometimes feels sorry that she is alive.

One of the neighborhood boys tells Pena she will feel better if she breathes some gasoline in a plastic bag. She has a supply of gasoline as her father keeps gasoline in a storage shed for an old lawn mower that he makes Pena use to mow the grass and weeds. She feels great for a short while after "bagging" gasoline fumes, then the old hopeless and worthless feelings return.

One day before school, after "bagging" gasoline, the boy who told her about the gasoline says he has something else they can use to feel better and gives her something else to breathe. He also touches her in some private places. Pena thinks about saying "no," but she does not care. She begins to feel euphoric. When she comes down from the high, she feels awful but goes to school because it is better than going home and she doesn't want the truancy officer visiting her home again. She hates to go to school because she can't concentrate and has little idea of what is going on in class. She is failing in school. Pena feels guilty about letting the boy touch her in private places, but he is the only one who talks to her and he has introduced her to inhalants that make her feel good, even if the feeling lasts only a short while.

Case Study

Pena passes out in the girl's bathroom at school. One of her classmates goes to get the school nurse. Pena has regained consciousness when the school nurse arrives. The nurse smells a chemical odor to Pena's breath. She seems lethargic, her movements are uncoordinated, her eyes are red, and her speech is slurred; however, Pena does begin to respond to questions. The nurse says: "Tell me what happened." Pena replies: "I just passed out because I forgot to eat supper last night and I got up late and didn't have time for breakfast this morning." The nurse notices some gold paint on Pena's face and hands.

A student comes into the bathroom with a nosebleed, and another girl says she has just started her first menstrual period and needs a pad. It is nearly time for the nurse to begin teaching a health care class, and the truancy officer has sent word that he wants to talk to the nurse before he goes out to visit one of the families.

Questions and Suggested Answers

1. **If you were the school nurse, would you say: "Tell me what happened"? Why or why not? What else would you say or do or avoid saying and/or doing when approaching this client initially? Based on the client's symptoms, what problem(s) could this client have instead of inhalant use? What are some clues that this student has been using inhalants?** "Tell me" is an open-ended therapeutic communication technique. It does not lead the adolescent client (plant ideas) or jump to conclusions about what is going on. Initially, you would want to tell/remind the child of who you are and stress that you are there to help (e.g., "I am Nurse Jones. Perhaps you remember me and know that I am here to help you?"). The nurse must avoid jumping to conclusions that the student has been doing drugs or inhalants. This student could be experiencing a medical problem. The client with diabetic ketoacidosis often presents with an acetone smell to the breath, lack of coordination, and an altered state of consciousness. The client who is diabetic and hypoglycemic, or who has hypoglycemia for any reason, may have an altered state of consciousness. A client who is anemic may also "pass out."

   Clues that the client may have been using inhalants include the gold paint on the student's body. The fumes from aerosol cans of spray paint can be used to get high. Gold and silver spray paint are particularly high in the chemicals used to alter mood. The client's bloodshot eyes are another good clue for inhalant use, but this redness could be due to crying and/or lack of sleep or allergies or other causes as well. When you combine the clues of gold paint, bloodshot eyes, and chemical smell to breath, along with altered state of consciousness and slurred speech, there is a stronger case for Inhalant Intoxication.

2. **What are the criteria for Inhalant Intoxication, and could Pena likely meet those criteria? What are the criteria for Inhalant Abuse, and does this client appear to meet any of those criteria?** The criteria for Inhalant Intoxification are:

   1. The client needs to have intentionally used or had short-term, large-dose exposure to volatile inhalants (exclusion: anesthetic gases and vasodilators of short-acting type).
   2. There must be maladaptive behavior or behavior indicating psychological changes, and it must be clinically significant and have developed during or just after being exposed to or using volatile inhalants. Examples of this behavior include being belligerent, demonstrating impaired judgment, having impaired functioning in social or work settings, and being apathetic.
   3. The client must have at least two signs from a list of signs. These signs must have developed during or soon after using inhalants or being exposed to them. These signs are: lethargy, tremor, euphoria, stupor or coma, blurred vision or double vision, overall muscle weakness, psychomotor retardation, unsteady gait, slurred speech, nystagmus. The signs and/or symptoms must not be due to a different condition (general medical disorder or mental disorder) (Adapted from APA, 2000).

   Although unknown by the nurse, Pena used inhalants this morning and has had some impairment in work (school) and could meet criteria 1 and 2. She has more than two signs under criterion 3: slurred speech, loss of consciousness, and an unsteady gait. The school nurse does not have enough information, nor is she qualified, to diagnose Inhalant Intoxication.

   The criterion for Inhalant Abuse is substance use in a maladaptive pattern that leads to clinically significant impairment or distress as demonstrated by at least one of the following, happening within a one-year period:

   1. Repeated substance use with a failure to carry out major role obligations at home, work, or school as exemplified by such behaviors as repeated work or school absences, suspensions, or expulsions and/or neglect of household duties or children

2. Repeated substance use in ways that are physically hazardous, such as driving a motor vehicle or operating machinery, while impaired by substance use

3. Repeated legal problems related to substance use (for example: arrests for disorderly conduct related to substance use)

4. Ongoing use of substance even when having persistent or repeated social or interpersonal problems due to or made worse by effects of the substance (for example, fights with spouse about consequences of substance use) (Criteria adapted from APA, 2000)

Pena's grades have slipped, and she continues to inhale harmful substances. She has only recently begun to inhale gasoline and paint fumes, so perhaps she does not meet the criteria or maybe she does and we don't have enough information. If we knew she was mowing the grass after inhaling, she might be able to meet criterion 2. She may or may not ever meet criterion 3 since the substance she is using is legal and easily attained. In regard to criterion 4, she already had social and interpersonal problems prior to using inhalants so it would be difficult to apply the criterion.

3. **You learn from one of Pena's classmates that several students are inhaling solvents. What are solvents? Are there different categories of inhalants that this client could have used? How are nitrites different from the other three types of solvents? Give some examples of nitrites. How are solvents used?** "Solvents are volatile substances that produce chemical vapors that can be inhaled to induce a psychoactive or mind-altering effect" (www.nid.nih.gov/ResearchReports/Inhalants/Inhalants.html).

The National Institute on Drug Abuse (NIDA) points out that exact classification of inhalants is not easy; however, they break inhalants down into four classifications: 1. Volatile solvents; 2. Aerosols; 3. Gases including medical anesthetics; and 4. Nitrites in a form found in some industrial and medical products. Volatile solvents are liquids that have vapors at room temperature. They include common items often found in the home garage or storage area (e.g., paint thinners, paint removers, gasoline, glues, as well as dry cleaning fluids and felt tip marker pens). Aerosols are sprays containing propellants and solvents (e.g., spray paints, deodorant, hair spray, fabric protector spray, and spray cooking oil). Gases include such products as ether, chloroform, and nitrous oxide. Nitrous oxide is said to be the most abused inhalant substance (National Institute on Drug Abuse, 2005). It is found in the following household items: whipping cream dispensers, butane lighters, and propane tanks.

The Consumer Product Safety Commission has prohibited nitrites from being sold, but they are still found for sale in bottles labeled video head cleaner, leather cleaner, or room odorizor.

Nitrites are used mainly as a sexual enhancer with a street name of "poppers" or "snappers." Nitrites act directly on the central nervous system, but other inhalants do not. The nitrites dilate blood vessels and cause muscle relaxation, while other inhalants mainly alter mood. The fumes of mothballs are also among volatile solvents inhaled. A recent report of concealed mothball abuse prior to anesthesia reveals that mothball abuse is another easily available household substance being abused that the medical team would not normally assess for in presurgery or other assessments (Kong and Schmiesing, 2005).

The fumes of some inhalants are sniffed or snorted from containers. Aerosols are sprayed directly into the nose or mouth. Some substances are sprayed or deposited on the inside of a plastic or paper bag and breathed in, a practice called "bagging." Some substances are sprayed on clothing and sniffed or soaked into a rag, which is stuffed into the mouth and inhaled (huffing). Some nitrous oxide is inhaled from balloons filled with the substance.

4. **Two students (one with a nosebleed and one starting a first menstrual period), the truancy officer, and a class that the nurse needs to teach compete with this client's needs for the nurse's attention. How would you prioritize and proceed, that is, what would you put on hold and/or delegate? Would you accompany Pena to the hospital if you were the nurse in this case?** If you or one of the students in the restroom have a cellular phone, you can call 911, then call for the principal and/or vice principal to come help you or send someone to help you. You can ask them to bring a pad for the student who has begun menstruation. If you do not have access to a phone, you can send the first student who comes past the restroom door or comes into

the restroom to the principal or vice principal's office. The principal or vice principal are both, no doubt, trained in first aid and one of them can manage the nosebleed or send someone who can. One of these administrators can also deal with the problem of the class that needs to be taught.

Pena will probably be transported by 911 paramedics to the local hospital emergency room. You have clues she may have been using inhalants (spray paint on her body and other signs and symptoms), but she could be having a different medical problem or two problems at once (e.g., hypoglycemia and Inhalant Intoxication). You can send for the janitor and ask that the restroom be closed if there is another restroom for students to use. It is best that other students not come into the restroom to see and interpret/misinterpret what is happening with Pena and the other two students needing help. This is a confidentiality issue. You can send word to the truancy officer that you cannot meet with him or her due to a crisis, and you will telephone or meet as soon as it resolves. Asking the truancy officer to come help you is a matter of judgment. Remember that Pena has already had problems with truancy and the officer has visited her home. You do not know what her reaction to seeing the truancy officer in the restroom would be. On the other hand, you need help, so if the truancy officer is the only one who can come help you, then you can deal with this.

Your first priority is Pena. People can and do die from Inhalant Intoxication. The National Institute on Drug Abuse (2005) points out that "even a single session of inhalant use can disrupt heart rhythms and cause death from cardiac arrest." You must keep your focus on Pena and getting her immediate help.

It would be therapeutic for the student if someone familiar to her goes with her to the hospital to help her feel safe and to talk with her parents. It may or may not be you, as other students need your attention. You can discuss, with the principal or vice principal, the question of who on the faculty or administrative staff is most appropriate to go to the hospital with the student, not only to help her feel safe, but also to advocate for her.

5. **Is it possible for the hospital emergency room staff to run a routine drug screen for inhalants on this or any client (i.e., does an inhalant like gasoline appear in the urine or blood)?** According to the APA (2000), direct assays for inhalants are generally not available and are not found in a routine screen for commonly abused drugs. Hippuric acid is a metabolite of toluene, and if this substance is found in a ratio higher that 1:1 compared to creatine, it suggests but is not proof of toluene use. Anderson and Loomis (2003) also point out that there is no specific lab test to confirm a suspicion of Inhalant Intoxication. A tentative diagnosis is based on the clinician's suspicion and a thorough history.

6. **The client receives care at the hospital and returns to school. You ask the client to stop by your office each day and check in with you. You try to discuss the harmful effects of solvent inhalation. The client says: "I don't care." Is this a typical response from inhalant users? What are the harmful effects of solvent inhalation that you would like to discuss with Pena?** Yes, apathy is a typical response from inhalant users/abusers. They do not perceive their life as good, and using inhalants is the way they cope with their lives. Pena will have to learn some new coping mechanisms and develop some strengths before she can hear what you are saying about the harmful effects of inhalants.

Pena has used gasoline and spray paint. Because the effects last only a short while, the tendency is to prolong by continuing inhalation and repeatedly inhaling over several hours. Prolonging inhalation can lead to convulsions/seizures from abnormal electrical brain discharges, coma, or death. Sudden death can occur from cardiac dysrythmias or other causes with a single short-time use of inhalants such as gasoline and/or spray paint. Sometimes people choke from inhalation of vomitus after use of inhalants or suffer fatal injuries from accidents while intoxicated. Inhaling volatile solvents also lessens inhibitions and can cause the person to do things that ultimately harm them, such as having unprotected sex. Inhalation of volatile solvents causes damage to areas of the brain that are involved in vision, hearing, cognition, and movement. The person can develop severe dementia, lose feeling, have vision and hearing loss, and become uncoordinated. There can be damage to the myelin sheath with symptoms similar to multiple sclerosis. Other organs of the body can be damaged, leading to impaired liver and kidney function.

7. If you were provided training and assigned by the principal to do a support group for this client and other children who are having problems, what would be the expected benefits of this group? One of the benefits of a support group for this client and others would be the discovery that she or he is not alone in having problems. Yalom and Leszcz (2005) describe the benefits of group psychotherapy, and although a nurse or a teacher who leads a school support group is not a psychotherapist nor doing psychotherapy, the benefits of group are similar if not the same. The benefits of group work, as identified by Yalom, would include instillation of hope, finding others have similar problems, gaining information, being able to help others, developing social skills in a safe setting, developing a sense of cohesiveness with other members of the group, getting things out and feeling better, and finding a purpose in life.

Note: In a number of high schools, the teachers are asked to volunteer to lead support groups for students. In some instances a strong peer volunteer is trained to assist the teacher. If teachers can do this, it is surely not beyond the scope of school nurses.

8. Would you put together a homogenous or a heterogeneous support group for children? What circumstances would warrant breaking confidentiality, and who could receive the information? How would you prepare the students to know about and accept the situations that could not be kept within the group? Typically, support groups in schools are made up of children with a variety of problems, such as dealing with the death of a parent, dealing with unsupportive parents, dealing with alcoholism or illness in the family, feeling alone and isolated, dealing with ADHD behaviors and medication, and dealing with personal medical problems such as diabetes. An important point to make in group is that what is talked about in the group stays in group, that is, confidentiality must be kept by members.

It is important to discuss the rules of the group up front. You can ask the group to help make the rules so they will help enforce and will more likely abide by the rules. The group members will likely contribute rules like "Don't interrupt others," "No cuss words," and/or "Be respectful of other people's feelings." You could ask: "And what rule do we need to have for situations in which someone is talking about hurting themselves and others?" You may have to make a point of explaining that a couple of things can't be kept confidential as well as who can receive this information: 1. Taking about hurting yourself and/or others will have to be shared with appropriate persons; and 2. Sexual and physical abuse or severe neglect will have to be reported to the authorities under the law if the authorities are not already aware of it.

9. If you were the school nurse, would you educate children in the classroom about Inhalant Abuse and the dangers of using inhalants? What are the signs and symptoms you could teach parents to look for that would indicate their child might be inhaling solvents? Your school district would probably have guidelines and policies, which could either mandate or prohibit nurses from educating children about the dangers associated with inhalant use. You may feel strongly about telling children about inhalants or may oppose it strongly. It is possible that you have never given this idea any thought. Some people who influence policies will think that telling children about inhalants will give them ideas that they would not have otherwise and lead them to experimenting with inhalants. Another group of people will be proponents of warning children about using inhalants and the damage it can cause to the brain and other organs of the body. Anderson and Loomis (2003) proposed education of youth and parents as essential to decrease experimentation with inhalants and "sudden sniffing death syndrome."

As a school nurse, you would probably find that you could at least provide pamphlets from the health department on abuse of inhalants to parents and direct them to web sites for information or hold drug informational groups for parents. In Pena's case, providing pamphlets to her parents and inviting them to come to a meeting might not work as they would probably refuse to attend meetings or to read literature.

You could tell parents to be alert to any chemical odor on a child's breath or clothing; major interest in using spray paint or model glues; paint on the face, hands, and clothes; finding chemically soaked rags or clothing; or unusual interest in maintaining a gasoline supply or other item that can be inhaled. You can tell the parent(s) that if their child reminds them to buy things like gasoline, paint thinner, or mothballs, or can't seem to get enough whipped cream of a specific kind (aerosol can), or asks for/buys substances containing inhalants, the parent(s) should observe the child closer for possible inhalant abuse, as this is generally considered to be unusual behavior in a child. Parents would also be told to be alert to possible Inhalant Intoxication or use if the child appears drunk or disoriented; has slurred speech, nausea, or loss of appetite; is inattentive; or is uncoordinated, irritable, and/or depressed ("A Parent Guide to Preventing Inhalation Abuse," 2004).

10. **Would you expect this client to have withdrawal symptoms if she stops using inhalants? If so, what symptoms would you expect?** It appears that Pena has just begun using inhalants and may not suffer withdrawal symptoms if she stops at this point, but we cannot be sure of this. The nurse must be aware of the possibility of withdrawal symptoms, which include: nausea, chills, muscle cramps, sweating, hand tremors, nausea, hallucinations, and DTs. Detoxification from inhalants can take as long as forty days (Lien Munson, 2002).

11. **What are the current treatment(s) for Inhalant Intoxication and for Inhalant Abuse?** There is currently no medical treatment to reverse the effects of inhalants when a person is experiencing Inhalant Intoxication. Treatment includes medical management of the problems associated with damage done by the inhalants to the organs of the body. After clients are detoxified, treatment is designed to meet individual needs and may include cognitive therapy; individual, group, and family therapy; and interventions designed to target underlying causes for use of inhalants, which in this case has to do with the worthlessness, hopelessness, and isolation felt by the client.

Sometimes teens who abuse inhalants are placed in residential treatment facilities where they can be treated by a team of professionals on a long-term basis. Parents do not always pay for this treatment option. The school district, scholarships, churches, or other organizations sometimes pays it for.

In some states (e.g., Texas) students who have used inhalants are found in larger percentages in Alternative High Schools, as evidenced in a study of 354 studies in 5 Alternative High Schools in Texas. The previous lifetime use of inhalants among students in Alternative High Schools in this study was 27.7 percent, which is much higher that the 2004 national MFT study and much higher than the 8 percent in a Texas school district in regular public schools (Fleschler et al., 2002). Did the Alternative High School somehow become a planned, or unplanned, treatment modality for inhalant users? These schools are designed to prevent students who are having difficulty in school from dropping out of school. The students in the five alternative schools in this study were found to be less likely to be financially supported by parents or guardians, more likely to use addicting substances, and more likely to carry weapons and consider suicide. The Alternative High School offers students options of times to attend school so the student can work around jobs and child care as a large percentage of these teens have children of their own to care for. These schools offer options of time frames for completion of graduation requirements. There is a focus on developing the students' talents and interests and making the student strong, goal oriented, and independent.

In some states with vocational high schools, the student who is abusing inhalants due to a difficult home life and feeling hopeless and helpless and isolated may improve when offered a chance to enter one of these high schools and learn how to make a living and become financially and otherwise independent of his or her parents.

12. **In writing a care plan for this client, what assessment data would you gather? What nursing diagnoses, goals, and interventions would you write for this client and share with the team mentioned above?** You want information about the physical and mental status of the client. Continued inhalation use will cause mental and physical problems. You need to assess for suicide ideation on an ongoing basis. You need to assess the client's strengths and limitations as well as those of the family. Problem-solving skills and family dynamics need to be assessed. At some point you may hear from Pena about the sexual abuse by her father, the neglect and physical abuse by the parents, and the sexual abuse by the neighbor boy, and you will have to report this suspected abuse to the state child protective agency.

You need to assess the client's perception of the benefits and harmful consequences of inhalant abuse. You need to assess her reasons for inhaling gasoline and other chemicals, as well as to get her to look at the harmful and possible harmful effects.

You will want to assess for any possible motives for quitting the use of inhalants. It is likely that there will be a meeting of several people on the school staff to discuss Pena's situation. The principal, vice principal, school psychologist, teacher, you, and the truancy officer will probably meet to pool assessment findings and discuss resources for helping Pena. The team will probably invite the parents to meet with them to discuss options for helping this student.

Nursing diagnoses could include one or more of the following diagnoses:

- Ineffective coping as evidenced by use/abuse of chemicals
- Altered role performance at school and home as evidenced by lowered grades and withdrawal
- Social isolation
- Knowledge deficit related to harmful consequences of inhalation of solvents
- Situational low self-esteem
- Powerlessness related to abuse
- Dysfunctional family processes: Alcoholism
- Impaired parenting
- Risk for suicide

Probable goals for this client would include the following goals.

Client will:

- Describe harmful consequences of inhalants
- Remain free of use of inhalants of all types (solvents, aerosols, gases, and nitrites) and other substance of abuse
- Agree to attend individual and family therapy sessions, education classes, support groups, and/or other classes or activities as scheduled 100 percent of the time
- State at least one positive self-affirmation
- Spend time daily in at least one appropriate activity with at least one other child who is not using inhalants
- Find at least one healthy area of interest

Possible interventions could include the following interventions:

- Build a trusting relationship with client
- Schedule one-to-one sessions with nurse and/or school psychologist on a regular basis
- Model and teach problem-solving process
- Enlist teacher's help to increase interaction with at least one peer in class (e.g., assign the same each time to work in pairs with Pena); select a peer who comes across kind and helpful
- Discuss with parents keeping Pena after school to finish homework before going home to ensure success
- Model positive affirmations and work with client to find one or more positive affirmations to apply to self
- Encourage and assist student to find an activity to participate in or an interest to develop
- Assign to a support group with other students
- Explore the possibility of getting a mentor from a group like the Big Brother-Big Sister organization
- Take client to an Alateen Meeting (support group for teens with alcoholism in the family) if appropriate or have someone from Alateen come and talk to students at school about the location, time, and benefits of the group

References

American Psychiatric Association. (2000). *Diagnostic and Statistical Manual of Mental Disorders, 4th ed.* Text Revision. Washington, DC: American Psychiatric Association.

Anderson, C.E. and G.A. Loomis. (2003). "Recognition and Prevention of Inhalant Abuse." *American Family Physician* 68(5): 869–874.

"A Parent Guide to Preventing Inhalation Abuse." (2004). *Brown University Child and Adolescent Behavioral Letter* 20(5): 9.

Fleschler, M.A., S.R. et al. (2002). "Lifetime Inhalant Use Among Alternative H. S. Students in Texas: Prevalence and Characteristics of Users." *American Journal of Drug and Alcohol and Drug Abuse* 28(8): 477–495.

Kong, J.T. and C. Schmiesing. (2005). "Concealed Mothball Abuse Prior to Anesthesia." *Acta Anaesthesiology Scandanavia* 49(1): 113–116.

Lien Munson, B. (2002). "How to Recognize and Treat Propellant Inhalation." *Dimensions of Critical Care Nursing* 21(1): 18–20.

National Institute on Drug Abuse. (2005). NIDA Research Report: Inhalent Abuse. NIH Pub. #00-3810 (Printed 1994, Revised 2005). Available at http://www.nida.nih.gov/PDF/RRInhalants.pdf. Assessed June 22, 2005.

Yalom, I. with M. Leszcz. (2005). *The Theory and Practice of Group Psychotherapy, 5th ed.* New York: Basic Books.

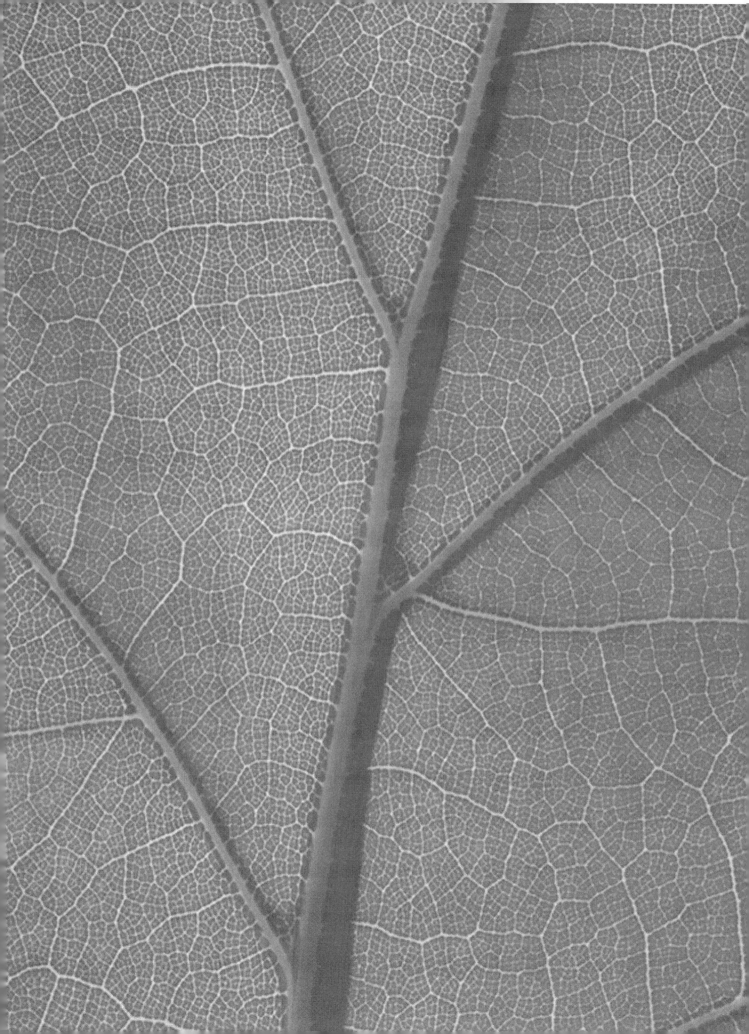

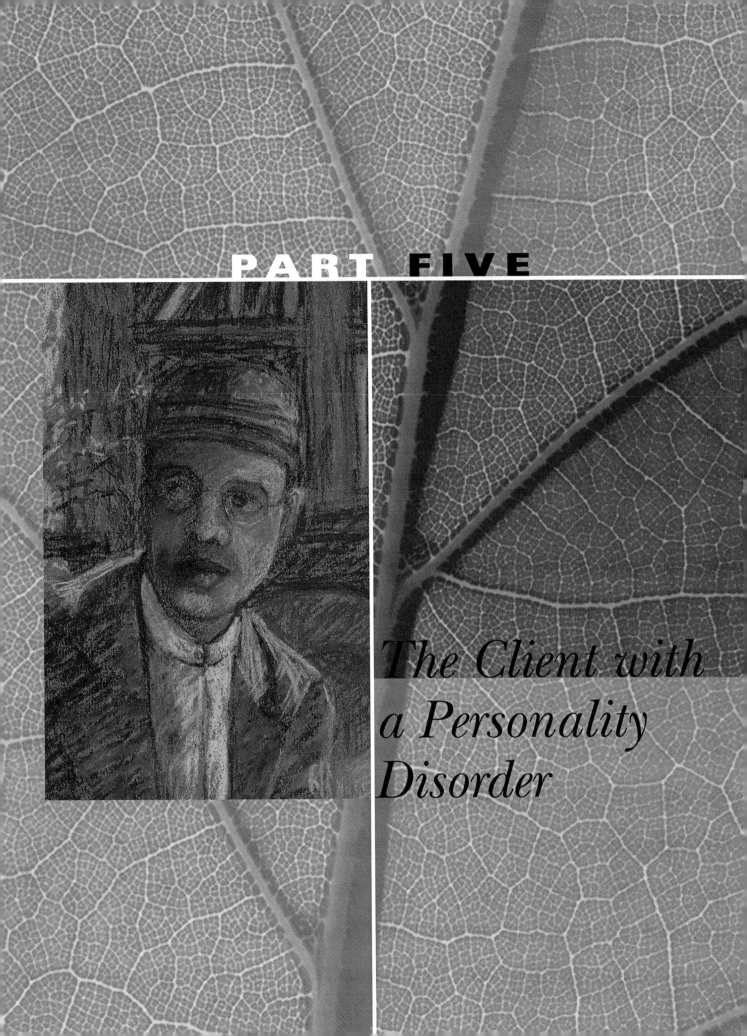

PART FIVE

The Client with a Personality Disorder

GENDER

Female

AGE

27

SETTING

- Company nurse's office

ETHNICITY

- White American

CULTURAL CONSIDERATIONS

- Midwestern farming culture; pioneer and Germanic influence

PREEXISTING CONDITION

COEXISTING CONDITION

COMMUNICATION

DISABILITY

SOCIOECONOMIC

- Upper-class professional

SPIRITUAL/RELIGIOUS

PHARMACOLOGIC

PSYCHOSOCIAL

- Desire for approval from father
- Perfectionism and control issues interfere with social relationships

LEGAL

ETHICAL

- Recommending one therapist: therapeutic or unethical?

ALTERNATIVE THERAPY

PRIORITIZATION

DELEGATION

EASY

OBSESSIVE-COMPULSIVE PERSONALITY DISORDER

Level of difficulty: Easy

Overview: Requires the nurse to use critical thinking to identify and understand the behavioral traits of Obsessive-Compulsive Personality Disorder (OCPD) and to determine effective therapeutic approaches. The nurse must differentiate OCPD from Obsessive-Compulsive Disorder. Requires the nurse to identify the role of the industrial nurse and to make decisions within that role.

Client Profile

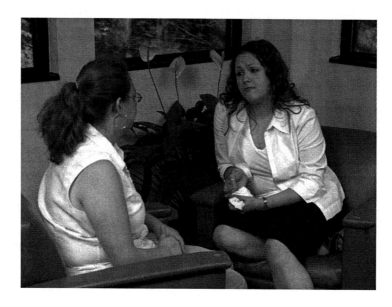

Vicky is a 27-year-old single woman who lives alone and works for a technology company. Vicky grew up on a midwestern small farm with frugal parents. An authoritarian father rarely said much to her except to criticize her behavior. She tried to be perfect at school, often recopying papers several times and thus failing to get them in on time, which meant only a B or C grade. Once when she got a 98 on a paper and was hopeful of getting praise at home, her father said: "What are you going to do about getting 100 next time?" By college Vicky was a straight A student, but her father still didn't praise her. Growing up, she was overly organized with everything in its place in her room and lists posted everywhere. Vicky resisted going to bed until work on the lists was done or she was exhausted and gave up. In the past few years, Vicky has had trouble getting rid of things. She tries to set things aside for charity, but eventually takes things out, one by one, and puts them back inside the house, thinking maybe she will use them some day. Although she is wealthy, she is frugal with her money.

Vicky spends hours trying to get projects at work perfect. When assigned to a project with a coworker, she does most or all of the work herself, because she thinks coworkers won't do it correctly. Sometimes she realizes coworkers are having fun on the weekend while she has no time for leisure activities. Once in awhile she misses a project deadline due to trying to perfect the work.

A former coworker and friend with a romantic interest in Vicky has repeatedly invited her to visit him in another city. Finally, Vicky accepts since she will have her own room and a housekeeper will be there. The friend takes her to a museum to see a European art collection on loan. Vicky insists on viewing the paintings starting at the entrance and going right to left, seeing each painting, reading each plaque, and making a note about it. By the time the museum closes, they have not gotten close to the collection they came to see. Before going out to eat, Vicky insists her friend change his shirt to match his pants and then change his tie. She organizes his ties by color and after some indecision selects one. Before Vicky leaves, her friend tells her he cares for her and gently asks her to see a therapist about her perfectionism and need to control.

Case Study

On Monday afternoon, Vicky presents in the nurse's office of the company where she works asking the nurse to take her blood pressure and complaining of feeling dizzy. The nurse notices that Vicky has rearranged the magazines in the office waiting area and has brought a large stack of what looks like work with her. The nurse asks her about the stack of papers. Vicky says she is behind schedule since she was out of town over the weekend. She shares that she thought maybe she would have time to do some work while waiting to see the nurse. Vicky's blood pressure is within normal limits, as are the rest of the vital signs. The nurse observes that the client looks thin and seems anxious. When the nurse assesses Vicky's heath practices and asks about diet, Vicky says: "Oh, I eat well, but sometimes I skip lunch to get some work done or I forget to eat breakfast when I get busy doing work before I come to work." She admits to getting four to five hours of sleep nightly. The nurse asks Vicky about turning some of this work over to her team members and going home to rest. Vicky seems anxious and even angry as she replies: "No one else can get it right." Then she bursts into tears and says: "A friend of mine says I am a perfectionist and controlling and I should get some help. He doesn't really understand. Do you think I should see a therapist? I really don't have time."

Questions and Suggested Answers

1. **If you were the nurse talking with Vicky, how would you respond to her statements about her friend's thoughts on her perfectionism, need to control, and need to see a therapist, as well as her question to you on whether she should see a therapist or not?** Keep in mind that people with Obsessive-Compulsive Personality traits or the disorder itself tend to resist entering therapy unless they feel they are in crisis or they receive an ultimatum from a significant other or someone in authority such as a supervisor. There are several good responses you can use in this situation, for example, saying: "Let's talk a little more and then get back to your question." You would then do some further assessment and follow up with a statement such as: "Earlier you asked me if I thought you should see a therapist and now that I have a better picture of what is going on with you, let's discuss this. It seems like you have given this idea of seeing a therapist some thought yourself and you no doubt have some ideas about how a therapist could help you sort some things out. I know you are aware that work with a therapist would be confidential." In using this approach you are planting an idea that the client has thought about seeing a therapist in a positive light. You can give the client the list of therapists/counselors approved by the company insurance. The client with OCPD traits may spend an inordinate amount of time selecting the best therapist and procrastinate making an appointment for fear the therapist selected won't be the perfect one. To avoid this procrastination, give Vicky the name of one good therapist you believe could work with her. Ask her to stop by your office or call you within a day or two to see if she needs further help in making an appointment with a therapist. The reality is that she may decide she does not have time to see a therapist or doesn't need to see one or just procrastinate and not call one. As you build a trusting relationship with this client, you may be able to help her see the benefits of talking with a professional counselor or therapist. Ethically you cannot make her accept therapy or change her behavior. Suggesting one therapist rather than suggesting several or asking her to select from a list may be questionable from an ethical standpoint but can also be viewed as therapeutic. It is important to give her the list of therapists approved by the insurance she carries through her employer and describe what it is while still focusing on one therapist for her.

2. **What behaviors did Vicky exhibit in the waiting room and nurse's office that might clue the nurse to assess further for behaviors matching traits of Obsessive-Compulsive Personality Disorder?** Many people carry work around with them these days. Some professionals tend to do this more than others (e.g., teachers with papers to grade and lawyers with briefs to read). However, carrying work around plus talking about not having enough time to do it and especially not being able to turn it over to others on the team because they are not capable are clues to possible OCPD traits. Rearranging the magazines in the waiting area provides another clue. The statement that her friend finds her perfectionistic and controlling offers an additional clue that this client could have OCPD traits or the disorder itself.

3. **If you were the nurse, what other assessments would you want to do at this time?** The client looks thin, so you definitely want to measure height and weight to determine if she is underweight or not. If she is underweight, you need to determine if this is due simply to high metabolism and skipping a few meals or if this could be a clue to an eating disorder or another clue to OCPD. Clients with anorexia and OCPD share some of the same perfectionistic behaviors. Serpell, Livingstone, Neiderman, and Lask (2002) state: "Several authors have suggested that anorexia nervosa has a considerable overlap with obsessive-compulsive disorder and that

this may reflect common neurobiological, genetic, or psychological elements." More recent studies suggest there may be a closer relationship between anorexia nervosa and OCPD. Anderluh et al. (2003) reported on a study of one hundred women, forty-eight of whom were diagnosed with anorexia nervosa, twenty-eight with bulimia nervosa, and twenty-eight healthy women without eating disorders. They found that "childhood obsessive-compulsive personality traits showed a high predictive value for development of eating disorders. . . ." They found that for every obsessive-compulsive personality trait present, the odds for eating disorders were estimated to increase by a factor of 6.9. In addition, they discovered that subjects who reported perfectionism and rigidity in childhood also were more likely to have OCPD or OCD along with the eating disorder.

You could informally assess for perfectionism by asking: "You mentioned your former coworker thinks you are perfectionistic. What do you suppose led him to think this?" You can also ask the client: "Would other people in your family think you are perfectionistic, and if so, why?"

It would be a good idea to assess for depression. Depression can accompany OCPD. You could ask the client about depression in her family and in her own life, and/or you could use a tool like the Beck Depression Inventory.

4. **What are the traits of Obsessive-Compulsive Personality Disorder? What behaviors does Vicky have that match these traits? What are the criteria for a diagnosis of OCPD by a professional qualified to make a diagnosis?**

Traits of Obsessive-Compulsive Personality Disorder	Client's Behavior Matching Traits of OCPD
1. Perfectionism: Sometimes unable to finish projects due to having overly strict standards.	Vicky has a history of recopying papers to make them perfect to the point of sometimes missing a deadline.
2. So focused on details, lists, rules, and organization that the purpose of an activity is forgotten.	Vicky made up rules about viewing the paintings and organized the way to view them to the point that the paintings she and her friend went to see were not seen. They were going out to eat and she didn't like his tie and, in selecting one, decided to organize his ties according to color.
3. Attends to work and productivity to extent there is little or no time for leisure activities and friendships.	Vicky was working so much that she was giving up sleep. No evidence she had any friends other than former coworker who was in another city.
4. When it comes to issues of morality, ethics, or values, is overly conscientious and not at all flexible.	We don't really have a sense of this with Vicky, except she agreed to visit her male former coworker because the housekeeper would be a chaperone of sorts and things would either be proper or look proper.
5. Unable to throw away or give away worthless or worn-out belongings even when they hold no sentimental value.	This client intends to give up belongings to a charity and places them in a box only to take them back one by one until only a few remain to be given away.
6. Difficulty delegating tasks to or working with others, unless they will do everything exactly his or her way.	Vicky cannot delegate to others and provides the rationale that they won't do it right or they don't know how to do it.
7. Hoards money and spends little on self and others. Thinks of money as something to use in the future.	Vicky is a saver and spends little on self or others.
8. Demonstrates stubbornness and inflexibility when it comes to giving up control, going along with the ideas of others, or considering changes.	We don't have a lot of evidence of this behavior, but we can suspect that she is inflexible and assess for this.

(Adapted from APA, 2000)

In order to be diagnosed with Obsessive-Compulsive Personality Disorder, a person has to exhibit five out of eight of the personality traits discussed above, and these traits must be "inflexible, maladaptive, and persisting and cause significant functional impairment or subjective distress" (APA, 2000). Vicky's OCPD traits have caused her to miss deadlines and have interfered with her social relationships.

5. **Obsessive-Compulsive Personality Disorder sounds a lot like Obsessive-Compulsive Disorder. Are they two different disorders or not? Discuss how OCPD and OCD are alike and how they are different.** Yes, these are two different disorders. They share some common symptoms, as persons with either disorder may have patterns of rigidity and may hoard clothing or other things.

   Obsessive-Compulsive Disorder (OCD) is an anxiety disorder that develops at various times in the life of those who are afflicted with it. It sometimes improves spontaneously or with therapy. Obsessive-Compulsive Personality Disorder is not considered an anxiety disorder but rather a personality disorder with enduring personality traits.

   In OCPD the person may be upset if items in the house are moved out of their usual order and is concerned with perfectionism, which is not a concern to people with OCD, who have obsessive thoughts and compulsive behaviors like checking door locks or washing their hands repeatedly. People with OCPD tend to be very rigid and inflexible in their expectations that others follow certain rules or patterns of behavior and become upset when these expectations are not met.. This is not true of people with OCD.

6. **Is there any difference in the reported prevalence of this disorder in males compared to females?** Males are diagnosed with this disorder twice as often as females (Bienenfeld, 2002; APA, 2000).

7. **If Vicky goes to a therapist, the therapist will probably ask about her family and her experiences growing up. Does childhood family environment possibly play a role in the development of Obsessive-Compulsive Personality Disorder? Was Vicky's father's behavior possibly culturally influenced in any way?** Frisch and Frisch (2006) point out that childhood family environment is believed to play a big role in the development of OCPD. When the developmental history of a person with OCPD is taken, the person typically grew up in a family in which they were expected to be perfect and adhere closely to rules with little or no emotional warmth in the home. The client often reveals having to strive for a correct performance just to escape criticism and yet never actually receiving praise if the performance was perfect or near perfect. It is interesting to note that when this child reaches adulthood, even if their parents are no longer present, they will still adhere rigidly to rules and expect a spouse or significant other to abide by their rigid rules of conduct. There is a tendency not to strive for an emotionally warm environment, but to stay with the familiar lack of emotional warmth. Even if the parents no longer demand perfection or provide criticism, the client does this for herself or himself.

   We already know that Vicky's father did not praise her and that he was authoritarian, implying that he had strict rules. Vicky, in talking with the therapist, could reveal more details, such as her father not letting her talk at the table and having to sit straight and chew each bite twenty times with her mouth perfectly closed and having to sit quietly during trips because if she said anything her father would turn around to go back home. She could reveal that her father would cut his food precisely and methodically as if doing surgery. Her father ate meals at precisely the same times each day and never deviated from his precise style of eating. Perhaps her father had some traits of OCPD and/or culture played a role in developing his behavior patterns. Part of the midwestern culture has been to be frugal, and this derives from both early pioneers coming from the East Coast and from German settlers arriving directly from Germany. Early settlers had to make the most of what they could bring with them, grow, gather, or make. The motto was to use it up, wear it out, or eat it up: nothing was wasted. The early settlers often had authoritarian male heads of the household, which remained as part of the culture perhaps until recently. The German settlers valued neatness, order, and precision and tended to raise children in an authoritarian manner. When Vicky visited her grandparents, she was careful not to talk but just to listen and try not to get noticed for anything. She knew that father's father (her grandfather) was a rule man who never hugged or praised anyone and complained about everyone's behavior. He once made Vicky's father open and close the door correctly five hundred times because he had slammed it.

Some children grow up in families like this and have OCPD traits, and some do not. Researchers continue to study other environmental influences that offset the family influences and if there is a biochemical component to this disorder.

8. **Are environmental factors the accepted cause of Obsessive-Compulsive Disorder?** There is controversy about the cause of personality disorders. Bienenfeld (2002) explains it this way: "Traditional thinking holds that these maladaptive patterns are the result of dysfunctional early environments that prevent the evolution of adaptive patterns of perception, response, and defense. A body of data points toward genetic and psychobiologic contributions to the symptomology of these disorders; however, the inconsistency of the data prevents authorities from drawing definite conclusions."

9. **Using Erickson's psychosocial development theory, what developmental stage is this client in and how could that play a role in her wanting to modify her behavior by working with a therapist?** Vicky is at the age of generativity versus stagnation (21 to 45 years), in which a person accomplishes productivity through caring for and guiding children; however, she has clearly not mastered the developmental stage of intimacy versus isolation (18 to 25). As you look at the other stages of development, you probably have doubts that she has mastered some earlier stages. You will recall that Vicky accepted an invitation from a male former co-worker with a romantic interest, and you can wonder what was behind her acceptance. Perhaps she just wanted to visit another city or get a break from work, but more likely she is trying to work on resolution of intimacy versus isolation. Vicky may want children and therefore feel a need to work on having a relationship. The desire for children can be a powerful motivator for change.

Vicky has provided a clue that she is concerned about what her former coworker thinks of her and their relationship as she breaks into tears in the nurse's office and shares what he said to her with the nurse. Her personality traits associated with OCPD may pull her in the direction of resisting the idea of therapy, but her developmental stage may help in this time of crisis to pull her in the other direction, provided the nurse gives her information and support.

10. **What nursing diagnoses would you write for this client?** The following nursing diagnoses, among others, would seem appropriate for this client:

   - Risk for imbalanced nutrition: less than body requirements
   - Disturbed sleep pattern
   - Risk for loneliness
   - Impaired social interaction
   - Anxiety
   - Chronic low self-esteem
   - Defensive coping

When determining what nursing diagnoses to choose, it is helpful to go to your assessment and circle signs and symptoms or behaviors that indicate a problem. Looking at these identified problems or potential problems, it is helpful to go to the current publication of NANDA *Nursing Diagnoses: Definitions and Classification* book and read the description of tentative nursing diagnoses. This is particularly helpful when you are deciding between two nursing diagnoses such as social isolation and impaired social interaction (NANDA, 2005).

11. **What interventions do professional counselors, therapists, or psychiatric nurse clinicians use in working with clients who have traits of OCPD or a diagnosis of this disorder? What interventions would be helpful on the part of the industrial nurse in this case?** The current main treatment for personality disorders is individual psychotherapy, which is directed to improving the client's perception of social and environmental stressors as well as improving responses to these stressors. Cognitive Behavioral Therapy and Interpersonal Therapy are two of the therapies used with clients with OCPD (Bienenfeld, 2002).

Psychiatrists and others qualified to prescribe medications may target symptoms associated with OCPD. For example, according to Greve and Adams (2002) some clients with OCPD who are prone to physical aggression or anger when others do not meet their standards may benefit from anticonvulsant medications such as carbamazepine (Tegretol) or phenytoin (Dilantin), which have a mood-stabilizing effect and decrease irritability and hyperresponsiveness.

Sadigh (1998), in reporting on a possible connection between chronic pain and OCPD, offered several suggestions for working with the client with OCPD and pain. These suggestions would seem helpful for working with the client regardless of accompanying pain or lack of pain. These suggestions included: 1. Avoid being overly enthusiastic; 2. Meet the client where they feel comfortable: the intellectual domain; 3. Offer specific and detailed exercises; 4. Avoid putting an emphasis on exploring feelings; 5. Include the client in creating the treatment plan, as they need to be in control; and 6. Do not take any criticism from the client personally.

Silly group therapy exercises help the person with OCPD to see that people can do things that are spontaneous and puts peer pressure on for the person with OCPD to do something less than perfect. The person with OCPD has great difficulty doing this exercise and may need to be assigned to a peer for help and support in coming up with a silly thing and actually doing it. These silly things consist of such acts as wearing a shirt backward or a name tag upside down.

The nurse needs to keep conversations with the client at an intellectual level, which is where the client is. In addition the nurse needs to avoid any joking content as it may be misunderstood. Instead of offering specific and detailed information related to OCPD, the nurse could give the client information about what the group insurance covers in terms of mental health, about insurance-approved clinicians, and about how to proceed in getting an appointment with a therapist or counselor or psychiatric nurse clinician. The industrial nurse could build a relationship with the client and encourage continuing therapy with her therapist rather than dropping out of treatment early. The industrial nurse's role is to be supportive and facilitative to help the client get into therapy and stay in therapy as long as it is necessary and not to do the therapy himself or herself.

References

American Psychiatric Association. (2000). *Diagnostic and Statistical Manual of Mental Disorders, 4th ed.* Text Revision. Washington, DC: American Psychiatric Association.

Anderluh, M.G., K. Tchanturia, S. Rabe-Hesketh, and J. Treasure. (2003). "Childhood Obsessive-Compulsive Personality Traits in Adult Women with Eating Disorders: Defining a Broader Eating Disorder Phenotype." *American Journal of Psychiatry.* 160(2): 242–247.

Bienenfeld, D. (2002). "Personality Disorders." Available at www.emedicine.com/med/topic3472.htm#section~workup.

Frisch, N.C. and L.E. Frisch. (2006). *Psychiatric Mental Health Nursing, 3rd ed.* Albany, NY: Thomson Delmar Learning.

Greve, K.W. and D. Adams. (2002). "Treatment of Features of Obsessive Compulsive Personality Disorder Using Carbamazepine." *Psychiatry Clinical Neuroscience* 56(2): 207–208.

Morey, L.C. et al. (2002). "The Representation of Borderline, Avoidant, Obsessive Compulsive and Schizotypal Personality Disorders by the Five-Factor Method." *Journal of Personality Disorders* 16(3): 215–234.

North American Nursing Diagnosis Association. (2005). *Nursing Diagnoses: Definitions and Classification 2005–2006.* Philadelphia: North American Nursing Diagnosis Association.

Sadigh, M.R. (1998). "Chronic Pain and Personality Disorders: Implications for Rehabilitation." *Journal of Rehabilitation* 64(4): 4–9.

Serpell, L., A. Livingstone, M. Neiderman, and B. Lask. (2002). "Anorexia Nervosa: Obsessive-Compulsive Disorder, Obsessive-Compulsive Personality Disorder, or Neither?" *Clinical Psychology Review* 22(5): 647–669.

GENDER

Male

AGE

39

SETTING

- Outpatient community mental health center

ETHNICITY

- White American

CULTURAL CONSIDERATIONS

- Girlfriend is Hispanic

PREEXISTING CONDITION

COEXISTING CONDITION

- Chronic depressed mood, possibly dysthymia

COMMUNICATION

DISABILITY

SOCIOECONOMIC

- Slightly above minimum wage

SPIRITUAL/RELIGIOUS

PHARMACOLOGIC

- Paroxetine (Paxil)
- Trasodone (Desyrel)

PSYCHOSOCIAL

LEGAL

- Legal obligation to provide secure e-mail if e-mailing with clients

ETHICAL

ALTERNATIVE THERAPY

PRIORITIZATION

DELEGATION

AVOIDANT PERSONALITY DISORDER

Level of difficulty: Easy

Overview: Requires recognition of the basic traits associated with Avoidant Personality Disorder and critical thinking to build a professional nurse-client relationship and keep the client engaged in treatment. Helping the client to slowly increase social contact requires careful planning, effective interventions, and patience.

Client Profile

George is a 39-year-old male who lives alone. He divides his time between work and being in his bedroom on the computer. He has rarely socialized with anyone because of a fear of being criticized or rejected. Recently George quit a day job because he thought the store owner was critical of him, when in reality the store owner wanted to promote him to day manager. George felt inadequate to be a manager, fearing he would embarrass himself in the job and be criticized more. George likes his new job better because he works nights at a convenience store and does not have to interact with many people. This job is also close to a bus stop; George cannot afford a car. He has difficulty sleeping whether he is working days or nights. When he can't sleep, he works on the computer.

George had one date with Maria, whose family is from Mexico. He went to pick her up and was greeted by her extended family. He felt totally inadequate around her family and felt he was embarrassing himself and Maria, especially after Maria told him she wanted to help him shop for clothes and offered him advice on losing weight. Now he only communicates with Maria by e-mail or telephone, telling her he is "resting up for work" or "busy" when she asks him to go somewhere with her. He fantasizes about relationships with Maria and with women he meets in chat rooms, but he does not meet with them except on the computer.

Members of George's own family criticize each other in a teasing but emotionally hurtful sort of way. He has always felt rejected and criticized by his family, but once or twice a year on special occasions, he attends a family gathering at the urging of his mother. George's father talked him into going to college, but George skipped many of the classes. His father thinks he is just a few hours short of a degree when in reality he has few credits.

Case Study

George comes to the community outpatient mental health center clinic saying his father asked him to see about an antidepressant because he is overweight and seems depressed. The nurse notices that George seems very shy, as evidenced by looking down, speaking softly, and blushing at times.

George is assessed for depression, and the nurse takes an extensive health history. George describes symptoms of a depressed mood nearly every day for several years with no episodes of deep depression or elevated mood. At one point, during the history taking, George says: "You seem busy today; perhaps I could come back another day." The nurse's reply is effective as George stays for the rest of the appointment.

During assessment, the nurse uncovers much of the information in the client profile above and does a complete review of systems and asks about past and current health problems. A head-to-toe physical assessment is postponed until the next visit. The nurse finds that in addition to being somewhat depressed in mood most of the time, George has some traits of Avoidant Personality Disorder. The nurse wonders if George has sufficient traits for a diagnosis of avoidant personality disorder

The nurse suspects that George could benefit from an antidepressant and consults with the community mental health center psychiatrist, who also talks with George and prescribes a two-week supply of samples of paroxetine (Paxil) and trasodone (Desyrel). The nurse does some education with George about the medications and gives George an appointment in two weeks' time. George responds: "My job keeps me pretty busy. I don't have much time off. Could I just e-mail and tell you how I am doing? You could mail the medication to me."

Questions and Suggested Answers

1. **Discuss possible reasons for George saying to the nurse: "You seem busy today; perhaps I could come back another day." What would be a good response on the part of the nurse to this statement?** George suggesting he could leave and come back another day is consistent with his usual avoidance of contact with others. He is avoiding developing a relationship with the nurse: a relationship in which he might be criticized. There

is also the possibility that George is being self-critical and self-deprecating and thinks he does not deserve treatment, or the nurse's time, as much as the other clients do.

Sadigh (1998) points out that clients with Avoidant Personality Disorder "tend to avoid relationships in order to safeguard themselves from the overwhelming pain of rejection." He points out that while these clients go out of their way to avoid relationships, they are starved for and crave attention and human contract. However, the nurse must keep in mind that these clients do not crave attention and contact as much as they fear criticism and rejection.

There are several therapeutic and helpful responses the nurse could use in responding to George, such as "Your care is important and I have time for you." This is a simple statement and does not allude to any new relationship, which might be frightening, but does let the client know that he is worthy of the nurse's time.

2. **Why did the client receive only a two-week supply of paroxetine and trasodone instead of a month or three months supply?** The doctor possibly gave the client only two weeks of medication to prevent the client having enough of this medication to overdose should the client become suicidal. The media has called attention to the possibility of increased suicide risk with Paxil as well as Prozac. Spratto and Woods (2006) list possibility of suicide attempt as one of the side effects observed with a frequency of up to one in one thousand clients. Another possible reason for dispensing cautiously is that this medication may not be well tolerated by George. In addition, George was given samples and the clinic has to use its limited supply of samples cautiously.

3. **Describe an acceptable response to George's suggestion that he could e-mail rather than keep a follow-up appointment.** In regard to e-mailing, the nurse could say something like: "While e-mailing could be easier, I need you to come to the clinic in person. This is important for several reasons. We can assess your response to the medication better and give you another supply of medication if you are responding well."

The nurse needs to see the client in person because it is important to observe the client's appearance and affect and assess the client for any side effects of the medication as well as any suicide ideation. In addition, the nurse needs to work on building a nurse-client relationship with this client. Having him come to the clinic provides an opportunity to work with him to decrease his fear of interacting in person. Yet another reason for the client to present in person is the difficulty in ensuring confidentiality in e-mails. If the client is periodically given the option of reporting in by e-mail to keep the client in treatment, a secure line must be provided and confidentiality ensured. Even if the client did not care about confidentiality, the clinic is legally obligated to ensure confidentiality.

The nurse can encourage the client to talk about any problems he foresees in coming to the clinic in person and teach problem-solving approaches to overcome these problems.

4. **What do you think was the rationale for delaying a head-to-toe physical assessment? Discuss the value of doing the physical examination versus delaying it.** In working with clients who have Avoidant Personality Disorder, the clinician may find that "because of their self-depreciating and vigilant tendencies, they may be resistant to being directly touched" (Sadigh, 1998). It may help the client accept the nurse's touch in physical assessment if there is a professional nurse-client relationship.

The nurse-client relationship is important in this case in order to keep the client engaged in treatment. If the client has had a physical examination within the last year and has no medical complaints, it is less important for the nurse to do a head-to-toe physical assessment. The client can be asked to sign a release of information form so copies of the findings on the earlier physical examination can be obtained.

On the other hand it is always a good idea for new clients to have a physical examination. A number of medical problems can present with symptoms that can be mistaken for a psychiatric disorder.

Clients in crisis may be more compliant with physical examination as they want help desperately. In this case, however, the father has asked the client to go to the community mental health center. The degree of commitment to treatment by the client needs to be assessed and interventions could be directed toward increasing compliance with treatment.

Whether the client receives a physical assessment or an examination on this visit is a matter of judgment and facility policy. Major considerations are obtaining accurate information about the cause of the client's symptoms, keeping the client in treatment as long as needed, and protecting the health care staff and clinic from being sued for not doing adequate assessment and providing appropriate treatment.

5. **The nurse observed some client behaviors that suggest this client might have Avoidant Personality Disorder. What traits does George have that match this disorder? What percentage of clients in the outpatient mental health clinic would likely meet the criteria for a diagnosis of Avoidant Personality Disorder?** The person with Avoidant Personality Disorder has "a pervasive pattern of social inhibition, feelings of inadequacy, and hypersensitivity to negative evaluation" that is evident by young adulthood and observed in a variety of areas of the person's life. To meet the criteria for this disorder, the client must have at least four of the seven behavioral patterns (APA, 2000).

Avoidant Personality Disorder Criteria	Client's Behavior that Matches Criteria
1. Avoids work activities having much interpersonal contact due to fear of being rejected, criticized, or experiencing disapproval.	Quit a day job to work nights partly in order to deal with fewer people and due to thinking his day job boss was critical.
2. Not willing to get involved with others unless sure others will like them.	Client thinks others don't like him and so does not get involved with other people.
3. Holds back or avoids intimate relationships due to fear of others shaming or ridiculing him (or her).	Interacts with females by e-mail or phone, but has used excuses to not accept invitations to meet in person.
4. Has frequent thoughts about being criticized or rejected in social settings.	Feels rejected and criticized by family and avoids family social events.
5. Inhibited when in a new interpersonal situation due to feeling inadequate.	Felt inadequate around Maria's family and thought he was embarrassing himself and Maria, especially when she said she wanted to help him pick out clothes and advised him on weight loss.
6. Holds opinion of self as that of a socially inept, unappealing, and/or inferior person compared to others.	Needs further assessment.
7. Usually shows reluctance to take personal risks or engage in new activities due to fear of possible embarrassment.	Needs further assessment.

(Adapted from APA, 2000)

While the prevalence in the general population is said to be 0.5 to 1 percent, the prevalence in outpatients in mental health clinics is thought to be about 10 percent.

6. **What approach or approaches by the nurse would most likely work best with this client?** Initially the focus needs to be on gaining cooperation and trust. A gentle approach is helpful. The use of criticism is to be avoided even if it is for educative purposes or in the form of advice. This client expects to be rejected by others and looks for this rejection, and advice is often seen as criticism and constructive criticism is seen as rejection. The nurse and other staff working with this client need to be supportive and somewhat reassuring. Techniques used by a therapist working with a client with APD, as described by Miloria (1998), have application for the nurse. Those techniques are listening, using silence, and encouraging to get the client to talk and explore issues.

Sadigh (1998) suggested that staff avoid touching the client, saying, "Because of their self deprecating and vigilant tendencies they [clients with APD] may be resistant to being directly touched."

Duff (2003) suggests three essential elements—training, support, and guidance—are needed to equip the nurse and other staff members to provide effective care and management of clients with personality disorders.

7. **What is the cause(s) of Avoidant Personality Disorder?** The cause of Avoidant Personality Disorder is not known. Like other disorders categorized as mental disorders, it could be multicausal and may be related to inherited temperament. In the literature, which is very limited on APD, this disorder is said to have overlapping characteristics with social phobia, which has been studied much more than APD. Social phobia or anxiety has been hypothesized to involve the amygdala and other areas of the brain's limbic system. Abnormal regulation in the brain's dopamine system has also been found to be associated with adult social anxiety disorder.

APD is usually not diagnosed in anyone under age 18. Many mental health professionals hesitate to, or just do not, put a diagnostic label on a child. People with APD often recall having characteristics of APD as a child (Rettew and Jellinek, 2003).

8. **Will paroxetine and/or trasodone change the traits of Avoidant Personality Disorder as well as the symptoms of depression?** More research needs to be done to determine the effect of paroxetine and trasodone on the behavioral traits of APD. The uses listed for paroxetine in drug handbooks (e.g., Spratto and Woods, 2006) includes, in addition to depression, the following conditions/disorders: Obsessive-Compulsive Disorders, panic attacks, Social Anxiety Disorder, and Generalized Anxiety and PTSD. The Food and Drug Administration (FDA) has not approved any medications to treat APD. Paroxetine is the only medication approved by the FDA to treat social phobia, which may turn out to share some genetic similarities to Avoidant Personality Disorder. Although not approved, paroxetine is considered by some psychiatrists as a first-line treatment for APD as well as for social phobia in adults (Rettew and Jellinek, 2003).

Trasodone has "drowsiness" as one of its side effects. Since George has had trouble sleeping, he was probably given the trasodone not only to alleviate symptoms of depression, but also to help him get adequate rest and sleep. Day workers often take trasodone only at night to help them sleep as well as to alleviate depressed mood. A night worker would likely take it before going to bed, whatever that time might be.

9. **What education does the nurse need to do with George in regard to paroxetine?** The nurse needs to make George aware that the full beneficial effects of this drug may not be seen until after one to four weeks and to allow four weeks for therapeutic effects. Some clients quit the drug early thinking it is not helping when it has not yet taken effect. The client also needs to be taught that if he experiences relief of symptoms, he should not stop the drug. George needs to be taught to check with the nurse or health care provider before discontinuing the drug or about experiencing any side effects. The client is to be told to avoid alcohol and OTC products. The client must be made aware that there needs to be at least fourteen days after stopping an MAO inhibitor and starting paroxetine or after stopping paroxetine and starting on an MAO inhibitor. Side effects reported by one in one thousand people are numerous, including: somnolence and insomnia, agitation, seizures, dizziness, drugged feeling, confusion, and/or impaired concentration. There may be increased risk of a suicide attempt.

The National Institutes of Mental Health (2002) *Medications Booklet* advises that if the client experiences side effects such as headache, nausea after a dose, or trouble falling asleep or waking during the night, time or a reduction in dose will resolve this. If the client feels jittery or agitated and did not have this feeling before taking the drug for the first time and it persists, the health care provider should be notified.

This drug can cause sexual dysfunction such as ejaculatory delay or impotence, including failure to achieve erection or failure to achieve orgasm. This side effect is fairly common, but reversible. It is interesting to note that this drug is given to some clients for treatment of premature ejaculation. All indications are that this client is not sexually active and therefore the adverse effects of male ejaculatory disturbance are probably not a worry. Clients who experience this adverse effect are often changed to a different antidepressant such as Welbutrin, which has less risk of sexual dysfunction.

10. **What is the most likely reason that this client stopped seeing Maria, the girl he once dated and now only e-mails? Would her Hispanic culture present any special challenges/problems in a relationship with George and his Avoidant Personality Disorder traits?** The most likely reason that this client did not ask Maria out on a date again or accept any of her invitations is that he perceived that Maria was being critical of him in wanting to help him dress better or suggesting he lose weight.

Dating a Hispanic woman would present a problem to George with his tendency to avoid most people and social settings because a typical Hispanic family tends to have large family gatherings. Extended family members usually have a close relationship with the nuclear family. George's fear of new relationships and his vigilance for detection of criticism would make it difficult for him to assimilate into a Hispanic family.

11. **What treatment(s) has been found to be helpful to the client with Avoidant Personality Disorder?** Phillip Long (1990) wrote, "Psychotherapeutic treatment must first be directed at solidifying an alliance with the therapist to prevent early termination of therapy. Unlike the schizoid personality, the avoidant personality may find assertiveness training useful. The therapist should be cautious when giving assignments to exercise new social skills outside of therapy, because failure may reinforce the patient's already poor self-esteem." Long believed that group therapy could desensitize the client to the exaggerated threat of rejection.

The work of cognitive therapy developed by Aaron T. Beck (Beck, Freeman, and Associates, 1990; Beck and Rush, 1995) is delineating and modifying dysfunctional beliefs. In this therapy the client learns to replace destructive, nonhelpful thoughts with those that are helpful. An example of the application of Beck's Cognitive Therapy can be found in a case study involving a client who feels inadequate (www.geocities.com/ptypes/beckcasestudy.html).

Miloria (1998) describes the successful use of psychoanalytic theory and techniques in working with a client with Avoidant Personality Disorder over a ten-year period. Miloria describes the client with Avoidant Personality Disorder as "reluctant to form a mirroring self-object transference because of the dread of being seen by the therapist as defective and flawed, a dread that derives from the person's childhood," and because of this and a desire to be accepted, the client plays "hide and seek" with the therapist. The therapist helps the client through self-object transference to gradually develop the "capacity to hold unpleasant emotions within the self rather than look to the therapist as a container without limits for deposit of the client's anxiety." At some point into the therapy Miloria seems to describe the therapist helping the client to gain insight as the therapist shares with the client her (the therapist's) empathetic understanding that the client was reluctant to trust the therapist because of experiences from her early childhood.

12. **What nursing diagnoses would you write for this client? What goals would you likely write in collaboration with the client? Describe one or more interventions and identify how you would apply the evaluation part of nursing process.** Nursing diagnoses would likely include but would not be limited to:

- Chronic low self-esteem
- Impaired social interaction
- Anxiety
- Ineffective coping
- Deficient diversional activity

Examples of possible goals are:

- Will keep 100 percent of outpatient clinic appointments
- Will remain in treatment for at least six months
- Will have in-person social contact with at least one other person twice a week for at least one hour
- Will describe at least two ways of dealing with thoughts that others are critical and he is inadequate
- Will try one new diversional activity

Interventions to improve self-esteem could include asking the client to state a positive affirmation, in other words, a positive statement about himself. Early in treatment, the client may not be able to come up with positive affirmations if asked to do so. In a group setting where everyone is expected to come up with one positive self-affirmation, this is the client who is likely to say: "I can't think of one." The nurse may help the client come up with a positive affirmation. These clients often have pets as they relate better to animals than people. The nurse might ask: "Do you have a pet?" The client will probably say "yes" or "I used to have one." The nurse might respond: "I suspect you are a person who takes good care of your pet."

The client with Avoidant Personality Disorder will tend to avoid group activities for fear of shame or ridicule or embarrassment, but will more likely participate in group activities if he or she receives frequent and abundant assurance of support and nurturance. Some outpatient therapy and nontherapy social groups are set up to serve this purpose. On an inpatient basis, the nurse is often in a position, as part of the treatment team or perhaps as a group co-leader, to assign the client to a supportive group or to facilitate support within the group.

The evaluation part of the nursing process will involve looking at the goals, which are written, in a measurable fashion to determine to what degree the goals have been met.

References

American Psychiatric Association. (2000). *Diagnostic and Statistical Manual of Mental Disorders, 4th ed.* Text Revision. Washington, DC: American Psychiatric Association.

Beck, Aaron T., Arthur M. Freeman, and Associates. (1990). *Cognitive Therapy of Personality Disorders.* New York: Guilford Press.

Beck, Aaron T. and A. John Rush. (1995). *Cognitive Therapy. Comprehensive Textbook of Psychiatry/VI, vol. 2.* Ed. Harold I. Kaplan and Benjamin J. Sadock. Baltimore: Williams & Wilkins.

Duff, A. (2003). "Managing Personality Disorders: Making Positive Connections." *Nursing Management* 10(6): 27–31.

Long, P. (1990). "Avoidant Personality Disorder." Available at www.mentalhealth.com. Accessed June 6, 2006.

Miloria, M.T. (1998). "Facial Disfigurement: A Self-Psychological Perspective on the 'Hide-and-Seek' Fantasy of an Avoidant Personality." *Bulletin of the Menninger Clinic* 62(3): 378–395.

National Institutes of Mental Health. (2002). *NIMH Medications Booklet: Index of Medications.* Available at www.mental-health-matters.com/articles/article.php?artID=237. Accessed November 1, 2005.

Rettew, D.C. and M.S. Jellinek. (2003). "Personality Disorder: Avoidant Personality." Available at www.emedicine.com/ped/topic189.htm. Accessed November 2, 2005.

Sadigh, M.R. (1998). "Chronic Pain and Personality Disorders: Implications for Rehabilitation Practice." *Journal of Rehabilitation* 64(4): 4–9.

Spratto, G.P. and A.L. Woods. (2006). *2006 Edition PDR Nurses Drug Handbook.* Clifton Park, NY: Thomson Delmar Learning.

www.geocities.com/ptypes/beck_case_study.html. Accessed November 1, 2005.

Jim

GENDER

Male

AGE

55

SETTING

- Client's home

ETHNICITY

- White American

CULTURAL CONSIDERATIONS

- Military culture
- Wife is Japanese

PREEXISTING CONDITION

COEXISTING CONDITION

- Chronic back pain
- Diabetes Type II

COMMUNICATION

DISABILITY

SOCIOECONOMIC

- Middle class: retired military and disability pay; wife has no income

SPIRITUAL/RELIGIOUS

PHARMACOLOGIC

PSYCHOSOCIAL

- Death of mother

LEGAL

- Confidentiality

ETHICAL

ALTERNATIVE THERAPY

- Massage; chiropractic treatments

PRIORITIZATION

DELEGATION

DEPENDENT PERSONALITY DISORDER

Level of difficulty: Easy

Overview: Requires identification of effective ways to work with an individual who not only has traits of Dependent Personality Disorder, but also has chronic pain. Requires critical thinking to determine what culturally influenced behaviors of the spouse are enabling the husband's dependence and how to work with the spouse to modify her behavior.

Client Profile

Jim is a 55-year-old male who has both psychological and medical problems. He sees a nurse psychotherapist, goes to a pain clinic, a massage therapist, and a chiropractor for help with what he describes as uncontrollable back pain; he sees an internist for his diabetes; and he has a visiting nurse working with both him and his wife with a goal of increasing his independence in activities of daily living, exercises, and diabetes control.

In individual therapy Jim reveals a nanny cared for him for six months when he was separated from his mother at age two, due to his mother's hospitalization for treatment of major depression. Jim's father was overly protective as Jim was adopted and his father feared social services would find a reason to take Jim away. When Jim's mother returned home, Jim felt anxious when away from her.

Jim married young and joined the army. He turned every responsibility he could over to his wife whether he was home on leave or away on duty. Shortly before he retired from the army, his wife "burned out" from doing so much for him and left him for another man who paid attention to her needs. Jim immediately married Mari, a Japanese woman who seemed willing to take care of him. He then separated from the army with retirement and disability pay for a back injury. Jim's mother died two years ago, and he is still depressed about her death. He fears his wife and caregivers will reject him because he is not worthy of their attention. Jim's wife wants to go to Japan to visit her family, but when she mentions it, Jim becomes "clingy." Jim says he can't make a trip due to his bad back, which gets worse when Mari mentions a trip. Jim won't let her go, fearing something will happen to her and he'll have no one to care for him.

Case Study

The visiting nurse arrives at the client's home. Earlier in the day, the client's wife had called the nurse and described Jim becoming dizzy while shopping with her. She shared that she is now pushing Jim in a wheelchair. She stated she could do the shopping alone, but her husband insists on going with her. She said Jim often becomes angry with clerks in the stores and berates them, and this embarrasses her. She thinks he is on too much pain medication and it is causing him to be forgetful and dizzy at times. Mari said that Jim won't make decisions, has her pick out his clothes for the day, and won't do any tasks on his own initiative. She has to remind him to do his blood sugar testing and then he wants her to do it. Before the conversation ended, Mari added: "Jim needs constant care. I am getting tired. I am worried that he will get worse."

Jim greets the visiting nurse and says he needs help deciding what to do about his back pain. It is not getting better, and he has to take more pain medication and anti-anxiety medication. He can't do the exercises the doctor prescribed because it hurts too much; maybe if she would give him a massage and help him exercise, he could do a little exercise. He asks the nurse: "Would you also check my blood sugar before you do the massage?" The nurse recalls that Jim has been taught to check his own blood sugar.

Questions and Suggested Answers

1. **Why would the visiting nurse need to discuss this client's case with his other care providers as well as Jim and his wife? Does the nurse need to get a release of information signed by the client before discussing his case?**
   The nurse needs to coordinate Jim's care with others providing his care to determine what his true medical and psychiatric situation is and what he needs help with as well as how to best foster independence in some areas of his life. Working in concert will prevent some providers working toward independence and others fostering dependence.

   If all care providers work for the same employer, they can discuss the client's case without a signed consent form. If any of the health care providers do not work for the same employer, which is likely, the client needs to sign release of information forms so that the visiting nurse, psychiatric nurse clinician, internists, massage therapist, and chiropractor can share information.

The client may not wish to share information between care providers. When a caregiver asks a client to sign a release of information form, the client may choose to sign it or not.

2. **What is a person with Dependent Personality Disorder like?** Sadigh (1998, 4) describes the person with Dependent Personality Disorder as having "an insatiable desire to have things done to them instead of learning to take care of themselves." He pointed out that these individuals may "easily become dependent on passive, physical modalities such as massage and may develop symptoms of withdrawal if treatment is discontinued." The essential feature of this disorder as described by the APA (2000, 721) is "a pervasive and excessive need to be taken care of that leads to submissive and clinging behavior and fears of separation." People with Dependent Personality Disorder have a hard time starting projects or doing things by themselves. These folks are likely to function adequately when assured another person is supervising and approving. They tend to fear looking, or being, more competent. Their perception is that if they could do things for themselves, their supervisor, caregiver, spouse, or significant other would leave them. Millon and Davis (1996) describe persons with Dependent Personality Disorder as showing dichotomous thinking in regard to independence, as they believe either that a person is completely dependent and in need of help or totally independent and alone. The ultimate goal of therapy is not viewed as complete independence but the flexibility to operate on a continuum between self-reliance and a healthy mutual dependence. Millon and Davis describe subtypes of Dependent Personality Disorder including: 1. The accommodating dependent characterized by submissiveness and agreeableness; 2. The disquieted dependent who is anguished and fearful of loss; this type may vent tensions in outbursts of anger directed to others whom they perceive as not appreciating their need for security and nurturance; 3. The immature dependent who remains childlike throughout life; and 4. The ineffectual dependent. This subtype discussion provides a possible explanation for why the client in this case vents anger at store clerks.

3. **If you were the visiting nurse and had all the information available about Jim from other health care providers, as well as your own observations, what traits of Dependent Personality Disorder would you identify in this client?**

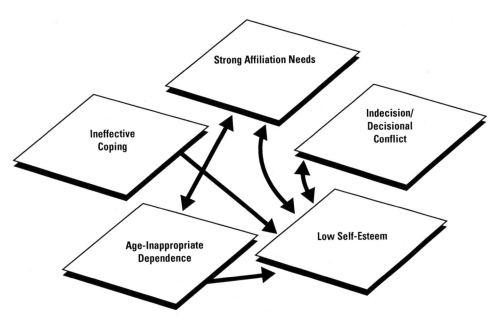

Concept map of issues and problems associated with Dependent Personality Disorder.

Traits of Dependent Personality Disorder	Client's Traits
1. Has a need for someone else to assume responsibility for a good many of the important areas of his or her life.	Yes. Jim turned over all responsibilities he could to his wife. When his wife divorced him, he quickly remarried a woman who would take care of him and these responsibilities.
2. Exhibits difficulty making day-to-day decisions, seeking more reassurance and advice than the average person.	Yes. Spouse says client will not make simple decisions (e.g., what to wear).
3. Trouble verbalizing disagreement with others they are dependent upon, due to fear of withdrawal of support or approval (excludes realistic fears of retribution).	Needs further assessment. No evidence that Jim expresses disagreement with his wife or that he fears support or approval will be withdrawn if he disagrees.
4. Goes to excessive lengths, even volunteering for unpleasant jobs, to get desired nurturance and support.	No evidence of this.
5. Experiences discomfort or feeling of helplessness when alone due to exaggerated fears that he or she will not be able to care for themselves.	Yes. Jim has admitted to being uncomfortable and/or feeling helpless when alone due to fear he may not be able to care for himself.
6. Exhibits difficulty starting projects or doing things on own initiative due to lack of confidence in judgment or abilities and not due to insufficient motivation or energy.	Yes. Wife has said that she has to remind client to test his blood sugar and then he wants her to do it. She says he won't start any task on his own.
7. Looks desperately for another relationship to provide care and support when a significant relationship closes.	Yes. Jim married young and immediately sought and found a new spouse after his first wife divorced him.
8. Unrealistically fearful of being abandoned to take care of self.	Yes.

(Adapted from APA, 2000)

The client must have five or more traits for a diagnosis of Dependent Personality Disorder using criteria from APA (2000). It appears than Jim may have as many as six of the traits. The visiting nurse cannot make a diagnosis of Dependent Personality Disorder, but can assess for behaviors associated with traits of this diagnosis, share findings with the psychiatric nurse clinician and the internist, and develop a nursing care plan that helps the client become more independent.

4. **What causes Dependent Personality Disorder?** The cause of Dependent Personality Disorder is unknown. One theory is that overly protective primary caregivers/parents didn't let the toddler do things on his or her own. As the child aged, the child began to think he or she could do nothing on his or her own. The child did not master the stage of autonomy versus shame and doubt. The caregivers or parents were very controlling, and the child became submissive.

The diathesis-stress model theorizes that children with an anxious temperament and difficulty with peer relationships may be overprotected by caregivers and parents. This combination of anxious temperament and overprotective parenting leads to dependent personality traits.

The cause of Dependent Personality Disorder may involve several factors, such as genetic factors, brain biochemistry, and environment, or it may be simply a matter of genetics and biochemistry or simply a matter of early family environment.

5. **What would be a helpful response on the part of the visiting nurse when Jim asks her to check his blood sugar?** The visiting nurse wants to empower and not enable the dependent client. The nurse could use active

guidance, modeling, and positive reinforcement with Jim. She could say something like: "Jim, let's go over the steps for taking a blood sugar. I'll write them down as you come up with them. Tell me the first step you would take." The nurse could actively guide Jim through a review of the steps for testing blood sugar. If Jim says: "I can't recall," the nurse can give him two possible options, one of which is correct. When he gives the correct answer, give positive reinforcement (e.g., "That's right. You know this well"). The nurse can either have Jim do each step, looking at his list of steps, or demonstrate a step and have him do it. The wife needs to be where she can observe the nurse and learn ways to get Jim to do some things for himself. The nurse needs to have patience and not become frustrated because the client doesn't exhibit age-appropriate independence.

6. **What nursing diagnoses would you write for Jim if you were the visiting nurse?** Chronic low self-esteem and fear are two common nursing diagnoses for Dependent Personality Disorder. The person with DPD may also have anxiety or depression due to fear of rejection and abandonment. Jim also has pain as a nursing diagnosis, and he appears to have dysfunctional grieving over his mother's death.

7. **The visiting nurse and others caring for the client, including the spouse, are scheduled to meet for a planning conference. What goals or outcomes do you think the team might come up with? Should Jim meet with the team?** It would be helpful to have Jim meet with the team to get his input and for the team to present information to him. The team might first go over their various assessment findings, impressions, thoughts about what the problems are, and ideas for the treatment goals and interventions. The team then has the client join them to get the client's input. The team will then determine short and long term goals. When dealing with behaviors related to lifelong personality traits, it is important to select small goals with the hope that the client will continue to change due to experiencing success in meeting small goals.

Nursing Diagnosis Common to Dependent Personality Disorder	Short-Term Small Goals
Chronic Low Self-Esteem	• State one positive self-affirmation daily. • Practice positive self-affirmations in the mirror while doing grooming in the morning.
Fear	• Share feelings about fear of abandonment and other fears with the psychiatric nurse clinician. • Spend thirty minutes alone each day with wife in house for one week, then thirty minutes alone with wife gone on shopping trip.
Anxiety	• Practice relaxation exercises for five minutes twice a day. • Recognize and rate anxiety on scale of one to ten.
Depressed Mood	• Name one activity that elevates mood. • Identify one thought that depresses mood. • Practice negative thought suppression each day (e.g., erasing thoughts like the mind is a blackboard or replacing a negative thought with a positive one).
Additional Nursing Diagnoses for Client in This Case Study	
Chronic Pain	• Find one means of increasing comfort (reducing pain) other than pain medication and use it daily (e.g., watching a funny movie, doing exercises to strengthen muscles as prescribed by the internist, or sitting in a spa or warm tub of water). This method is to be active and not something done by someone else. • Begin a chart of the pain levels, medication taken, and any symptoms other than pain such as dizziness. Share this chart with the visiting nurse and the internist.
Dysfunctional Grieving	• Spend time with someone who knew the mother and share stories about her. • Write in a journal for ten minutes each day about experiences with the mother.

8. **Would Mari's cultural background have an impact on how she relates to Jim's dependency needs? How would you work with her in terms of culturally generated behavioral tendencies?** The nurse needs to assess Mari's cultural beliefs and practices, as they may not be typical of Japanese women her age. We don't know if her parents were both Japanese or not or if she grew up in Japan or not. In other words there might have been non-Japanese cultural influences in her life. In addition she may have become somewhat Americanized. While the nurse must keep an open mind as to Mari's cultural background, it is helpful to know something of Japanese culture. In the Japanese culture, women typically manage the family finances, taking responsibility for this family duty. Women view the husband as needing to receive not only attention but respect as well. Girls grow up learning to expect first their father then their husband to be a strong decision maker. For example, when a young girl asks her father if she can visit overnight at a friend's house, the father will call the friend's father. If not satisfied with the conversation, he will tell his daughter "no" and neither daughter nor mother is to question his decision.

Mari's cultural background would have her respecting her husband, caring for him as he asks, and expecting him to make decisions. In the American culture, Jim appears weak with Mari doing everything for him.

Mari values her family and wants to make a trip to Japan to see her elders and visit the ashes of her ancestors. She cannot go because her cultural upbringing tells her to respect her husband's decision that she not go. While Jim has trouble making decisions, the one decision he has no trouble making is that he will not be left alone.

To work with Mari's cultural tendencies, you would not ask her to disrespect her husband or to go against his decisions, but to follow your modeling of ways to get Jim to do little things for himself and to feel confidence in his abilities. You might teach her to do such things as offer him a choice of two sets of clothing for the day. You would model appropriate responses when he refuses to choose and appropriate positive reinforcement for making the decision.

As you work with Mari's cultural beliefs, you may wonder if Jim selected Mari because of the manner in which Japanese women typically respond to their husbands. Many dependent individuals tend to look for someone with an inner strength, a powerful helper or partner in whom to place their trust and depend on to protect them from having to assume responsibilities (Millon and Davis, 1996). Mari is suffering caregiver role strain. The nurse can educate Mari about respite care, but her cultural beliefs may not let her accept this source of help.

9. **What general approaches do you think might be helpful for the nurse to use in working with Jim or any other client with Dependent Personality Disorder? What types of treatment modalities have been found to be helpful in working with clients with Dependent Personality Disorder?** The visiting nurse may have limited visits approved to work with this client, based on third party payer rules and regulations, and if so, it will be essential to talk about when termination will occur and to talk about this up front. Clients with Dependent Personality Disorder tend to try to hold nurse-client relationships longer by increased complaints about physical symptoms since getting better often causes an end to care by health care professionals.

The nurse will want to build as much structure into her visits as possible because this structure tends to reduce anxiety in clients with DPD. The nurse will try to avoid passive activities in which he or she does things to the client instead of guiding the client to do things for himself, as the client will tend to become dependent on passive treatment modalities.

There is somewhat of a controversy over whether clients with Dependent Personality Disorder benefit from psychotherapy. Coen (1997), looking at pathologically dependent patients and psychoanalysis, says: "These patients remain in treatment sometimes contentedly, sometimes amid rebuke and complaints, but they do not profit from it." While Coen seems to find these clients gaining some insight, he says that "their ability to use insight especially in the transference is matched by a proclivity for sadomasochistic enmeshment. In analysis, this tendency translates into a continuing dependent attachment to the analyst." On the other hand, Millon and Davis (1996) state that the prognosis for clients with Dependent Personality Disorder is relatively good.

Obviously for individual psychotherapy to be therapeutic, the personality of the therapist and the approaches utilized must not result in a continuing attachment to the therapist. While the therapist must build a trusting relationship with the client, the therapist must avoid being the only one the client can trust, or who can help the client, or the only resource in any area of the client's life. The relationship between the therapist and the client must not mimic or reestablish the dominance-subordination relationship pattern. The therapist is to help the client separate and differentiate self from others. The therapist will receive from the client much of the same behavior that the client had in dealing with one or both parents and with his wife as well. The therapist will carefully plan the therapeutic response to the client's behavior: a response that is different and hopefully is reassuring and encourages independent behaviors from the client. What is true for the therapist-client relationship is also true for the visiting nurse working with this client.

Millon and Davis (1996) discussed the following treatments, which are still in use today: 1. Assertiveness training as people with this disorder are often reluctant to stand up for themselves; 2. Teaching client skills that allow expression of negative feelings in constructive way; 3. Communication skills training; 4. Role playing as it helps the therapist learn about the client's relationships and allows the client to practice increasingly assertive behavior; 5. Cognitive therapy to enhance self-image and encourage the use of the problem-solving approach in dealing with problems of life; 6. Identification of distorted thoughts, which are then monitored and subsequently changed; 7. Guided discovery and Socratic type questioning rather than providing answers for the client; 8. Antidepressants and antianxiety medications to promote vigor and alertness and reduce anxiety, which may temporarily increase as the clients tries new more independent behaviors; 9. Group therapy sessions where the client can learn autonomous skills, develop self-confidence, test assertiveness skills, get feedback from peer equals, and learn that these behaviors don't lead to abandonment; and 10. Family or couples therapy.

10. **What interventions would you write and utilize in regard to one or more of this client's nursing diagnoses?** A long-term goal for improving self-esteem is the client's report that his self-esteem has improved or that he will no longer put himself and others down. Interventions could include: modeling the use of self-affirmations, encouraging the client to identify positive things about himself, and asking the client what he says to himself as he looks in the mirror. If it is negative, use this response: "Tell me how that makes you feel better." When he says: "It doesn't," the nurse can respond: "Think of one thing you could say that would be honest and make you feel better about yourself."

In regard to fear of abandonment, one intervention would be to explore those fears with the client and to get the client to face these fears by spending a small amount of time alone and gradually increasing this time. Relaxation exercises would also help the client reduce anxiety associated with this fear. The nurse can teach the client some relaxation techniques and help the client obtain relaxation tapes.

An intervention to deal with reducing the amount of pain would be to use the word "pain" less and substitute "comfort level." The wife can be taught some basic behavior modification techniques, such as giving more attention when the client is comfortable and engaged in distracting and appropriate activities and ignoring some requests for help with things he can do himself. The nurse and client need to assess carefully what the client can and cannot do for himself. He may ask for help tying his shoes. Ignoring this may cause him to fall. The reality may be that he cannot physically reach his shoes to tie the shoestrings.

11. **Is Dependent Personality Disorder common in clients with medical disorders in general and with chronic pain specifically?** According to a number of sources, including the American Psychiatric Association (2000), Dependent Personality Disorder is one of the most common psychiatric disorders seen in mental health clinics. It is also commonly seen in a variety of other treatment settings, psychiatric and medical.

Several studies have found a relatively high percentage of personality disorders in clients with chronic pain, and one of the most prevalent personality disorders is Dependent Personality Disorder. Sadigh (1998) reported on a number of these studies. One study concluded that preexisting personality variables and dependency in relationships may be important contributing factors in chronic low back disability. Another concluded there is a clinically significant prevalence of personality disorders in the chronic pain population especially those with anxiety features. Finally, another found that disability due to chronic pain is a complex phenomenon that encompasses physical, emotional, psychological and socioeconomic factors. They found personality disorders the most useful determinants of disability.

Latvala, Janhonen, and Moring (2000) videotaped ten different nursing situations and interviewed clients and nurses involved in the situations and found 65 percent of the clients were passive recipients of care, 22 percent were responsible recipients of care, and 14 percent were responsible participants in their care. These researchers suggested that in general, psychiatric clients need to participate more in their own care.

12. **Do clients with Dependent Personality Disorder seek treatment, and if so, under what conditions?** Most people with Dependent Personality Disorder do not seek or get treatment specifically for the personality disorder. They do not come into a treatment setting saying: "I have Dependent Personality Disorder and I want treatment." If this disorder is treated, it is often due to a caregiver having left the client through divorce or death, prompting the client to seek help to deal with anxiety and/or depression associated with abandonment, or because of a physical condition such as back pain, diabetes, or some other chronic medical condition or chronic psychiatric condition. A health care professional in their assessment then identifies traits of Dependent Personality Disorder.

References

American Psychiatric Association. (2000). *Diagnostic and Statistical Manual of Mental Disorders, 4th ed.* Text Revision. Washington, DC: American Psychiatric Association.

Coen, S.J. (1997). *The Misuse of Persons: Analyzing Pathological Dependency.* Hillsdale, NJ: Analytic Press.

Latvala, E., S. Janhonen, and J. Moring. (2000). "Passive Patients: A Challenge to Psychiatric Nurses." *Perspectives in Psychiatric Care* 36(1): 24–32.

Millon, T. and R.D. Davis. (1996). *Disorders of Personality: DSM IV and Beyond, 2nd ed.* New York: John Wiley and Sons.

Sadigh, M.R. (1998). "Chronic Pain and Personality Disorders: Implications for Rehabilitation Practice." *Journal of Rehabilitation* 64(4): 4–9.

Brad

GENDER

Male

AGE

62

SETTING

- Private psychiatric hospital outpatient clinic

ETHNICITY

- White American

CULTURAL CONSIDERATIONS

PREEXISTING CONDITION

- High blood pressure
- High cholesterol

COEXISTING CONDITION

COMMUNICATION

DISABILITY

SOCIOECONOMIC

- Affluent
- Professional

SPIRITUAL/RELIGIOUS

- Attends a church with prestigious upper-class members

PHARMACOLOGIC

PSYCHOSOCIAL

- Seeks relationships with people viewed as special or important

LEGAL

- Keeping information provided by a spouse confidential from the other spouse

ETHICAL

ALTERNATIVE THERAPY

- Chiropractic
- Massage therapy
- Health club workouts with trainer

PRIORITIZATION

- Needs of client with Narcissistic Personality Disorder vs. needs of partner

DELEGATION

MODERATE

NARCISSISTIC PERSONALITY DISORDER

Level of difficulty: Moderate

Overview: Requires knowledge of Narcissistic Personality Disorder and the use of therapeutic communication skills to work with the client. The nurse will need to help the client identify the needs he has to meet for himself and those that cause distress in his relationships.

Client Profile

Brad is a 62-year-old married male whose recall of growing up includes a feeling of feast or famine in terms of attention or lack of attention by his mother. She either smothered him with too much attention or was too busy to give him any attention. His father's business was also unpredictable, resulting in the family having lots of money most of the time with occasional periods of having to move to less pretentious housing or change from private school to public school for a semester or two, both traumatic events to a young boy. When Brad started high school, he was back in private school and his father had bought a boat. Having a boat made Brad popular with the girls, and he learned the importance of having special possessions that would attract desirable people into his company and make him feel important. He went to law school and became a lawyer. He studied finance and became a stockbroker and later began managing large financial portfolios. All these activities helped lessen his fear of losing special status and brought him into contact with prestigious people.

Brad married Mary, a girl with money and family prestige. After many years, Mary has developed health problems and is concerned that Brad had no empathy for her health situation. She is irritated at Brad frequently asking her to drop whatever she is doing and meet him somewhere or do something for him. She suspects he has had a number of affairs. After a trip to a local prestigious private psychiatric outpatient clinic, Mary tells Brad she expects him to get therapy at the clinic or she may divorce him.

Case Study

On hearing from Mary that she has been to the outpatient clinic and is thinking about divorce, Brad agrees to go alone and do a preliminary intake meeting with the staff nurse. The threat of Mary leaving him, rather than him leaving her, distresses him. Brad presents himself at the outpatient clinic. He is well-dressed and well-groomed and appears somewhat arrogant and haughty in wanting to check the credentials of the staff and dropping some names of important doctors that he knows. He states that he expects to be seen on time, as time is money in his business. He wants to use the center telephone to make some important business calls even though a sign says the telephone is for staff use only. He displays a money clip with a large number of bills and flashes a large diamond ring. He gives the impression that he is someone important and is entitled to special privileges. He calls and has a large gift basket delivered to the health care provider's home.

As the staff nurse begins the intake process, she recalls that Brad's wife, Mary, described Brad as lacking empathy and consideration and probably having affairs in the past, but the nurse is determined to keep an open mind as she gathers data from Brad. The nurse notices that Brad answers questions briefly, then asks questions about the nurse's qualifications. Brad seems to know a lot about the medications he is taking for elevated blood pressure and cholesterol and tests the nurse's knowledge about these medications and seems to enjoy any time the nurse knows less than he does about the medication.

Brad manages to mention that he owns a vacation home in an exotic location. He describes important people that he has taken there and mentions he might take the nurse to his vacation home. The nurse replies: "Let's get back to the questions on the assessment" and asks about Brad's relationship with his wife. Brad paints a picture of being very generous with his wife and her being stubborn, unloving, and unappreciative. Brad does not reveal a series of affairs throughout the years or that there is a woman he fantasizes about as an ideal lover and mate. The nurse notes that Brad seems concerned that he is aging, and this seems to be a major stressor for him. He reveals he is spending time and money seeing chiropractors and massage therapists and working out in the most prestigious health club in town. At the end of the session, the nurse suspects Brad meets a number of the criteria for Narcissistic Personality Disorder. Before Brad leaves, he says to the nurse: "I would love to know what my wife told you about me." The nurse will present the intake information to the team, and a therapist or therapists will be assigned to Brad and his wife, Mary.

Questions and Suggested Answers

1. **When the nurse hears Brad say he might take her to his vacation home, she replies: "Let's get back to the questions on the assessment." What technique is she using, and what is a rationale for this reply? What is a likely rationale for Brad suggesting the trip to the nurse and for sending the health care provider a large gift basket?** The nurse is using a therapeutic communication technique called refocusing. Brad has digressed from the topic and is now trying to make the nurse feel ingratiated to him (i.e., to make her feel indebted to him for taking her to his special vacation home in the future). Having the nurse in his debt makes asking for and getting special favors and a bending of the rules more likely to happen. Brad is probably sending the health care provider a large gift basket for the same reason. It could also be possible that he is trying to start a personal relationship with the nurse. The nurse needs to refocus the client to keep the client on task, avoid becoming ingratiated to him, and avoid a social relationship with the client.

2. **What are the criteria for a diagnosis of Narcissistic Personality Disorder (NPD), and which criteria does Brad seem to meet?** There are nine criteria associated with a diagnosis of Narcissistic Personality Disorder (APA, 2000). A person must have five or more of the nine for a diagnosis of NPD. A person can have traits of NPD and not meet the diagnosis when less than five of the criteria are met.

   The first criterion is the presentation of a grandiose sense of self-importance. The person with this diagnosis may exaggerate talents and achievements. Brad presents with what appears to be a sense of self-importance. The staff nurse and later the nurse therapist will have to assess further to get a sense of whether Brad exaggerates his talents and achievements.

   The second criterion involves "preoccupation with fantasies of unlimited success, power, brilliance, beauty, or ideal love." Brad has fantasies about ideal love with a women he is having an extramarital affair with, and he has fantasies about being just as or more powerful as the people with whom he associates.

   The third criterion is a belief of being "special," or unique and of being understood by or needing to associate with other special or high-status persons or places. Brad is working hard to associate with special or high-status persons. He takes this type of person to his vacation home, which is seen by Brad as a place of high status. He takes them to exclusive and expensive restaurants and often picks up the bill.

   The forth criterion involves requiring excessive admiration. The staff nurse and the nurse therapist will probably find that Brad does need to be admired.

   A sense of entitlement is the fifth criterion. Brad definitely seems to feel entitled to special treatment in all settings. He is entitled to the best seat, the best food, and a shorter waiting time even though others have waited longer.

   The sixth criterion is being interpersonally exploitative, in other words, taking advantage of others to get his own needs met. As the nurse therapist assesses Brad on this behavior, she may find Brad taking advantage of his wife and mistress to get his needs met. He may be interpersonally exploitative when he sends a gift basket to the health care provider's home. He may expect special treatment in return for favors.

   The seventh criterion is a lack of empathy. Brad's wife has accused him of not being empathetic to her health needs or her needs in general. The nurse and the therapist will further assess this dimension of Brad's behavior.

   Envy of others or believing that others are envious of him or her is the eighth criterion. Brad may believe others are envious of his status and belongings, and he could even set up some envy by bragging. He may also be envious of others. The nurse will need to further assess this area.

   The ninth and last criterion is showing arrogance and haughty behaviors or attitudes. You will note that he appeared at the clinic giving the impression of being haughty and arrogant while checking out the credentials of the staff (Adapted from APA, 2000).

   The *Diagnostic and Statistical Manual* (APA, 2000) points out that many successful persons have narcissistic personality traits, and that only when the traits are inflexible, maladaptive, and persistent and cause significant impairment in functioning or subjective distress is the person considered for a diagnosis of Narcissistic Personality Disorder.

3. Most persons with a diagnosis of Narcissistic Personality Disorder are of what gender? How often are persons diagnosed with Narcissistic Personality Disorder hospitalized specifically for treatment of this disorder? Males make up 50–75 percent of persons diagnosed with NPD. People with this diagnosis are rarely, if ever, hospitalized to deal with problems associated solely with a diagnosis of Narcissistic Personality Disorder. Samples of outpatient psychiatric populations find that clients with NPD make up less than 1 percent of this population (Links and Stockwell, 2002). They come into treatment usually when the spouse or significant other has difficulty with their behavior and brings them into therapy, or when the threat of losing the spouse or significant other causes the person with NPD distress and this distress brings them to seek help.

4. Describe Kohut's and/or Kernberg's theory of causation of Narcissistic Personality Disorder. Heinz Kohut first used the term "narcissistic personality disorder" in the literature in 1968. Kohut theorized that the self is polar with one pole in early life involving the self as confident self-superiority with immature grandiosity that can evolve into forms of ambitiousness in adulthood. The opposing pole is associated with the tendency to admire and even idealize the superiorities of others, and this pole may evolve into an internalized system of ideals. In NPD, Kohut saw the development of healthy self-esteem being arrested. Kohut and others have looked at nurturing parenting as essential to transforming childhood narcissism into healthy ambition and ideals. Lack of consistent parental nurturing has been proposed as a possible contributor to the development of narcissistic traits (Watson and Hickman, 1995). Otto Kernberg wrote about narcissistic personality as a defense mechanism, seeing the narcissistic person as having been left with emotional needs unmet by a cold, unempathic mother. He saw the child feeling bad and unloved defending himself by narcissism and thus being unable or less able to love others, having a lack of empathy and a feeling of emptiness and boredom, and needing to search for power and being overdependent on acclaim (Lachkar, 1992).

5. What possible motivation is behind Brad calling Mary to meet him at a moment's notice? How would you feel and what would you need if you were Mary? Brad's motivation in calling Mary and expecting her to drop what she is doing and meet him immediately may be to get his immediate needs met without concern for her needs. A deeper, more subconscious need may be a need for power and autonomy. Control and self-importance may be served by getting Mary to drop everything and be where he dictates when he dictates.

A person in Mary's place may feel "used," "controlled," "like a servant," like a "doormat," and/or "unappreciated." At other times, she may like and appreciate associating with important people and doing things that she would not get to do otherwise, as a result of Brad's desire to be with important, special people and to be admired.

6. What would it feel like to be Brad? How would Brad and others with NPD likely react to changes associated with aging? Many nurses may have difficulty imagining what it would be like to be Brad. He puts his needs first, but nurses are taught to take care of others. If you were Brad, you would feel entitled to special treatment. The world revolves around you and the special people you associate with. You would feel important. Yet there is something vulnerable about being Brad. Underneath all this bravado, you may feel insecure, not worthy enough, and there may be a sense of not being loved enough, a fear of abandonment and a fear of anything that threatens your being important and others admiring you.

You fear illness and dying. Adjusting to the physical and occupational limitations associated with aging may prove difficult and distressing to the person with NPD (APA, 2000).

You fear losing your social status, and you must take great risks to get what you want. If you are not a risk taker, it may be hard for you to put yourself into Brad's place and feel what he would feel.

7. What will the nurse therapist most likely need to do to keep Brad engaged in couples therapy? Would there be any advantages to the nurse therapist bringing in a second therapist or cotherapist to work with this couple? What does Brad need to gain from therapy? To keep Brad engaged, he would have to feel like his needs are getting met. He will likely have a low tolerance for other people getting their needs met first, especially early in therapy. Links and Stockwell (2002) describe work with a couple similar to Brad and Mary in which the cotherapists and the wife agreed to the husband getting his concerns and needs addressed first in therapy sessions in order to keep him working in therapy.

The nurse therapist may bring in a second therapist to participate in the therapy work with this couple. One advantage of the nurse bringing in a second therapist is that one therapist could focus primarily on Brad's needs while the other could focus on Mary's and the work could involve individual and/or couple's marital work. Marital therapy with this couple could prove challenging. Links and Stockwell (2002) pointed out that some couples, in which one person has narcissistic traits or NPD, benefit from couples therapy while others may do better in individual therapy. Having his own therapist would facilitate Brad working on his own issues and lessen any attempts to manage Mary's issues or dominate her in sessions. Having a separate or cotherapist would provide additional and different insight into the dynamics of this particular relationship. The two therapists processing after sessions can lessen the chance of the therapists' own issues impeding progress and can facilitate therapeutic use of transference or counter-transference in future sessions as well as facilitate other strategies to help Brad and Mary develop some healthy behaviors individually and as a couple.

To save his marriage, Brad will need to learn to listen to Mary as she communicates her needs and gradually learn to meet more of her needs in addition to meeting his own needs. There may be areas in which he can meet her needs first and then his own. One of her needs will most likely be for Brad to give up his extramarital affair and to find some way to get his need for intimacy met by Mary. Brad also will need to learn to accept and nurture Mary's need to be more assertive and to have clearer boundaries. Brad needs work to improve his self-esteem and feel secure about his own actual accomplishments rather than relying on associations with important or special people to prove he is worthwhile. His fear of aging will need work. The psychiatric nurse therapist can look at where he is in terms of Erickson's developmental tasks (integrity versus despair) and do some work to help Brad accomplish what he needs to accomplish.

8. **What will the therapist most likely need to do to help Mary get her needs met in this relationship?** Mary most likely needs work on learning how to express her own needs to Brad. She may need work on setting boundaries, being assertive, and improving her self-esteem. Mary needs to set some goals for herself and to set some goals with Brad for the relationship. At the same time, if Mary wants to preserve the relationship, she will need to help Brad feel power and autonomy while in the relationship. Campbell, Foster, and Finkel (2002) conducted five studies investigating links among narcissism, self-esteem, and love. In all studies "narcissism was associated primarily with a game playing love style," which was "the result of a need for power and autonomy." Narcissism is also "linked with lesser commitment." It is more in keeping with the narcissistic personality to idealize a fantasized love at a distance than one at hand.

9. **How does the staff nurse need to respond to Brad's statement: "I would love to know what my wife told you about me"?** Brad may try to manipulate the nurse into revealing something his wife said in confidence. He probably feels entitled to know. The nurse therapist needs to emphasize that whatever he says in individual sessions is confidential and whatever his wife says in individual sessions is also confidential. The nurse must be careful not to reveal a confidence. She can say also something like: "I really need to hear more about you from you," which conveys that the nurse recognizes the importance of what he has to say. If Brad needs to know something that Mary said in confidence to the nurse therapist, the nurse therapist will work with Mary to see if Mary is willing to tell Brad and how best to tell Brad. The revealing will be done by Mary or at the very least with Mary present and giving verbal consent. This also holds true for Mary learning something that Brad has said in confidence.

10. **If you were a nurse in a health care provider's office or on a medical unit in the hospital and your assessment of a client revealed some narcissistic personality traits, would you plan your care differently to work more effectively with this client, and if so, how?** If you encountered someone with NPD or some of the personality traits of NPD, you would keep in mind that this person does need to feel special and does need to have their needs met and is not really willing to wait until others get their needs met first. If the client is demanding, you may feel some passive-aggressive need to ignore him or make him wait even longer than his turn, but this tactic usually does not work well. The client could leave and/or write complaints about you and the service. A better tactic would be to tell this person that it is important to you and/or the health care team to

take care of his needs; however, you have some rules that you must follow and outline these rules briefly. You might meet some other need of the client within the rules if his demands present a break with the rules. If he feels his needs are being met and/or that he is admired or special, he may stop demanding. You might give him a few minutes of conversation on a topic he is interested in, something to drink, or something to read to help pass the time while he is waiting. You might want to compliment him on his attire or some area with little room for misinterpretation. Convey that he will get taken care of and that this is important to you.

References

American Psychiatric Association. (2000). *Diagnostic and Statistical Manual of Mental Disorders, 4th ed.* Text Revision. Washington, DC: American Psychiatric Association.

Campbell, W.K., C.A. Foster, and E.J. Finkel. (2002). "Does Self Love Lead to Love for Others?: A Story of Narcissistic Game Playing." *Journal of Personality and Social Psychology* 83(2): 340–354.

Lachkar, J. (1992). *The Narcissistic/Borderline Couple: A Psychoanalytic Perspective on Marital Treatment.* New York: Brunner/Mazel.

Links, P.S. and M. Stockwell. (2002). "The Role of Couple Therapy in the Treatment of Narcissistic Personality Disorder." *American Journal of Psychotherapy* 56(4): 522–533.

Watson, P.J. and S.E. Hickman. (1995). "Narcissism, Self-Esteem and Parental Nurturance." *Journal of Psychology* 192(1): 61–73.

CASE STUDY 5

Leah

GENDER

Female

AGE

22

SETTING

- University health center

ETHNICITY

- White American

CULTURAL CONSIDERATIONS

- Sorority house culture

PRE-EXISTING CONDITION

CO-EXISTING CONDITION

COMMUNICATION

DISABILITY

SOCIOECONOMIC

- Affluent

SPIRITUAL/RELIGIOUS

PHARMACOLOGIC

PSYCHOSOCIAL

LEGAL

- Providing female nurse presence during physical examination of female client by male health care provider to avoid a false claim of sexual misconduct.

ETHICAL

- Protecting female client from misconduct by male physician during physical examination.

ALTERNATIVE THERAPY

PRIORITIZATION

- Nurse decision to accept phone call versus remaining present during physical examination.

DELEGATION

- Male nurse delegates assisting male health care provider with physical exam to female nurse peer.

HISTRIONIC PERSONALITY DISORDER

Level of difficulty: Easy

Overview: Requires understanding of Histrionic Personality Disorder (HPD). Requires critical thinking to avoid legal ramifications for the professional staff, especially for the male health care provider and male nurse. The nurse must also identify effective techniques for working with the client with HPD.

Client Profile

Leah is a 22-year-old female college student who has always seemed to be the center of attention in her family, in school, and in her peer group. Although Leah's sister has many material things from their affluent family, she can't seem to get any attention from their parents. When Leah enters a room, it is with great dramatic flair. She spends a great deal of energy, time, and money on her appearance and dresses seductively. Leah has been known to fish for compliments. She is flirtatious and sometimes insinuates that she is intimate or close to important males when there is not a close relationship at all. Leah appears uncomfortable when she is not the center of attention and goes to great lengths to regain status. Leah says things like "He is such a difficult person." She gives no details and leaves the recipient of this statement wondering what she meant. Leah frequently goes through a variety of emotions rather quickly.

Case Study

Leah comes to the student health center seeking care for the "very worst cold" she has ever had. She tells the male nurse that it may be pneumonia or worse. She wonders if she should get an important close friend to fly her to Florida in his private plane. She says she feels like she will die if she does not get some sun. Later Leah mentions she might need to go to the Mayo Clinic and see the chief of the medical staff who is a close friend of her father's.

The male nurse asks the health care provider to wait a few minutes before the physical examination on Leah. He asks a female nurse peer to assist the male health care provider. The female nurse is with the health care provider when he examines Leah. The nurse thinks Leah is engaging in seductive behavior around the health care provider. Leah suggests she might need the health care provider to make a house call. Leah has obviously spent a lot of time grooming for the occasion but says to the health care provider. "I am so sick. I must look awful. Do you think I look dreadful?" The female nurse receives a message that she has an urgent telephone call, and she wonders if she can leave the examining room. The health care provider is almost finished with the examination and ready to tell Leah to get dressed.

Before Leah leaves the clinic, she dramatically approaches the male nurse saying that she is horribly depressed and maybe that is why she got a cold. Her boyfriend broke up with her and she is "just devastated." She then says: "Maybe, darling, you would be willing to make a house call to my sorority house?" The nurse responds: "I would be glad to sit and talk with you for a few minutes here at the clinic." Leah responds: "Oh well, if you don't make house calls, perhaps you would take me to the football game. I think you could make me feel much better."

Leah goes to the football game with a friend and tells the friend that "Bill" the health care provider at the clinic wanted to take her to the game, but he had to work. She suddenly yells out a girl's name and runs down the steps in the middle of the ballgame, struggles across a row of people, and hugs a girl in the middle of the row. Leah then turns to the crowd during a play that most people are trying to watch and yells out dramatically, "This is my old roommate and I haven't seen her for a month."

Questions and Suggested Answers

1. **What personality trait of a person with a diagnosis of Histrionic Personality Disorder (HPD) is usually most noticeable? Which of Leah's behaviors make you suspect she has this personality trait?** Probably the most noticeable trait of HPD is the constant seeking of attention through a variety of means and the lack of comfort in situations in which the person with HPD fails to be at the center of attention. Leah became the center of attention at the clinic by saying she was going to faint. Even during the ball game, she managed to be the center of attention.

2. **Could Leah or anyone else have personality traits of Histrionic Personality Disorder and not have the disorder itself? If yes, what behaviors would Leah have to have to get this diagnosis and does she have these behaviors?** Sometimes student nurses and others read the criteria for the various psychiatric disorders described in the current American Psychiatric Association *Diagnostic and Statistical Manual of Mental Disorders* and begin to think they have several of the diagnoses they are reading about. The reality is that all of us have some personality traits that can be found in some mental disorders, but most of us don't have a disorder. Leah or anyone else could have some personality traits of Histrionic Personality Disorder and not have the disorder itself. In order to be diagnosed with Histrionic Personality Disorder, a person has to have five of eight specific behaviors. In addition to being uncomfortable when not the center of attention, which we already discussed, the other seven behaviors are: lack of comfort when in situations that do not provide a center of attention experience; frequent, inappropriate sexually seductive or provocative behavior; shifting and shallow emotional display; drawing attention to self through physical appearance; impressionistic speech style with content lacking in detail; suggestible or easily influenced; and views relationships with others as more intimate than they are (APA, 2000).

You will recall that the female nurse thought that Leah acted seductively with the health care provider. She also said some things that could be considered sexually seductive to the male nurse.

In regard to shifting and shallow emotional display, Leah went from being devastated at her boyfriend leaving her to smiling and trying to get the male nurse to come to her sorority house or take her to the ball game.

We don't have any evidence of her being suggestible or easily influenced. The client with Histrionic Personality Disorder who is suggestible and easily influenced is gullible and overly trusting. They frequently follow the latest trends and beliefs with little evidence.

Leah does give us clues that she believes her relationships are more intimate than they are. Her dear friend could fly her to Florida. Her father's friend is an important health care provider at an important hospital. She says the health clinic care provider wanted to take her to the ball game and calls him by his first name.

There are very good clues that Leah's behavior would match most of the criteria for a diagnosis of Histrionic Personality Disorder; however, only when the traits are "inflexible, maladaptive, and persisting, and cause significant functional impairment or subjective distress do they constitute Histrionic Personality Disorder" (APA, 2000). She won't get diagnosed with this disorder unless her personality traits cause her enough distress to seek out professional counseling.

3. **Why did the male nurse delegate the task of assisting the health care provider with the physical examination to a female nurse? If you were the female nurse in the examining room with the health care provider while he examined Leah, what would you do if someone came and told you that you had an urgent telephone call? Give a rationale for your decision.** Female clients can, and do on occasion, accuse health care providers of improper touching or sexual acts. If it is only the health care provider and client in the room, it is his word against hers. Having a female nurse in the examination room with the male health care provider and client protects the health care provider against false charges and usually makes the client more comfortable.

Telephone emergencies are seldom life and death if not answered within one minute. The female nurse needs to stay in the room with the health care provider and client unless another female nurse can relieve her. The nurse can ask that a message be taken and even relayed back to her. The health care provider needs a female nurse in the examining room with him to verify that nothing improper or unprofessional happened between the health care provider and the female client. Since Leah is attractive as well as engaging in seductive behavior and possibly easily led, a health care provider could behave in a sexually inappropriate manner with the client. The nurse's presence in the examining room assures that the client is protected against improper sexual contact and that the health care provider is protected in case of a false legal claim.

4. **Did the male nurse respond appropriately when Leah suggested he make a house call? Why or why not?** The male nurse responded appropriately when he offered to sit with Leah for a few minutes at the clinic and talk with her. This is within the range of professional behavior. Visiting Leah at her sorority house is not likely within his job description nor is it professional to make a social call.

5. **If you were the male nurse, how would you have responded when Leah asked you to take her to the football game?** One option would be to say something like: "Leah, you are a client at the clinic and I am a professional nurse. It is not professional to date clients. I can help you with your health problems here at the clinic, but I cannot take you to the football game."

6. **Based on your limited knowledge of Leah's behavior, what nursing diagnoses do you suppose would most likely apply in her case?** Nursing diagnoses include:

   • Impaired social interaction
   • Ineffective coping

   Long (1990) points out that people with histrionic personalities have their self-esteem "heavily centered in perceptions of their body image." Physical attractiveness is so important that it is conceivable that an illness might bring a diagnosis of situational low self-esteem related to a particular illness or a diagnosis of disturbed body image.

7. **What nursing interactions might be of help to Leah?** Setting limits and boundaries have already been discussed above. The nurse should display empathy and maintain a matter-of-fact, nonjudgmental approach at all times. If the client makes a provocative statement, the nurse can confront the client by saying something like: "That statement seems provocative. I want you to tell me what you mean; explain it to me." The nurse can also confront the client about familiarity and ask the client not to refer to him or her by terms of endearment such as "sweetie" or "darling."

   The nurse can use some techniques of behavior modification. The nurse will realize the client needs attention and can give positive feedback and attention for anything the client does that is appropriate and can ignore some of the behaviors that need to be diminished.

8. **What treatment interventions are currently being used in the treatment of Histrionic Personality Disorder?** While little is written in the current literature about the treatment of Histrionic Personality Disorder, it is evident that medication is not usually used for these clients, as they have no symptoms that medication will target. The main treatment is individual psychotherapy. The lack of insight and dependency needs of persons with HPD was addressed by Bornstein (1998) in a comparison of dependency needs in persons with Dependent Personality Disorder and persons with Histrionic Personality Disorder. Bornstein found that those with HPD had less insight than those with Dependent Personality Disorder. While some clients with HPD may need and receive longer, insight-oriented psychotherapy, others will respond to periodic brief psychotherapy. Brief therapy may include training in problem solving and education on how to develop a meaningful relationship. Nurses can model and teach problem-solving and interpersonal skills.

   The therapist may help the client find ways to tap into talent and to achieve satisfaction in ways other than being the center of attention. Long (1990) pointed out that clients with HPD may not be aware of their own feelings and may need help in clarifying their inner feelings as part of the therapeutic process. He cautioned the therapist not to reward "sham" emotion (Leah and her feeling devastated one moment and happy the next). Long also mentions "Patients of both sexes may attempt to draw the physician into a rescuing, admiring role in order to ward off anxiety associated with the threat to self-esteem that is posed by the illness" (Leah trying to get a compliment out of the health care provider by saying; "I am so sick. I must look awful. Do you think I look dreadful?"). Long cautions the health care provider to provide as much emotional support and interest as possible to reduce the client's anxiety but to avoid a close personal relationship or "fostering magical expectations of a cure." He tells the health care provider to adopt a kind, objective stance and to provide clear explanations of the disorder and plans for treatment, as this fosters trust and counteracts any denial of illness on the part of the client. This advice can well apply to the nurse.

   Lively (2005) does not address HPD specifically, but for all personality disorders he stresses a collaborative relationship between the professional person and the client. Lively states: "The most important stance for treating personality disorder is to provide support, empathy, and validation (for the client)."

Group therapy can also be beneficial to the person with Histrionic Personality Disorder as it presents an opportunity for peers to give feedback and the client with HPD to get feedback in a supportive climate. Group therapy could present a challenge in getting the histrionic client to stay out of the center of attention and let others talk. Sometimes this is done by going around the circle of clients and having each one tell or ask something. The nurse can use this technique when working with a group that includes a client who has HPD or HPD traits (e.g., in any education group provided by the nurse).

9. **Do clients with Histrionic Personality Disorder get better?** Most references talk about personality traits being deeply engrained and difficult to change. Lively (2005) reiterates the difficulty in working with clients with personality disorders but says they can and do get better over time. Long (1990) alludes to clients with HPD getting better. Seivewright, Tyrer, and Johnson (2002) report on a study they did of 202 clients who had a neurotic disorder, dysthymia, panic disorder, or generalized anxiety. (When the study began, the diagnostic and statistical manual was DSM III, which included neuroses. Histrionic fell under neurosis. Later editions of the DSM did not use the term "neuroses.") When the study ended twelve years later, the researchers found that of all groups studied, antisocial and histrionic personality disorders were the ones to show improvement. The author's conclusion was that, contrary to popular assumptions, those personality characteristics actually do change with time.

10. **What causes Histrionic Personality Disorder?** The cause is currently unknown and may be due, like many other psychiatric disorders, to a variety of factors, which could include a biochemical imbalance as well as environmental factors. Little research, if any, is being done currently to find the cause. Gunderson (1988) described one theory of causation in which the child has had his or her feelings negated by his or her mother and as a result of this, he or she then turns to the father for nurturance. The child finds the father responding better to his or her need for nurturance when he or she uses dramatic emotional behaviors. Since dramatic emotional behaviors get him or her what he or she wants, the behaviors are repeated whenever he or she feels the need for nurturance.

References

American Psychiatric Association. (2000). *Diagnostic and Statistical Manual of Mental Disorders, 4th ed.* Text Revision. Washington, DC: American Psychiatric Association.

Bornstein, R.F. (1998). "Implicit and Serf-Attributed Dependency Needs in Dependent and Histrionic Personality Disorders." *Journal of Personality Assessment* 71(1): 1–14.

Gunderson, J.G. (1988). "Personality Disorder." In *The New Harvard Guide to Psychiatry*, ed. A. Nicholi. Cambridge, MA: The Bellnap Press.

Lively, W.J. (2005). "Principles and Strategies for Treating Personality Disorders." *Canadian Journal of Psychiatry* 50(8): 442–451.

Long, P.W. (1990). "Histrionic Personality Disorder." www.mentalhealth.com. Accessed November 3, 2003.

Seivewright, H., P. Tyrer, and T. Johnson. (2002). "Change in Personality Status in Neurotic Disorders." *Lancet* 359(9325): 2253–2254.

GENDER

Male

AGE

36

SETTING

- Emergency room

ETHNICITY

- White American

CULTURAL CONSIDERATIONS

PREEXISTING CONDITION

COEXISTING CONDITION

- Fractured arm

COMMUNICATION

DISABILITY

SOCIOECONOMIC

- Low-paid, white-collar government worker with good health benefits

SPIRITUAL/RELIGIOUS

- Is not a "joiner"
- Prefers to worship alone

PHARMACOLOGIC

PSYCHOSOCIAL

LEGAL

ETHICAL

- Nurse's spouse has relationship with client
- Nurse has potential for dual relationship with client
- Strict confidentiality vs. selective breach to nurse's spouse

ALTERNATIVE THERAPY

PRIORITIZATION

DELEGATION

SCHIZOID PERSONALITY DISORDER

Level of difficulty: High

Overview: Requires critical thinking to assure confidentiality in a situation in which the nurse and the nurse's spouse each have a professional relationship with the client and the nurse has potential for a dual relationship. Requires critical thinking in determining effective means of communicating with a client who prefers to be alone and does not enjoy interacting with others.

DIFFICULT

Client Profile

Howard is a 36-year-old male who was raised by his father after his mother died when he was 6 months old. The father was absent a lot from Howard's life due to his work and dating the same woman for twenty years before he suddenly died. Howard only met the father's girlfriend a handful of times and was raised by a strict grandmother. Howard stayed away from grandmother as much as he could so he would not be punished.

As Howard grew up, he became fascinated with computers and now calls himself a computer "geek." He works in a remote office inputting computer data and doing research for a state agency. He keeps track of the milk production of cows by county throughout the state. The pay is fairly low, but he does not have to go to meetings or interface with anyone except for meeting twice each month with his supervisor. Howard's work earned an award in his state agency, but he would not go to the dinner to accept the award. His supervisor picked the award up for him.

Howard is described by others as pretty much a "loner": living alone, never trying to make friends, and never joining any group. He does not attend a church, preferring to read the bible and pray alone. A first cousin and childhood playmate of Howard recalls that Howard has stayed away from family activities ever since he was old enough not to require a babysitter. Once in awhile the cousin goes to visit him, but Howard never initiates a visit to the cousin. The cousin recalls that Howard's facial expression has always been somewhat flat, and as a child he did not mimic her when she would smile or make faces. The cousin has never noticed any behavior that would indicate Howard is interested sexually in women or perhaps men. A neighbor once tried to start a relationship, but she noticed that Howard became anxious whenever she came near him and he was somewhat cold and aloof.

Case Study

Howard has been brought to the emergency room by EMS. The emergency medical technician (EMT) reports that Howard had apparently been riding his bicycle to work when the driver of a car, claiming to have been blinded by the sun, hit him. The EMT further reports that Howard wanted to go home when he talked with the policeman on the scene, but finally agreed to come to the ER to get checked out for injuries.

When the ER receptionist asks Howard if she can call any of his family or a friend for him or if he would like to call them, he responds: "No." He hides behind a book in the corner of the ER until the x-ray technician comes to x-ray his arm, which he has said hurts and has some pins-and-needles-like feeling.

When the health care provider views the x-ray, it is clear that the ulna is broken. The provider shares with the emergency room nurse that he wants to reset the broken bone, cast the arm, and keep Howard overnight. The nurse goes to tell Howard what the provider plans to do.

After surgery, Howard is taken to his room. It is late in the evening shift when he arrives at his room. When the nurse gets her assignments and receives report, she goes to do the initial assessment on Howard and finds him wide awake. She introduces herself. Howard says: "That is an interesting and unusual last name. My supervisor at work must be related to you. His name is Mark." The night nurse realizes that Howard's supervisor is her husband and that she may see Howard in the future when she attends activities at her husband's workplace.

Questions and Suggested Answers

1. **Does Howard demonstrate traits of Schizoid Personality Disorder (SZPD), and if so, what traits?** The person with this disorder will have a strong pattern of lack of attachment with others and their emotional expression will be limited starting in early childhood. They will exhibit four of seven traits:

   - Not wanting or enjoying close relationships, which includes family relationships
   - Nearly always selecting activities that can be done alone
   - Having little or no interest in sexual activities with another person

- Finding few activities, if any, that provide pleasure
- Having no close friends or people to confide in other than first-degree relatives
- Seeming to be uncaring about the praise or criticism of others
- Showing emotional coolness, flattened affect, or inability to attach to others (Adapted from APA, 2000; www.mentalhealth.com/)

Howard exhibits many of these traits. You will recall that he has not wanted to be with his family since he was old enough not to need a babysitter. He is in the hospital after an accident but does not initiate calls to his cousin or anyone else. Howard has chosen to work on computers and works alone, and there is no evidence of anything that gives him pleasure. We have no evidence that he selects any activities done with someone else. He has no close friends. There is no evidence that he has ever had an interest in sexual activities, and he was anxious around the neighbor who wanted to start a relationship.

He did not pick up his award. This may have been because he is not interested in praise or he could have not wanted to be around people. While many of these areas could be assessed more, on what information we have, Howard looks like he has many of the traits of a Schizoid Personality Disorder.

2. **Can a person described as a "loner" with all or most of the traits of Schizoid Personality Disorder still not meet all the requirements for a diagnosis of SZPD? If so, what additional requirement has to be met?** Yes, it is possible that a person can have all the traits of Schizoid Personality Disorder and not meet the requirements for a diagnosis, because to be given this diagnosis the traits must be "inflexible and maladaptive and cause significant functional impairment or subjective distress" (APA, 2000). Clients with four or more of the traits required for diagnosis of SZPD rarely seek psychiatric help as they adjust their life around their traits and do not often exhibit functional impairment or subjective distress. If the client with traits of SZPD presents with another problem such as Howard has, the professional staff may be able to piece together enough history to warrant a diagnosis of Schizoid Personality Disorder.

3. **Looking at Howard's behaviors, what makes you more certain they are those associated with SZPD and not those of Avoidant Personality Disorder?** If he had Avoidant Personality Disorder or simply a number of traits from this disorder, then Howard would avoid social contact due to fear of being rejected, being embarrassed, or just not measuring up to expectations of others in some way. Howard's behavior more closely matches the detachment associated with lessened and limited desire for intimacy with others.

4. **If you were the female nurse going to tell Howard about the health care provider's plans to set his arm and cast it and keep him overnight, what would you keep in mind as you plan your approach? What would you say to this client, and how would you say it?** You need to keep in mind that Howard is anxious just being around anyone and possibly more so around females. He will no doubt be even more anxious if you make any remarks that could be taken as seductive or intrusive into his personal life. You must strive to come across as professional and talk to him very straightforwardly about his medical needs and what the doctor has in mind. Use concrete, simple language rather than abstract terms, so the chances of any misinterpretation of your communication are minimized. You should avoid any gestures or facial expressions as well as words that could come across as flirting or seductive in any way. Any touch must be strictly professional, necessary, and the client must be warned before the touch. You should realize that dress is a means of communication too, and you should be dressed professionally and similarly to other nurses in the ER. Schools of nursing have dress codes and nursing instructors are strict about how students dress for clinical experiences. One of the reasons is that certain types of clients, such as the elderly or a client with any psychiatric disorder and this disorder in particular, don't respond well to female nurses in a uniform or street dress that is too short, too low-cut, or made of see-through material worn without undergarments. You should proceed with professional dress, professional expressions, and professional language.

5. **If you were the female nurse ready to do the initial assessment of this client and he discovered that you were the wife of his supervisor, what options would you have and which one would you select?** One option is to talk with the client, assuring him that he will receive professional nursing care from you and that everything will be kept strictly confidential and that his supervisor/your husband will not hear about him from you.

Once promised, you must keep your word. In fact it is never a good idea to share information about clients you care for with your family or others outside the workplace, as your breach of confidentiality can be discovered by the client when this information is passed from person to person. Another option is to tell the client that you were unaware your husband was his supervisor and you make it a practice not to care for anyone who has any ties to your husband or that you know in some other relationship and that you will have another very good nurse to care for him. In this case as in the first case, you would assure him that confidentiality would be kept.

A third option would be to leave the decision as to whether you care for this client or not up to your supervisor. Ward (2004) stresses that the client with Schizoid Personality Disorder has a "need for interpersonal distance" and the professional working with this client needs to "avoid overinvolvement in personal and social issues." Having a potential outside past and/or future involvement with you outside the professional role may be threatening to the client and/or may hinder development of a therapeutic relationship.

Licensed therapists are most often bound by their licensing rules not to engage in therapy with a client with whom they have another relationship. Nurse practice acts are usually less clear about situations like caring for one of your husband's employees or one of your former teachers or one of your current students if you teach nursing and work part-time at a hospital. It is often a wise move to excuse yourself from caring for these people with whom you have another relationship. For example, a nurse on the children's unit was reassigned to the adolescent unit when one of her neighbor's children was admitted. The mother later accused the nurse of spreading the word about her child's admission. The nurse denied this breach of confidence charge and stated the mother herself had told someone who had told someone else. When administration learned it was the nurse herself who asked to be reassigned to avoid caring for the child or knowing anything about the child's case, it was clear that the nurse had taken steps to avoid knowing information about the young client's condition and care, steps indicating the nurse planned to respect confidentiality. It also became clear that being reassigned was a great idea.

6. **What nursing diagnoses, in addition to acute pain and impaired skin integrity for his broken arm, would you write for this client in relation to traits of SZPD?** Some possible nursing diagnoses include:

   - Impaired social interaction
   - Deficient diversional activity

7. **How would you go about writing goals for this client, and what goals might you write if the client is to stay in the rehabilitation hospital for several days or weeks?** After assessing the client and identifying some strengths and interests, as well as some problems that translate to nursing diagnoses, you would likely ask the client what his goals are for hospitalization and try to come up with some goals that are attainable and measurable and pertain to his nursing diagnoses. If the client has no goals, you can suggest: "Perhaps you would like to learn one new diversional activity while you are here." The client may be interested in learning the guitar and now has time to do it. There may be a staff member who can teach him to play. You will recall one of the traits of SZPD is finding pleasure in few or no activities, so working on a new diversional activity is appropriate.

   Another appropriate nursing goal is that of building a trusting relationship with the client and getting the client to then build a relationship with a hospitalized peer. To successfully meet this goal, you will have to be exceedingly patient and start slowly with limited short contacts building to slightly longer contacts and gradually introducing contact with another person.

8. **What interventions might the nurse implement?** The nurse can teach the client a card game or have the client teach her one and then get the client to play the game with a hospitalized peer. The nurse in these instances does not sit close to the client but maintains a respectful distance and patiently and slowly tries to help the client take one step toward having an activity that brings joy or making one friend. Ingrained personality patterns can change, but it takes patience and usually a lot of time.

   The nurse needs adopt a respectful, somewhat distant professional stance to avoid causing anxiety in the client that could lead to further distancing.

9. **What are some theories of causation of Schizoid Personality Disorder?** McAllister (1999) states that "detachment is the chief defense for the schizoid individual." The schizoid individual has developed a long-standing expectation that relationships always lead to disappointment and it is not good to depend on others as they will always disappoint you. Detachment offers a feeling of safety for the client, and it derives from meeting his own needs. It is not too difficult to imagine that when the client in this case looked to others to meet his needs, he was disappointed time after time. His mother had died. His father was often gone with his girlfriend who did not have a relationship with the client. The grandmother had carried on the strict and stoic behavior of her parents and grandparents who came from Germany.

Blum (1997) did a study that he claimed was the first to support a strong association between a D2 receptor allele and schizoid avoidant behavior. He also found some weaker associations between schizoid avoidant behavior and a specific dopamine allele transporter. This study suggests that genetics, in addition to environment, could play a factor in the development of Schizoid Personality Disorder.

10. **What is the current treatment for Schizoid Personality Disorder?** The usual treatment is individual psychotherapy. If the client has a talent involving art or music or any interest that can be developed and shared with others, the therapist might get the client to gradually share this in individual therapy and then with one other person and finally a small group of peers. Gradually increasing exposure to others is a form of behavior therapy, which is called systematic desensitization, and it can increase a client's confidence in a social environment (Wolff, 1999). The nurse can also use this technique. The therapist and/or nurse would encourage the client to start with activities involving very little socialization and move up to those requiring a little more socialization. Skills are gradually built, although the client will still prefer solitary activities. Some groups can be helpful to the client as a safe place to learn and practice socialization (e.g., art therapy group where clients work in the same space but interact less intensively than in psychotherapy groups). Clients with family ties could possibly be seen in family therapy, which can be helpful in some, but not all, cases.

References

American Psychiatric Association. (2000). *Diagnostic and Statistical Manual of Mental Disorders, 4th ed.* Text Revision. Washington, DC: American Psychiatric Association.

Blum, K. (1997). "The Dopaminergic System and in Particular Dopamine D2 Receptor Implicated in Reward Mechanisms." *Molecular Psychiatry* 2(3): 239–246.

McAllister, M.J. (1999). "Mohawks and Combat Boots: The Schizoid Dilemma of Punks." *Bulletin of the Menninger Clinic* 63(1): 89–102.

Ward, R.K. (2004). "Assessment and Management of Personality Disorders." *American Family Physician* 70(8): 1505–1517.

Wolff, S. (1999). *Loners: The Life Path of Unusual Children.* New York: Routledge Press.

www.mentalhealth.com. Accessed October 21, 2005.

Stan

GENDER

Male

AGE

32

SETTING

- Outpatient mental health center clinic

ETHNICITY

- Black/White American

CULTURAL CONSIDERATIONS

- White American father, Black American mother

PREEXISTING CONDITION

COEXISTING CONDITION

- Hypertension

COMMUNICATION

DISABILITY

SOCIOECONOMIC

SPIRITUAL/RELIGIOUS

PHARMACOLOGIC

- Captopril in combination with hydrochlorthiazide (Capozide)
- Lorazepam (Ativan)
- Olanzapine (Zyprexa)

PSYCHOSOCIAL

- Paranoia limits and distorts interactions with others

LEGAL

ETHICAL

ALTERNATIVE THERAPY

- Over-the-counter vitamins, minerals, and enzymes

PRIORITIZATION

DELEGATION

PARANOID PERSONALITY DISORDER

Level of difficulty: High

Overview: Requires critical thinking and decision making in regard to who is going to be most effective in interacting with the client when the client's paranoia worsens. The nurse is required to work collaboratively with other team members and to provide supervision for the client's nonnurse case manager who works with the client in his independent living situation. The nurse is required to work with physical problems as well as mental health problems and to look at possible connections between psychological and medical problems and the medications used to treat them.

DIFFICULT

Client Profile

Stan is a 32-year-old single male. Stan lives alone in a government-subsidized apartment and receives social security disability income (SSDI). He says he stays away from his neighbors, as they are not to be trusted and could turn against him for no reason at all if he were to let them into his apartment.

Stan holds grudges against his mother and has not attempted to contact her for a couple of years. He talks about his mother trying to control his mind and his life and working against him to get him into treatment when he did not want or need it. He carries a grudge over his mother not giving him a birthday party ten years ago when his brother got a party: "Not that I wanted one, but it just was not fair of my mom to do that." Stan is also angry at his mother for giving him a White American father so Black American peers did not accept him and for her being Black American and causing him not to be accepted by White American peers when he was growing up. He was married briefly to Yvonne, a Black American woman he met in group therapy. He was extremely jealous of Yvonne talking to other people and thought she was unfaithful when he heard her talking to a "Bobby" on the phone. Bobbie was a girl his wife had met when she was an inpatient in the psychiatric hospital. This prompted him to follow his wife everywhere she went and to try to keep her home whenever he could to prevent her from meeting this "other man." Stan was verbally hostile to his wife at times, thinking she was criticizing him when in fact she was complimenting him. Stan was jealous every time Yvonne went for psychiatric treatment. He thought she was "hogging all the therapy" (i.e., getting more than her share of psychiatric care).

Stan gets psychiatric care through the county outpatient mental health center clinic. He has a nonnurse case manager who takes vital signs, supervises him in taking his daily medication, helps him with managing his money, and transports him to appointments at the clinic where he sees a psychiatric mental health nurse for all his medication reviews and health assessments. He sees the psychiatrist only if the nurse refers him, and this usually happens only if he is experiencing a significant change in his mental health, has medical problems or problems with his medications, or needs to have additional medication prescribed. Stan currently has prescriptions for two medications: a pill for hypertension (captopril [Capozide 25/15]) and a multivitamin. His medicine cabinet is full of various kinds of vitamins, minerals, and enzymes.

Case Study

Stan reports in at the reception desk at the mental health center clinic. The nurse is walking out to call him into her office about the same time he notices two women talking across the waiting room. He calls out a derogatory name and tells them to stop talking about him. When he sees the nurse, he puts his hands on his hips in a threatening kind of stance and says: "You think you are so smart, but I know what you put in those pills. Don't think you fooled me. And don't put that in my chart." The nurse feels a great deal of energy coming from Stan and feeling threatened; she senses she needs to back away from him. The nurse says gently: "Please sit down and rest for just a few minutes. I'll have your caseworker sit with you, and in a little while when you are ready to talk she can come and get me."

The nurse alerts the psychiatrist that she is going to try to talk with Stan about his medication, but that if Stan is too paranoid, she may need the psychiatrist to discuss his medications with him. The nurse knows from working with Stan for a while and reading his chart that he has a diagnosis of Paranoid Personality Disorder.

When the psychiatrist sees Stan he notes that Stan's blood pressure is still elevated and that he is paranoid and somewhat psychotic. The psychiatrist continues the Capozide and vitamin and orders lorazepam (Ativan) and olanzapine (Zyprexa).

Questions and Suggested Answers

1. **How would you feel and what would you think if you were assigned to work with Stan or any client who has Paranoid Personality Disorder?** It is important to stop and think about your feelings and thoughts before actually attempting to work with clients with Paranoid Personality Disorder or any personality disorder. A client with this diagnosis presents an interesting challenge. Some nurses like this challenge and some do not,

preferring to see the client cured after a brief treatment or preferring to work in an area such as surgery where they do not have to dialogue with the client or the dialogue is limited. In the journal *Mental Health Practice* (Tyrer, 2002) a book by Len Bowers called *Dangerous and Severe Personality Disorders* is reviewed, and Bowers is quoted as saying that personality disorder patients have a "perverse view of society and create special problems in all settings and are generally seen as the people no one wants." In a research study in three high security hospitals in England, Bower found that many nurses did not like to work with clients with personality disorders, although there were some who did. Clients with personality disorder traits and even diagnosed disorders are found in all settings in health care. You need to take the time and effort to learn more about people with Paranoid Personality Disorder, and how to work with these clients more effectively, as you will likely find yourself assigned to someone with Paranoid Personality Disorder at some time in your career. Knowledge about this disorder can increase your enthusiasm for, as well as your ability to, work with people with this disorder or with traits of this disorder.

2. **If you were the nurse and Stan said to you: "You think you are so smart," and you felt threatened, what would you think is going on with Stan?** Stan is probably feeling threatened by the ladies talking and transfers this feeling to the nurse or maybe he feels threatened both by the ladies and the nurse. His threatening words, stance, and energy may be a way of frightening the nurse off as a means of self-protection. In other words, this seemingly threatening behavior on his part is an attempt to get people to back away. He is afraid of the nurse and what she might do to him and in a sense "hisses" at her, much like we see various animals doing to get others out of their territory. People who are paranoid sometimes say to others directly: "Get out of my face," which means others are too close for comfort.

3. **What concept or rationale did the nurse possibly have in mind when she alerted the psychiatrist that she might need to have him go over Stan's medications?** The nurse may have felt so threatened that her rationale was to maintain her own safety and to protect the client from the consequences of harming her; however, there is another good rationale for wanting Stan to talk with the psychiatrist instead of the nurse. Clients with Paranoid Personality Disorder, while appearing aggressive, often feel fear and insecurity inside. Akhtar (1990) points out that the "classical triad of symptoms associated with paranoid persons: suspiciousness, feeling persecuted, and grandiosity as well as their demanding, arrogant, mistrustful, unromantic, acutely vigilant outer behavior is a strong contrast to an inner frightened, self-doubting, timid, gullible, inconsiderate person who is unable to understand the totality of actual events." People with all this inner insecurity don't respond well to empathy or compassion. They tend to respond better to someone they recognize as being in a position of power. They may refuse to take direction from the nurse and docilely follow instructions from the health care provider (Akhtar, 1990).

4. **What behaviors does Stan have that match those of someone with Paranoid Personality Disorder?** Beginning by early adulthood, the person with Paranoid Personality Disorder (PPD) has a deep, pervasive lack of trust of others and views the motives of others as malevolent. The person exhibits four of seven listed behaviors:

Paranoid Personality Disorder Characteristics	Stan's Behavior
Thinks others may be out to deceive, do harm, or take advantage of him or her even though insufficient evidence for thinking so.	Accuses the nurse of altering his medication.
Has preoccupation with thoughts that friends or associates are disloyal or not trustworthy.	Thought his wife was disloyal and not trustworthy. He won't let any neighbors into his apartment because they are not trustworthy and could turn against him if he let them in. Either one of these thoughts could be based in reality or they could be part of his pathology. His mother is also thought to be disloyal and out to harm him by getting him into treatment that he thinks he does not need.

(Continued)

Paranoid Personality Disorder Characteristics	Stan's Behavior
Resists confiding in others due to unwarranted fear anything said could be used maliciously against him or her.	Does not want the nurse to chart something about him. He does not confide in the neighbors as they might turn against him.
Translates benign remarks or events into demeaning or threatening messages.	On various occasions, is reported to have taken his wife's compliments as criticisms.
Holds on to grudges (e.g., does not forgive perceived insults, injuries, or slights).	Perceives that his mother slighted him in giving his brother a birthday party one year and not giving him one, and he holds a grudge against her even though he admits he did not want a party. He won't speak to his mother because of this slight and because she caused him to be hospitalized at times for treatment.
Thinks people are attacking his or her character or reputation even when others don't think this and often reacts angrily or counterattacks quickly.	Thinks two women across the room are talking about him and reacts angrily.
Without proof, questions the fidelity of sexual partner or spouse.	Questioned his wife's fidelity. Thought she was having an affair with Bobby when Bobbie was a girl she was in group with.

(Adapted from APA, 2000)

The APA (2000) points out that individuals with PPD "may be pathologically jealous" with this jealousy associated with suspecting the spouse or sexual partner of infidelity. One of the diagnoses for patients admitted to state hospitals in the mid to late 1800s was "jealousy" and often involved a wife committed to the state hospital by her husband. Tyrer (1994) reports that on a random sample of 600 men and women in New Zealand, every one of the 351 subjects returning the questionnaire admitted to jealousy at some time. Many stated it was inappropriate, and half said it was without good cause. Behaviors described by respondents included searching a significant other's belongings looking for incriminating evidence, checking on the partner by phone, and showing up unexpectedly, hoping to catch the partner in some amorous liaison. Tyrer suggests that jealousy may be ubiquitous and that suspecting the spouse or partner of infidelity without cause may not be an effective discriminator of those who have the disorder and those who do not.

5. **Is Paranoid Personality Disorder apparent in childhood and adolescence, and if so, what behaviors would clue the family and/or clinicians that a child has this disorder?** Yes, PPD can be apparent in the early years of life with parents noticing some or all of the following in their child: appearing odd or eccentric and being teased for this, hypersensitivity, poor relationships with peers, even solitariness, social anxiety, and underachievement (APA, 2000). You can see that perhaps having odd behavior and being teased might lead to hypersensitivity unless mediated by a teacher or relative. These behaviors could lead to poor peer relationships, which could lead to solitariness. The question arises as to whether some of the behaviors might come out of structural and biochemical differences in the brain or as part of a response to a somewhat hostile environment. In this case, we need to note that the client's early poor relationships with peers, solitariness, social anxiety, and underachievement could have been partially or totally caused by his perception, or the reality, that others did not accept him since he was of a mixed race.

6. **Some of the behaviors that qualify a person for a diagnosis of Paranoid Personality Disorder seem similar to other personality disorders. How can a person differentiate between PPD and other personality disorders, especially Schizotypal Personality Disorder (SZPD)?** Paranoid Personality Disorder and Schizotypal Personality Disorder do share some common behaviors including "odd, "eccentric," or "strange" behaviors;

suspiciousness; distancing from interpersonal relationships; and paranoid ideations. What helps differentiates Schizotypal from PPD is that persons with SZPD will usually have magical thinking and unusual perceptual experiences. One group of researchers (Farmer et al., 2000), in an experiment comparing persons with SZPD to those without the disorder, put an advertisement in the newspaper for people who have telepathic minds or feel like people are around when they are not, which indicates that one major differentiating factor for SZPD is that people with this disorder believe they have telepathy, or a sixth sense, or are clairvoyant.

Persons with Schizoid Personality Disorder are not paranoid so this is one way Schizoid Personality Disorder is differentiated from Paranoid Personality and from Schizotypal as well.

Persons with PPD are different than those with Antisocial Personality Disorder (APD) in that they don't tend to exploit people for personal gain, though they sometimes act out of revenge. People with APD or traits of APD are not paranoid unless the paranoia comes from a different cause.

People can have traits of more than one personality disorder, but not meet the criteria for any one disorder. If the person has several traits of more than one personality disorder and if the personality traits cause the client sufficient distress or impairment in social, occupational, and/or other areas of functioning, then the client can be classified as having Personality Disorder Not Otherwise Specified.

7. **How does Paranoid Personality differ from Schizophrenia, Paranoid Type?** While persons with Schizophrenia, Paranoid Type as well as persons with PPD all have symptoms of distrust and suspiciousness, the person with Schizophrenia, Paranoid Type has periods of psychosis in which they often have persecutory hallucinations and delusions and are often potentially violent or act out paranoia through violence. Examples of the hallucinations of a person with Schizophrenia, Paranoid Type include hearing voices saying: "We are going to kill you" or "We are going to kidnap your wife," or seeing the devil or a thousand policemen on the lawn coming after the person.

Delusions might involve thoughts about some group plotting to harm or kill the client in some way. An example of a delusion would be thoughts that a group of outer space spies had taken over the kitchens of all restaurants with red in their signs so they could drug diners and take them to another planet.

The person with PPD may or may not have periods of brief psychosis under stress, but does not have elaborate delusions and long periods of hallucinatory behavior. The person with PPD tends to be verbally aggressive rather than physically aggressive like the person with Schizophrenia, Paranoid Type.

Another major difference between PPD and Schizophrenia, Paranoid Type is that the traits of PPD are noticed when the person is a child. Although the client with Schizophrenia can display symptoms as a child or teen, the behavior associated with Schizophrenia is usually not seen until young adulthood.

8. **What is the current treatment for Paranoid Personality Disorder?** Medications are not a first-line treatment and are not often prescribed for Paranoid Personality Disorder per se; however, if the client becomes agitated or anxious, an antianxiety medication may be given for short-term crisis management. If the client gets even more anxious and psychotic for a short period of time, an antipsychotic might be given on a short-term basis.

The *Psychology Today* website (www.psychologytoday.com/htdocs/prod/PTOInfo/ptotermparanoid .asp) provides the following information on medication for PPD: "Medications for paranoid personality disorder are generally not encouraged, as they may contribute to a heightened sense of suspicion that can ultimately lead to patient withdrawal from therapy. They are suggested, however, for the treatment of specific conditions of the disorder, such as severe anxiety or delusion, where these symptoms begin to impede normal functioning. Medications prescribed for precise conditions should be used for the briefest interval possible to successfully control them."

Group insight-oriented or group for support therapy would not initially be a treatment of choice since misinterpretation of group members' statements and suspiciousness of others in the group tends to make the client worse. The client might at some time be able to benefit from a small group in which he mainly worked alongside others but was still independent, such as in an art therapy group. He would probably be started in individual art therapy, then work with one peer and work up to a small group.

Individual therapy on a long-term basis can be helpful. It is difficult to engage clients with this diagnosis in a therapeutic relationship and even more difficult to maintain a therapeutic relationship. People with

Paranoid Personality Disorder tend not to initiate therapy, and they tend to want to terminate early. It is a challenge to keep them in therapy. Being insecure and fearful, these clients want reassurances but misinterpret reassurances. Since they respond better to people in power, the therapist needs to project confidence and manage control issues carefully. Much thought is given to the approach to use and what responses to use. One goal for therapy sessions would always be to establish and/or maintain trust. The nurse clinician therapist or any therapist working with this type of client needs to be well trained and would be well advised to have an expert peer providing supervision. Some psychotherapists who have done psychotherapy for years continue to pay another therapist to provide supervision. Nurses managing care of clients or doing therapy in agencies have an assigned supervisor who goes over the management of their caseload with them.

9. **What does the nurse need to know about the antihypertensive, antianxiety, and antipsychotic medications the client is on? Is there any connection between the client's race and taking one or more of these medications? What do these three medications have in common?** The risk of hypertension has been found to be higher in five groups of adults in the United States: men, Black Americans, Hispanics, people with less education, and older adults (CDC, 2002). The Black American male may have a genetic difference or lifestyle factors that could account for elevated blood pressure (systolic 140 or greater and diastolic 90 or greater). Some researchers are exploring the possibility that elevated hypertension among Black Americans is a result, or partially the result, of "social stress and in particular exposure to racism" (Stewart, 2002).

   Antipsychotics, antianxiety, and antihypertensive medications all have the ability to lower blood pressure. It is important for the case manager to check the blood pressure and pulse before supervising the client taking this medication. The nurse must instruct the case worker as to the parameters for withholding the medication and notifying the nurse. The nurse must periodically review the client's blood pressure readings and check the blood pressure. Blood pressure and pulse needs to be taken after the client is supine five minutes and then after arising for two minutes. This is a check for orthostatic hypotension, which is a possible side effect of the antipsychotic medication.

10. **What assessment would you want/need to do if you were the nurse in this case? Given the information you have on this client, what nursing diagnoses would you write?** You are assured the client is taking his prescribed medication as it is supervised by the case manager. What you don't know is whether he is taking any over-the-counter medications that might interact with his prescribed medication or be in excess of what he needs. You must ask the client specifically about over-the-counter medications, including herbs, vitamins, minerals, and enzymes. You must assess whether the client is taking any street drugs or drinking alcohol, as these could potentiate his prescribed medications or cause serious reactions.

    There are many other things you could assess, including if he has one or more persons he trusts such as the case manager, the strengths and limitations he has, his interests and any hobbies, his goals for himself, his ability to abstract, his short-term and long-term memory, health problems if any, and his religious practices, if any, as well as his spiritual needs.

    Possible nursing diagnoses for this client include but are not limited to:

    - Anxiety
    - Fear
    - Disturbed thought processes
    - Defensive coping
    - Social isolation
    - Chronic low self-esteem

11. **What goals would you write for this client? What interventions would be helpful?** Having at least one trusting relationship may be a short-term and two or more such relationships a long-term goal. Another long-term goal is for the client to state that he is comfortable with his race (mixed White American and Black American). A third long-term goal could be to for the client to have a conversation with his mother in family therapy.

    Nursing interventions include, but are certainly not limited to: teaching the client about medication; presenting medications for the client to take in packages that are unwrapped and letting the client remove them from the packaging; providing clear directions in simple, concrete terms; avoiding any reference to client's race that could be misinterpreted; helping client find leisure time activities; and helping client learn problem-solving skills and work on positive affirmations to raise self-esteem.

References

Akhtar, S. (1990). "Paranoid Personality Disorder: A Synthesis of Developmental, Dynamic, and Descriptive Features." *American Journal of Psychotherapy* 44(1): 5–25.

American Psychiatric Association. (2000). *Diagnostic and Statistical Manual of Mental Disorders, 4th ed.* Text Revision. Washington, DC: American Psychiatric Association.

CDC. (2002). "State Specific Trends in Self Report Blood Pressure Screenings and High Blood Pressure, United States, 1991–1999." *MMWR Morbidity and Mortality Weekly Report* 51(2): 456–460.

Farmer C.M. et al. (2000). "Visual Perception and Working Memory in Schizotypal Personality." *American Journal of Psychiatry* 157(5): 781–786.

Psychology Today Staff. "Paranoid Personality Disorder." http://www.psychologytoday.com/conditions/paranoid.html. Accessed June 9, 2006.

Stewart, S.H. (2002). "Racial and Ethnic Disparity in Blood Pressure and Cholesterol Measurement." *Journal of General Internal Medicine* 17(6): 405–411.

Tyrer, P. (1994). "The Ubiquity of Jealousy." *Lancet* 343(8904): 992.

——. (2002). "New Book Takes Lid Off Nurses' Attitudes to Personality Disorders." *Mental Health Practice* 1(3): 3.

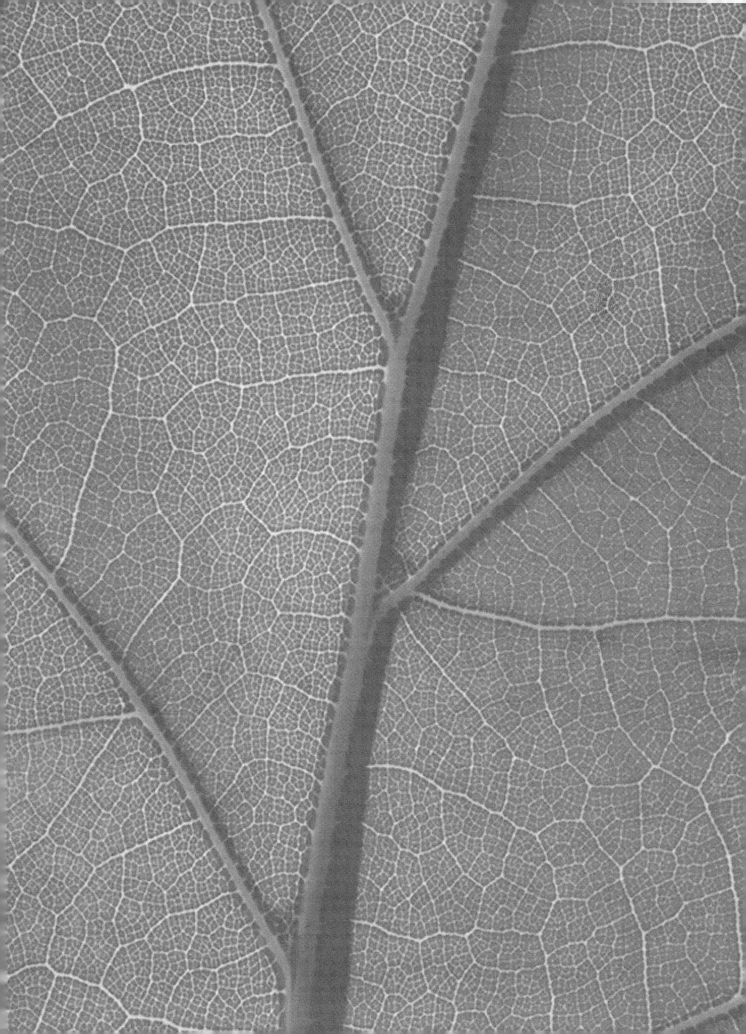

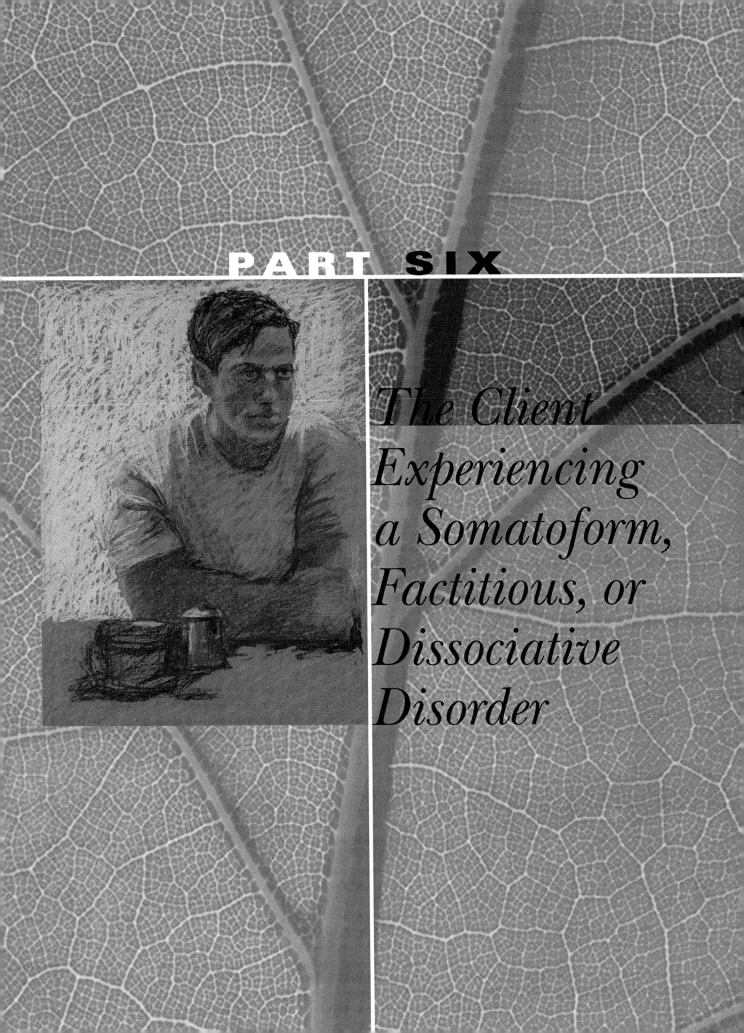

PART SIX

The Client Experiencing a Somatoform, Factitious, or Dissociative Disorder

GENDER	**SOCIOECONOMIC**
Female	
AGE	**SPIRITUAL/RELIGIOUS**
15	
SETTING	**PHARMACOLOGIC**
■ Emergency room	
ETHNICITY	**PSYCHOSOCIAL**
■ White American father and Chilean American mother	**LEGAL**
	■ Possible lawsuit if Conversion Disorder is misdiagnosed and treated in error as a medical or neurological condition
CULTURAL CONSIDERATIONS	
■ Germanic and Hispanic	**ETHICAL**
PREEXISTING CONDITION	
	ALTERNATIVE THERAPY
COEXISTING CONDITION	
	PRIORITIZATION
COMMUNICATION	
	DELEGATION
DISABILITY	

EASY

CONVERSION DISORDER

Level of difficulty: Easy

Overview: Requires realization that Conversion Disorder results from a subconscious defense mechanism and is not something within the client's control. Effective interventions will need to convey caring and empathy for the client without alienating the client's parents. Requires anyone working with the client to set aside any negative feelings or desire to confront the client.

Client Profile

Sarah Jane is a 15-year-old adolescent whose mother was born and raised in Chile and whose father's family was from Germany three generations back. She and her parents live on a small rural northern farm. She has wanted to play the piano like her paternal grandmother, but her mother has insisted she learn to play the violin. Her father, who is very authoritarian, told her: "Do as your mother asks." Now after eight years of violin lessons twice a week after school and on Saturday, Sarah Jane believes she is not very good at playing the violin. Sarah Jane practices hard to learn a lengthy and complicated piece of music for an important recital coming up. At the recital, Sarah Jane begins to play with her music teacher accompanying her on the piano. Sarah Jane looks up and sees her mother, who has seldom left the house because of agoraphobia and who has never come to a recital before, coming in late. Sarah Jane has forgotten which notes come next. She stops playing, and her teacher has her start over. Suddenly Sarah Jane realizes she cannot hold the violin up with her left hand. Her arm is paralyzed from the elbow to the fingertips.

Case Study

Sarah Jane has been taken to the emergency room in the small town hospital where she was playing her recital. The health care provider has completed a number of neurological tests, taken x-rays, and gotten an MRI. The physical assessment and vital signs were within normal limits. Sarah Jane is admitted to the hospital for observation. The primary nurse assigned to her does an admission assessment and finds it remarkable that this client does not seem concerned about her loss of the use of her left arm from the elbow to the fingertips. The doctor comes in and raises the client's paralyzed arm directly above the client's head. The client's arm remains above the head for a few seconds and then falls out to the client's side. The doctor writes in the client's chart: "Rule Out Conversion Disorder."

Questions and Suggested Answers

1. **What is Conversion Disorder? What symptoms does this client have that are consistent with Conversion Disorder?** The client with Conversion Disorder (CD) has symptoms that are caused unconsciously by psychological factors. Conversion Disorder is one of several disorders in a group of disorders called Somatoform Disorders. The symptoms cannot be explained by known medical or neurological conditions. The common symptoms of CD include, but are not limited to: loss of one of the senses, limb paralysis, paresthesias such as numbness or tingling of a hand or foot or both hands and feet, seizures, and impaired balance.

Criteria for Conversion Disorder	Does Client Match Criteria for this Disorder?
At least one symptom or deficit that affects voluntary motor or sensory function, suggesting a neurological or general medical condition.	Yes, the client has a paralysis from elbow to fingertips of one arm.
Psychological facts believed to be associated with the symptom or deficit as the start or exacerbation of symptom or deficit is preceded by stressors such as conflict.	Yes, the client has had a conflict in having to play the violin to please her mother. Another stressor was her mother showing up unexpectedly at the recital just as the client is playing.
The symptom or deficit is not feigned or intentionally produced.	To be assessed further. Nothing suggests that the client made up this symptom of paralysis or is feigning it intentionally.

(Continued)

Criteria for Conversion Disorder	Does Client Match Criteria for this Disorder?
After assessment and investigation, the symptom or deficit is not explained sufficiently by a medical condition, by taking a substance, or by a behavior or experience that is tied to and sanctioned by the culture of the client.	This is being assessed and investigated.
The symptom or deficit brings clinically significant distress or impairment or warrants medical evaluation.	Yes, the client could not continue playing the violin and/or use her arm for hygiene and other activities of daily living, which warrants medical evaluation.
Symptom or deficit is not only pain or sexual dysfunction and has not occurred only during Somatization Disorder course and cannot be better explained as caused by another mental disorder.	Yes, pain and sexual dysfunction are not present. Further investigation will rule out Somatization Disorder and other mental disorders.

(Adapted from APA, 2000)

2. **What are the current theories about what causes Conversion Disorder?** One theory of the origin of conversion symptoms comes from psychoanalytic ideas about what happens when a person is caught between conflicting needs, demands, or desires on some level of unconsciousness. The physical symptoms are believed to keep the unconscious conflict from reaching the conscious mind. Babin and Gross (2002) adhere to the idea of Conversion Disorder triggered by stress or conflict. They discuss the importance of keeping the stressor or conflict in mind when treating the client with Conversion Disorder even though the client may discount the importance of stressors or conflicts.

   Some neuropsychologists view "La belle indifference" (the beautiful indifference attitude)—not seeming concerned in a situation that would be alarming to others and which is associated with clients with Conversion Disorder—as similar to that of medically ill clients who are in strong denial about their symptoms. Some neuropsychologists suspect that the indifference comes from CNS inhibition of sensory inputs. The client is thought to not recognize the seriousness of the symptom or symptoms due to a dysfunction in the brain affecting sensory perception (Frisch and Frisch, 2006; Lezzi and Adams, 1993).

3. **If this client had symptoms of Conversion Disorder, why did the health care provider order more tests? Why did the provider put the client's affected arm above her head and leave it unsupported?** It is not easy to determine if the client has Conversion Disorder or a neurological or medical problem of some sort. Even in this case the client could have some organic problem rather than a psychological problem, or there could be an overlay of Conversion Disorder over another organic problem. Taking time and making effort to get an accurate diagnosis is very important since erroneous medical or neurological diagnoses may mean the client is exposed to unnecessary treatments with the possibility of serious side effects (Heruti, Levy, and Ohry, 2002; Heruti et al., 2002). On the other hand, diagnosis of Conversion Disorder or malingering may mean in some cases that the insurance company does not pay for hospitalization or doctor's fees. Misdiagnoses can cause legal problems for the health care provider should the client get care they don't need or be denied insurance. In clients with more complicated histories and symptoms, it is often more difficult to differentiate between Conversion Disorder and malingering. Malingering involves the intentional production of medical symptoms for the purpose of secondary gains. There are a number of psychological tests designed to identify clients who are malingering from those with a psychological disorder (Babin and Gross, 2002). In more complicated cases, consultation with a psychologist trained in testing might be indicated.

   The doctor put the client's arm above her head and left it unsupported because he wanted to see if the arm would fall and hit the client's head as it would in the case of a paralyzed arm or if it would remain suspended a short while and then fall to the client's side, which is more in keeping with Conversion Disorder.

4. **Do people with Conversion Disorder deliberately produce the symptoms for secondary gain?** Clients with Conversion Disorder do not deliberately produce symptoms for secondary gain. "Conversion Disorder involves the unintentional and unconscious production of medical symptoms as a result of psychological factors" (Babin and Gross, 2002). A person who produces symptoms for secondary gain such as attention or a monetary settlement is more likely to be malingering.

5. **What subtypes of Conversion Disorder are there? Which subtype of Conversion Disorder does this client seem to have? Does this subtype always produce symptoms of paralysis, or could other symptoms be produced instead? If so, what symptoms?** The subtypes of Conversion Disorder are:

- With Motor Symptom or Deficit
- With Sensory Symptom or Deficit
- With Seizures or Convulsions
- With Mixed Presentation (APA, 2000)

This client is likely experiencing Conversion Disorder, and the subtype is "With Motor Symptom or Deficit." She cannot move her lower arm. This subtype could involve any motor symptoms or deficits, such as gait problems, and would not necessarily involve paralysis.

6. **Does this client's onset of symptoms fit within the general onset of Conversion Disorder? What will be this client's course if she follows a typical course associated with Conversion Disorder?** This adolescent client's onset of symptoms does fit within the usual range of onset, which is between age 10 and age 35.

Symptoms will probably disappear within two weeks if the client follows the usual course. About 20–25 percent of people who have an episode of Conversion Disorder will have a reoccurrence within a year. A reoccurrence predicts future episodes. The client who has an acute symptom, has identifiable stress at onset, gets treatment quickly, and is of more than average intelligence has a good prognosis. Tremor and seizures have a poorer prognosis than paralysis, aphonia, and symptoms of blindness, according to the APA (2000).

7. **What stage of development, according to Erickson, is this client trying to master? What roles might stage of development and culture play in this client's development of Conversion Disorder?** This client at age 15 falls into the 11- to 20-year-old group in which the stage of development is identity versus role confusion. The client is trying to develop her own identity, but not without difficulty. Her father is authoritarian, which is associated with the Germanic culture as well as other cultures, and he demands the client please her mother by playing the violin rather than the piano she dreams of playing. The mother comes from the Chilean culture in which mothers play a strong role in deciding what an adolescent can and cannot do. This adolescent client is in an American culture and sees peers rebelling against parental authority, and she cannot do this. The task of adolescence is to question the ideas of parents and to separate from parents, and when the client cannot separate from her parents, she has conflicts that may come out subconsciously in physical symptoms.

8. **What information in data gathering or assessing would be helpful to the treatment team as well as the nurse?** It would be helpful to further assess the family dynamics and how and where the parents see their daughter five years from now. Is she to be independent at some point or always living with her parents? How much control will they try to exert over her choices of what she will do in life? It would be important to assess this client's needs on Maslow's hierarchy of needs. Where is she in terms of safety and security, love and belonging, and what is her level of self-esteem? What is her self-concept and what is her body image? What are her strengths and talents and what are her goals for the future? Is there a family history of Conversion Disorder or any psychiatric disorder? Is there any history of physical or sexual abuse in the family?

There is often a need for health care or treatment team meetings, so a team approach can be developed to assure consistency of team members in what they say and do with this client. There is a need for a primary nurse or case manager to ensure consistency.

9. What nursing diagnoses would you likely write for a client with Conversion Disorder?

- Powerlessness
- Anxiety

It is possible that the client feels powerless and/or experiences anxiety when dealing with her parents.

10. What treatment goals would you likely write for this client? What interventions do you think would likely work well with this client? Client goals can include:

- Will attend 100 percent of scheduled individual counseling sessions
- Will attend family therapy for two or three sessions with a mental health professional

Nursing interventions can include:

- Approach client with positive, caring attitude without confrontation
- Build a trusting therapeutic relationship
- Encourage client to identify likes and dislikes in food and other areas
- Give client as much control as possible, such as choice of two shower times, choice of some foods to be served, and choice of activities
- Teach parents and client about normal adolescent growth and development
- Encourage client to get individual counseling and family to also get counseling

11. What treatment approaches are reported in the literature? Treatment approaches reported in the literature include negative reinforcement techniques. Campo and Negrini (2001) report using negative reinforcement in the case of a 12-year-old boy who developed pain in an arm one month after a vaccination and three weeks later had a transient diffuse rash with arm and shoulder pain and soon claimed he was unable to move the arm. The family had endured some crises such as the mother having been treated for cancer and the father losing his job. The boy was in special education class. Tests revealed good muscle and nerve function and no apparent reason for his inability to move his arm. The health care providers decided on provisional diagnosis of Conversion Disorder, and negative reinforcement was recommended to the parents. The boy was not permitted to leave his bed except to go to the bathroom and for meals with his family. He was told he had to rest and use all his energy for getting well. After a few hours he reported his arm was feeling better, and he was sent back to bed to get well. Within twenty-four hours he reported his arm was well. A similar approach has been used with children with eating disorders. The child cannot go home on pass or discharge or play games until they are well. Negative reinforcement is not as popular as positive reinforcement, and it necessitates a strong alliance between the treatment staff and the parents or guardians.

Zeharia et al. (1999) reported on the diagnosis and management of forty-seven children with "conversion reaction" seen over nine years in their outpatient department. Forty of the forty-seven patients were diagnosed by detailed histories and physicals without additional tests. These pediatricians pointed out that when diagnosis was made early and presented to parents with certainty and stressing that the symptoms were not intentional, it was easier both for parents to accept the diagnosis and for the child to recover. Most of the children recovered within one session or a few days. The ages of the children were 9 to 15, with twice as many females as males. In the history taking, the search was on for school and social difficulties, poor peer relationships, family crises or stressors, and possible secondary gains. Treatment often involved dealing with the stressor. For example a 10-year-old girl had developed blisters on her feet after long hikes during the summer. Weeks after the blisters were gone, she claimed she had such pain she could not walk on her feet. The history revealed the girl had a conflict with a teacher and thoughts of the conflict kept her awake at night. With the pediatrician's reassurance that she would be able to walk soon and the mother's promise to help the girl work out the conflict with the teacher, she began to walk. Another girl who would not walk because of a complaint of bilateral knee pain was found to be assigned a good many household chores and child care of a brother. With the pediatrician's assurance she could walk and the mother decreasing the chores, the child began to walk. Zeharia et al. believe that pediatricians who have a good relationship with the family and the child can treat mild cases of Conversion Disorder in children rather than referring them to a psychiatric mental health professional. The pediatric nurse might well play a role in taking the history and in looking for stressors that might be a source of conflict leading to the conversion symptom(s).

References

American Psychiatric Association. (2000). *Diagnostic and Statistical Manual of Mental Disorders, 4th ed.* Text Revision. Washington, DC: American Psychiatric Association.

Babin, P.R. and P. Gross. (2002). "Traumatic Brain Injury When Symptoms Don't Add Up: Conversion and Malingering in the Rehabilitation Setting." *Journal of Rehabilitation* 68(2): 4–14.

Campo, J.V. and B.J. Negrini. (2001). "Innovative Treatment Approach Combats Conversion Disorder." *Brown University Child and Adolescent Behavior Letter* 17: 1–3.

Frisch, N.C. and L.E. Frisch. (2006). *Psychiatric Mental Health Nursing, 3rd ed.* Albany, NY: Thomson Delmar Learning.

Heruti, R.J. et al. (2002). "Conversion Motor Paralysis Disorder: Analysis of 34 Consecutive Referrals." *Spinal Cord* 40(7): 335–340.

Heruti, R.J., A. Levy, and A. Ohry. (2002). "Conversion Motor Paralysis Disorder: Overview and Rehabilitation Model." *Spinal Cord* 40(7): 327–334.

Lezzi, A. and H.E. Adams. (1993). "Somatoform and Factitious Disorders." *Comprehensive Handbook of Psychopathology,* 2nd ed. Ed. P.B. Sutker and H.E. Adams. New York: Plenum.

Zeharia, A. et al. (1999). "Conversion Reaction: Management by the Paediatrician." *European Journal of Pediatrics* 158(2): 160–165.

GENDER

Female

AGE

51

SETTING

- Home with visiting nurse

ETHNICITY

- African

CULTURAL CONSIDERATIONS

- African

PREEXISTING CONDITION

COEXISTING CONDITION

COMMUNICATION

DISABILITY

SOCIOECONOMIC

SPIRITUAL/RELIGIOUS

PHARMACOLOGIC

PSYCHOSOCIAL

- Socialization altered by client's focus on physical symptoms

LEGAL

- Possible lawsuit for unnecessary surgery, especially if complications from surgery or if an actual medical problem occurs and is missed

ETHICAL

ALTERNATIVE THERAPY

PRIORITIZATION

DELEGATION

SOMATIZATION DISORDER

Level of difficulty: Moderate

Overview: Requires critical thinking and decision making about when to listen to symptoms and when to refocus the client on the task at hand. Involves critical thinking in terms of assessing and identifying problems that are current and need to be the focus of interventions.

Client Profile

Melba is a 51-year-old married female of African birth who immigrated to the United States with her parents when she was 15 years old. She has a history of numerous physical complaints and several surgeries. She is presently recuperating at home from exploratory surgery. She had complained of abdominal pain, changes in bowel habits, abdominal bloating, nausea, and vomiting, and after numerous trips to a variety of health care providers who prescribed a number of medications for the pain, nausea, and constipation, she found a surgeon who thought an exploratory laparotomy was warranted. No pathology was found during this surgery. Melba's hospital stay was extended due to an infection at the incisional site and then she was sent home on antibiotics and wet to dry dressings. On discharge, instructions included no sexual intercourse until the incision heals. Her husband's response to the nurse was, "My wife has not thought about sex in years." Melba is to have home visits from a registered nurse.

Case Study

The home health agency nurse arrives at Melba's home. After introducing herself, the nurse begins to take Melba's vital signs, but finds it hard to concentrate as Melba wants to talk about her prior health problems and surgeries. Melba describes a series of surgeries and complaints going back several years beginning at age 26 with back surgery, although she is somewhat lacking in details of what was found or done in the surgery. Then there was the time she could not seem to empty her bladder: "It would fill up with nearly a gallon before I could get somewhere to be catheterized." Melba describes excruciating pain when urinating, bladder infections, and high fevers off and on for several years. Her health care provider has not diagnosed any bladder problems. She also talks about years of impaired coordination and balance keeping her from being able to work. Melba says sometimes she can't sleep at night because it feels like ants are crawling under her skin. She currently complains of knee pain keeping her from walking. X-rays and an MRI of the knee were negative. From Melba's story, the nurse feels certain that there have been few or no periods of time in Melba's life that she has been symptom-free. The nurse finishes the vital signs, which are normal, and suggests Melba learn to do the wet to dry dressings for her abdominal incision. Melba says her husband will do the dressings and to teach him. The nurse recalls an old lecture from nursing school and realizes that some of Melba's behavior sounds like it matches what she learned about Somatization Disorder.

Questions and Suggested Answers

1. **What is Somatization Disorder? What symptoms does Melba have or has she had that caused the nurse to think she might have Somatization Disorder? Could a person have some symptoms of this disorder and not meet the criteria for the diagnosis?** Somatization Disorder has been referred to as hysteria or Briquet's Syndrome in the past. This disorder involves multiple symptoms beginning before a client is age 30, continues over years, and involves a combination of symptom areas including pain, gastrointestinal, sexual, and symptoms of a pseudoneurological nature (APA, 2000).

   The following table provides the criteria for diagnosis of Somatization Disorder and the client's signs and symptoms that seem to match the criteria.

Criteria for diagnosis of Somatization Disorder	Do the client's signs and symptoms match the criteria?
Numerous physical complaints starting before age 30 and occurring over several years with treatment sought or significant impairment in important areas of functioning such as social, educational, and occupational.	Yes, back surgery at age 26 and occurring over the years since that time. Frequently sought treatments. Illnesses are a major focus in her life. Has not been able to work outside the home. Has impairment in sexual aspect of marriage.

(Continued)

Criteria for diagnosis of Somatization Disorder	Do the client's signs and symptoms match the criteria?
Four types of symptoms must have occurred sometime during the course of the disturbance. • Four pain symptoms at four or more different sites or functions including various parts of the body and during menstruation, sexual intercourse, or urination • Two GI symptoms excluding pain (bloating, nausea or vomiting, diarrhea, intolerance of certain foods) • One sexual symptom or reproductive symptom besides pain • One pseudoneurological symptom excepting pain (e.g., blindness, urinary retention, seizures, impaired coordination or balance, loss of touch or pain symptoms, loss of consciousness, difficulty swallowing).	Pain symptoms include back pain, bladder pain, abdominal pain and knee pain, and she has other problems with the bladder. GI symptoms include bloating, changes in bowel habits, and nausea and vomiting. Loss of libido or interest in sexual aspect of her marriage. Has urinary retention, impaired coordination and balance, and feeling of ants crawling under her skin.
One of the following is true: • Symptoms the client has from each of the four groups above cannot be explained by a known medical condition or a drug or medicine • Symptoms are not feigned or intentionally produced.	To date, symptoms from four groups above not explained by medical condition or drug or medicine. As far as has been determined to date, symptoms are not feigned or intentionally produced by this client.

(Adapted from APA, 2000)

There are many clients who have fewer symptoms than needed to meet the criteria for a diagnosis of Somatization Disorder but who still have troublesome transient, variable symptoms of the disorder. They are less impaired but still a challenge to the nursing staff and other health care providers. This type of client is said to have traits of Somatization Disorder or said to be displaying somatization behaviors.

2. **How do you think you might feel if you were working with Melba or a client with a similar history of physical complaints for which no medical explanation can be found?** Often nurses feel frustrated and irritated, angry, and/or inadequate when working with clients who have somatization behaviors and who convert their emotional distress into physical problems. Maynard (2004) has said that clients with this diagnosis "are probably able to produce more feelings of frustration, irritation, and concern" than clients with other diagnoses. Part of the frustration may come from not being able to apply the usual diagnostic tests/procedures and come up with something that can be readily fixed.

You could become frustrated because the client is focused on past medical problems and not on the current problems that you are trying to help the client resolve or manage. You might feel yourself becoming impatient with the client because she never seems to say that she has gotten better or will be getting better. As you try different ways to get the client to participate in her own care and she resists your efforts, you may feel yourself getting angry.

Having these negative feelings is a human response. It is all right to have these feelings, but recognize them immediately, then quickly set them aside to use more therapeutic types of thinking and feeling to assist the client in changing their behaviors. You must remind yourself to stay in your professional nurse role and to be persistent, patient, and calm.

3. **What are the current theories about the causation of Somatization Disorder?** The cause of Somatization Disorder is not known, although researchers are working hard to find the cause and have discovered some

evidence for biochemical or structural origins as well as evidence for environmental causes or influences. It may be a combination of psychosocial and biological factors.

Some theories link somatization to a problem in the central nervous system in regard to regulation and interpretation of sensory input or a failure in communication between the right and left brain (Maynard, 2004; Frisch and Frisch, 2006). Eleven patients from a Somatization Disorder Unit in Spain who did not meet criteria for any other DSM disorder and who had normal computerized tomography and MRI were studied with single photon emission computed tomography (SPECT) scans. Seven of the eleven subjects demonstrated hypoperfusion in SPECT images, some (four) in the nondominant hemisphere and some (three) in bilateral hemispheres. The region of hypoperfusion in one hemisphere or both varied. Although this was a small study and a number of improvements could be made in research design, it was remarkable that there were eleven subjects without other psychiatric pathology who could be studied, and the authors recommend additional controlled studies to confirm or refute the hypothesis that a communication problem between the left and right hemispheres of the brain plays a role in development of SD (Garcia-Campayo, Sanz-Carrillo, Baringo, and Ceballos, 2001).

Servan-Schreiber, Kolb, and Tabas (2000) present four psychological mechanisms, one or more of which might be evident in individuals with somatization or panic attacks:

- Mechanism 1: Amplification of Body Sensations. Client worries about physical disease and focuses attention on common variations in their body sensations to the point these sensations become "disturbing and unpleasant." The client's perception of the sensations causes an increase in the client's concerns, increasing anxiety and heightening the sensations.
- Mechanism 2: The Identified Patient. When a family system is under stress, having one member identified as the sick one may provide a focus for family members that serves to stabilize the system and decrease feelings of anxiety among family members. When one family member takes on a sick role, the family dynamic may be dysfunctional, and the health care provider can reinforce it by treating the person assuming a sick role as if they are medically ill.
- Mechanism 3: The Need to Be Sick. Subconsciously or unconsciously, the client on their own seeks the sick role to get relief from "stressful or impossible interpersonal expectations (primary gain)" and may get secondary gains such as attention and caring. The person does not consciously carry this out.
- Mechanism 4: Dissociation. In the absence of physical stimuli, there is activation of feelings of pain similar to phantom limb.

Some studies have found that SD tends to occur in clusters in families. Growing up with a mother or father who somaticized might tend to make some offspring more likely to somaticize as well.

Hurwitz (2004) states, "Somatic symptoms are a psychological defense against mental instability." Intrapsychic distress is relieved by the formation of somatic symptoms. Hurwitz theorizes that major affective disorders are often the mental instability that produces the somatic symptoms as a defense.

4. **What is the incidence of Somatization Disorder?** This disorder is said to be relatively rare, with estimates of the incidence of the disorder ranging from 0.13 to 2 percent (APA, 2000). What is no doubt less rare are cases of somatization behaviors not quite extensive enough to meet the criteria for diagnosis. Servan-Schreiber, Kolb, and Tabas (2000) state in a two-part article in *American Family Physician* that "somatization is common" and "as a process ranges from mild stress-related symptoms to severe debilitation."

It is generally agreed that more women than men meet the diagnosis for Somatization Disorder, with men rarely diagnosed with this disorder in the United States. There are higher frequencies of men with Somatization Disorder in Greece and Puerto Rico (APA, 2000).

5. **Do nurses other than psychiatric nurses need to know about this disorder, and if so, where would nurses encounter a client with this diagnosis or some of the traits of this disorder?** Nurses working in any setting are likely to eventually encounter a client with Somatization Disorder or one who somaticizes. Nurses are more likely to encounter the client in medical settings. These clients seek medical care, not psychiatric/mental

health care. These clients often move around to a variety of health care providers in an attempt to get a physical diagnosis. Nurses encountering these clients include nurses volunteering to do health screenings at senior centers or the visiting nurse doing home visits, the nurse in a long-term care setting or assisted living, the nurse in a variety of providers' offices, and nurses working in hospitals. You might begin to suspect somatization in a stranger when you say, "Hello. How are you?" just to be polite to someone on the street, in a store, or at a gathering and the person starts a long dialogue about his or her medical symptoms, some of which seem a bit out of the ordinary.

6. **If you were Melba's nurse, how would you respond when she tells you that she is not going to learn to do the dressing change and that you can teach her husband to do it?** You might say something like: "I'd like to teach both of you how to do it. Perhaps your husband will be unable to change the dressing sometime and you will be prepared to do it or to teach someone else to do it." You do not want to get into a control battle with the client by telling her she has to do it herself. In the suggested reply, you have included her in the learning and given her a bit of control in agreeing to teach the husband. You will notice that the suggestion does not assume the husband is willing. The nurse is simply stating a willingness to teach and providing a reason for why the client needs to learn. The nurse can interview the husband and find out his perspective on family dynamics, his needs, and his wife's needs.

7. **What assessment areas would you like to assess if you were this client's nurse?** As with any other client, you want to assess or gather data on the client head to toe and covering all body systems. You need to assess this client's abdominal incision and the amount and type of drainage if any. You will be hearing a variety of complaints from the client, but you need to gather objective data as well as subjective data from the client.

It is important to do a good psychosocial assessment. You will want to assess the family dynamics and assess for caregiver strain, which is common in those caring for clients with Somatization Disorder or traits of the disorder.

You also want to assess this client's complaint of "feeling like ants crawling under the skin."

8. **What impact might culture have on a client's symptoms?** Escobar (2004), writing on transcultural aspects of Somatization Disorder and dissociation, states that dissociation and somatization are perhaps the most common results of psychological trauma. He states that it is a well-accepted belief in cross-cultural psychiatry that the changing of personal or social distress into some physical complaint is the norm in most cultures. Escobar describes a number of various examples of people from other cultures turning distress into somatic complaints. One example is in India and Nigeria, people may complain of feelings of heat, peppery and crawling sensations, burning hands and feet, and the hot peppery feeling in the head. A feeling of ants crawling under the skin is sometimes elicited from people that are African. You will recall that Melba was born and raised in Africa. Nurses need to find out the symptom norm for the country a client comes from. What seems strange to nurses in this country may be a common complaint and not viewed as strange or psychotic in another country.

9. **What nursing diagnoses would you most likely write for this client? What would be some treatment goals of the nurse and client? What interventions would seem indicated for this client and possibly for the majority of clients with Somatization Disorder?** Ineffective coping, chronic pain, social interaction impaired, and sexuality patterns ineffective are likely diagnoses. Assessment may verify caregiver role strain and role performance ineffective. "Ineffective sexuality patterns" was approved as a nursing diagnosis in 1986, and it involves the client reporting difficulty, limitations, and/or changes in his or her sexual activities/behaviors. Related factors include illness or medical treatments as well as body image disturbance and low self-esteem.

Therapeutic treatment goals of the nurse and other treatment team members might well include: establishing a solid therapeutic alliance with client, teaching the client about the manifestations of the disorder, and giving consistent reassurances to client (Frisch and Frisch, 2006). Client goals could include the following:

- Will identify feelings and share this with the nurse or significant other at least twice a day
- Will name at least one means of dealing with feelings of anger or resentment
- Will use the phrase "I need" to get needs met

- Will stay focused in some activity for at least one hour without mentioning a physical symptom
- Will interact in some activity with spouse for one hour without mentioning a physical symptom
- Will identify two ways to improve relationship with spouse

Note: numbers and times can be adjusted based on what nurse judges are suitable for client.

There are many interventions that would be helpful and correct. A priority intervention is to build a strong therapeutic alliance by building trust and including the client as part of the team. Helping the family locate some respite care might revitalize the husband. Encouraging the client to identify interests and to engage in them would be another intervention. The nurse might find that the client is interested in studying African history, learning new recipes, or listening to books on tape. Listen carefully to the client for a set amount of time and limit the amount of time the client can talk about physical complaints. Give the client regular time and attention that is not dependent on coming up with physical symptoms. Having the same nurse care for the client is helpful in building an alliance. Help the client to identify needs and ways to get them met.

10. **What are current treatment approaches to clients with this disorder?** A common thread among approaches to clients with SD is to have the same primary care provider each visit and to provide scheduled visits that are not dependent on developing or maintaining symptoms. Maynard (2004) describes a study in which clients who didn't see the same provider in a clinic were 1.8 times more likely to have somatic symptom complex. The primary care provider and the team accept the client as a partner in care making statements such as: "It won't be easy to treat your problems and therefore I need your help." Cognitive behavioral therapy is commonly used with clients with this disorder, but the client may be resistant in therapy due to believing they are physically ill and have no need for psychotherapy. A fairly common approach is to have a mental health consultant: a psychiatrist and/or a psychiatric mental health nurse clinician.

The nurse working with this client and others with Somatization Disorder or its traits, needs to keep in mind that occasionally what appears to be somatization by the client is not somatization at all, but a serious medical problem. For example, the client who has had an exploratory laporotomy with no unusual findings can develop internal bleeding, infection, and other problems. In one case a ureter was accidentally cut resulting in a number of symptoms that became life threatening before the health care team realized these symptoms were not part of the somatization behaviors, corrected the problem, and settled out of court. To reduce risks to the client and avoid legal action the nurse must carefully assess all client complaints in a professional manner.

References

American Psychiatric Association. (2000). *Diagnostic and Statistical Manual of Mental Disorders, 4th ed.* Text Revision. Washington, DC: American Psychiatric Association.

Escobar, J.I. (2004). "Transcultural Aspects of Dissociative and Somatoform Disorders." *Psychiatric Times* 21(5): 10–13.

Frisch, N.C. and L.E. Frisch. (2006). *Psychiatric Mental Health Nursing, 3rd ed.* Albany, NY: Thomson Delmar Learning.

Garcia-Compayo, J., C. Sanz-Carrillo, T. Baringo, and C. Ceballos. (2001). "SPECT Scan in Somatization Disorder Patients: An Exploratory Study of Eleven Cases." *Australian and New Zealand Journal of Psychiatry* 35: 359–263.

Hurwitz, T.A. (2004). "Somatization and Conversion Disorder." *Canadian Journal of Psychiatry* 49(3): 172–178.

Maynard, C.K. (2004). "Assess and Manage Somatization." *Holistic Nursing Practice* 18(2): 54–61.

Servan-Schreiber, D., N.R. Kolb, and G. Tabas (2000). "Somatizind Patients: Part I Practical Diagnosis." *American Family Physician* 61(4): 1073–1079.

GENDER

Female

AGE

34

SETTING

- Adult psychiatric unit

ETHNICITY

- White American

CULTURAL CONSIDERATIONS

- Rural southern farming and strong churchgoing culture
- Culture of abuse

PRE-EXISTING CONDITION

CO-EXISTING CONDITION

COMMUNICATION

DISABILITY

SOCIOECONOMIC

- Raised poor then lower middle class when married

SPIRITUAL/RELIGIOUS

- Subconscious resistance to church related to abuse history.

PHARMACOLOGIC

PSYCHOSOCIAL

- Alternates between being withdrawn and uninhibited based on what alternative personality ("alter") is in charge.

LEGAL

- Need to avoid causing false memories of abuse
- Confidentiality

ETHICAL

- Is it educational or is it inappropriate, exploitive, and unethical to ask a client with Dissociative Identity Disorder (DID) to appear in public to discuss or demonstrate alternative personalities?

ALTERNATIVE THERAPY

PRIORITIZATION

DELEGATION

DISSOCIATIVE IDENTITY DISORDER (FORMERLY MULTIPLE PERSONALITY DISORDER)

Level of difficulty: High

Overview: Requires knowledge of DID and critical thinking to respond therapeutically to the client and any "alters," which present with a variety of behaviors and attitudes. Requires critical thinking to avoid letting personal attitudes or feelings get in the way of working effectively with the client and to avoid leading the client to false memories.

DIFFICULT

Client Profile

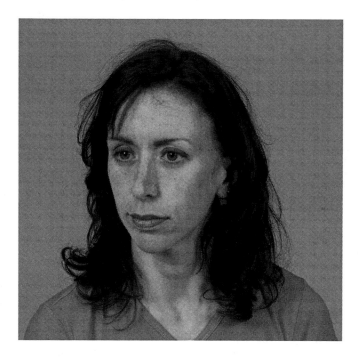

Amanda is a 34-year-old married female who was raised in a strong churchgoing family on a rural southern Bible Belt farm. Her grandfather as well as her father sexually, physically, and mentally abused her as a child. Each of them told her it would kill her mother if she found out and not to tell anyone or they would punish her. Her father, a deacon in the church, routinely abused her on Sundays after church and Sunday dinner when other family members took a nap. At first Amanda screamed, but no one seemed to hear. She began to dissociate: to mentally float above what was happening and feel like an observer. Her grandfather and her father died before she was 10 years old. Amanda repressed the abuse in her subconscious mind. At age 19 Amanda married Fred, a long-distance truck driver, who was kind to her but not often home. The marriage provided a means to get away from her mother who wasn't kind or supportive and who had actually known about the abuse and done nothing.

Recently Amanda noticed what she calls "trashy" clothes in her closet. She thought her husband had bought the seductive dresses until she found a charge receipt with her signature on it. Amanda has found herself in a store temporarily unable to recall what she came to buy or who she is. She has found herself talking in a strange childish voice or in a sultry seductive way: not like her real self at all. Amanda suspects she has different personalities within herself: one (Audrey) who likes to dress "trashy," tease men, and control; a small playful bear ("Bear"); "Sissy," age 5, who likes to play but is afraid of adults; Tom, who knows about "Sissy" and wants to protect her. Neither Tom nor Sissy know about Audrey, who seems to know everyone except Butch, who is angry about the abuse and wants Amanda to cut her arms. Amanda never has felt connected to the world and other people. She has little recall of her childhood and tries to deny flashbacks of the abuse.

Case Study

Amanda is admitted to the adult psychiatric unit. Her husband tells the nurse he fears his wife is "going crazy." Fred describes Amanda cutting her arms and having periods of time for which she has no memory. He relates that Amanda became very upset when he asked her to go to church with him. After the husband leaves, the psychiatric technician goes through the things Amanda brought to the hospital and removes items that she might hurt herself with, inventories them, and locks them up. The admitting orders provide a diagnosis of Dissociative

Identity Disorder. The psychiatrist's history and physical on Amanda states she has had one previous admission to the facility. The nurse orders and reads the old chart from medical records and becomes aware of some of the alters (alternative personalities) Amanda has revealed to her psychiatrist and therapists. The nurse offers to play checkers with Amanda after the evening meal. During the checker game one of the alters comes out and says in a child's voice, "I don't want to play with you."

Questions and Suggested Answers

1. **If you were the nurse on the unit, what would you say to the husband when he says that his wife (your client) is "going crazy"?** You can be empathetic, yet not agree that the client is "going crazy"(e.g. you can say something like: "This must be a difficult time for you, but our treatment team is very good and is here to help your wife.").

2. **Why is the diagnosis of DID controversial? Is this a real disorder, or do mental health professionals and clients misapply and misuse this diagnosis?** Dissociative Identity Disorder, as a diagnosis, became controversial when a number of lawsuits were filed and large settlements awarded in cases involving clients with various mental disorders who were thought to have been misled by mental health professionals into thinking they had repressed childhood abuse and multiple personalities. In some cases, family members and others had been falsely accused and imprisoned on the basis of the false abuse memories. One criminal trial involved charges against professionals and administration of a Houston DID unit: charges of misdiagnosing and falsely convincing people they had been abused by a satanic cult. The media described costly treatment in which patients were restrained in bed for abreaction sessions. While this case ended without a verdict, other cases followed against this Houston DID unit, including one resulting in a $5.8 million award to a client (Holmes, 2005). A case in Chicago brought a $10.6 million settlement, and across the country, lawsuits were filed against therapists for misleading clients into false memory recall. The American Psychiatric Association and other health care organizations warned their members not to mislead clients' into false memories. The International Society for the Study of Dissociation Guidelines for Treating DID in Adults can be found on the organization's website: http://mentalhealth.about.com/gi/dynamic/offsite.htm?site=http://www.issd.org/ (2005).

   No matter how many clients were misled into finding false memories, some psychiatric professionals such as Silberg (2000), as well as clients with the diagnosis, have written convincingly about dissociating and discovering numbers of distinct alternative personalities. West (1999), a psychologist, wrote a book about the other personalities within himself and his attempts to explore his childhood abuse. He was having flashbacks about things his grandmother had done to him and discovered from family members that his grandmother had sexually abused him. His mother was also a perpetrator, and there were other victims in the family, though no one wanted to talk about the abuse.

3. **What is the culture of abuse? What role did the southern, rural farm, Bible Belt culture possibly play in the abuse and dissociation?** A typical rule in a household of abuse is not to discuss what goes on in the family with outsiders or even among family members. People in the family know about the abuse, but they don't stop it. Abuse is often intergenerational. Abused children tend to try to hide from their abusers. Amanda's family and West's family, as described in his book, fit this description. There is often alcohol and other drug abuse and/or abandonment by one or more parents. Living in a rural farm culture made it easier for the client's family to isolate and keep the abuse secret. The strong church culture may have included beliefs about the male as head of the family with an obligation to control and discipline the children and women, who may be viewed as subservient to males. Amanda's abuse after church by her father, a church deacon, may have caused her anxious reaction to her husband asking her to go to church. According to Cook (2005), "Sexual abuse committed by clergy or other adults affiliated with the church may have additional ramifications because of deep violations of trust, honesty, and love. In addition, it can create spiritual distress in survivors of abuse."

4. **Are all clients who are diagnosed with DID survivors of sexual abuse, and are all sexual abuse survivors likely to have or to develop DID?** The literature supports the idea that most, but not all, people with DID were sexu-

ally abused as children and those who were not sexually abused likely suffered other forms of abuse or trauma. In a study of sixty-two people with a diagnosis of DID (Middleton and Butler, 1998), 87 percent of the subjects self-reported childhood sexual abuse, mostly by close family members. Some subjects reported sexual abuse on a daily basis for years, while others reported forced sex with animals and 23 percent reported someone inserting objects into their body parts. Some subjects reported that they were exposed to pedophile rings and child prostitution arranged by parents. Eighty-five percent reported physical abuse, 79 percent reported emotional abuse, and 21 percent reported being locked in rooms or cupboards as children. Thirty-one percent were subjected to gang rape on one or more occasions; 32 percent had witnessed a traumatic death.

Not all survivors of sexual abuse dissociate or have DID. Some survivors describe having dissociated but deny awareness of other personalities within themselves. Some survivors of rape will describe having felt like they were floating above the scene and are unable to recall the abuse details. Most don't believe they have several personalities who periodically take charge, however, the discovery of personalities or alters within seems, by the account of those who have DID, to have been made reluctantly over long periods of time.

5. **Discuss some characteristics and behaviors of a person with Dissociative Identity Disorder. What are the criteria for a diagnosis of DID, and does Amanda meet the criteria for this diagnosis?** DID manifests in two or more different personality states that alternately take charge for various time periods. When an alter takes charge, the person often does things totally out of character. Speech and behavior is different with each alter. Clients with DID can go for a long time without being aware of alternative personality states until clues arise, such as having strange clothing in the closet. A person with DID often experiences amnesiac effects and may feel like they are in a trance or have "out-of-body experiences." Headaches are not uncommon. Subjects have attributed headaches to arguments among the personalities in their head. Many with DID tend to engage in self-persecution, self-sabotage, and self-inflicted harm.

The DSM IV-TR (APA, 2000) criteria for a diagnosis of DID, as well as the client's behavior that matches the criteria:

Criteria for Diagnosis of Dissociative Identity Disorder

1. Has at least two distinct identities or personality states with each one having a separate and relatively enduring pattern of relating to the environment and the self as well as perceiving and thinking about environment and self.	**Yes.** Client has at least five distinct personality states as described in the case study: Audrey, Bear, Sissy, Tom, and Butch. Client's personality states appear to be separate and to have enduring patterns of relating to self and environment, and perceiving and thinking about it
2. Two or more of the personalities take charge of the person's behavior recurrently.	**Yes.** Audrey, Sissy, and others periodically take charge.
3. The client is not able to recall important personal information too extensive to be explained by just forgetting.	**Yes.** Amanda is unable to describe any memories from her childhood years.
4. Any disturbances are not related to effects of a substance or a general medical condition.	This must be assessed further.

Adapted from DSM IV-TR (APA, 2000)

6. **What is the cause of DID? What are the risk factors for DID?** No one knows what causes DID. Piper (2004) argues that this phenomenon is a "culture bound and often iatrogenic condition." Other clinicians and researchers suggest the disorder is a result of abuse as a child and possibly some genetic predisposition to dissociate. Spillman (cited in Silberg 2000) found that parental subjects who scored higher on dissociation tend to have children who were maltreated.

Object relations theory suggests that when children suffer abuse they can "split off" awareness and memories from the rest of their identity, as a survival mechanism. During the splitting off, different identities are formed, holding different memories and feelings and performing different functions. When someone who has learned to dissociate experiences a new trauma (e.g., a vaginal examination), the feelings of powerlessness, exposure, intrusion, and/or loss of control may bring about flashbacks and/or dissociation (McAllister, 2000).

Dissociation can be an effective defense against anxious anticipation of pain as well as actual physical and emotional pain. Defensive dissociation becomes an automatic defense whenever the person feels threatened or anxious, even if the situation is not abusive or threatening to the average person.

Wakeman (2002) describes four risk factors for DID which were identified by Kluft in 1984. These factors are: 1. Inherited predisposition to dissociate; 2. Repeated or chronic trauma that most often begins in childhood; 3. Severe trauma; and 4. Absence of positive nurturing and support.

7. **If you were the nurse playing checkers with Amanda and she said in a childlike voice, "I don't want to play with you," what therapeutic response would you make and why?** You must avoid being defensive or authoritarian in your response. The word "play" and the sentence "I don't want to play with you" suggest a child lashing out to avoid being hurt. As the nurse you need to have a gentle manner and tone. You can introduce yourself and ask: "Who are you?" If the alter gives a name (e.g., "Sissy"), the response might be: "Welcome, Sissy. I am happy to meet you." The nurse can choose from many words, but "happy" is a child-friendly word also appropriate for regressed or frightened adults.

The nurse has many choices of responses including a play on the person's ambivalence (e.g., "You don't want to play with me, but perhaps you will play anyway?"). If the alter's response is "No," you can say, "Maybe another day." If the alter withdraws, don't think you have failed. You have begun to build a relationship with an alter and opened the door for future interactions.

The nurse must keep in mind that he/she is part of the therapeutic team and any approaches to the client must be congruent with team approaches and goals. McAllister et al. (2001) state that all too often nurses and clients are left out of the team process and as a result have little needed information; however, they view nurses as important in "facilitating the group of alters to find their own strategies to strike deals between themselves."

8. **What should the nurse do if the treatment team doesn't want staff nurses to interact with the client's alters?** When the treatment team asks the nurse not to interact with alters, the nurse needs to meet with the team and listen to the team members' views. The nurse(s) can ask for in-service education and seek training in regard to the client with DID as well. It can be problematic to have untrained people working with complex clients. Sometimes the team does not want staff nurses to interact with client alters because the staff nurse may be overcome with curiosity and encourage the client to make up alters by giving the client too much attention. Not everyone agrees. Wakeman (2002) suggests that curiosity by the nurse models that it is acceptable to be curious about the parts of the person (alters). This curiosity may facilitate working agreements among alters and eventual integration, according to Wakeman.

The International Society for the Study of Dissociation Guidelines for Treating Dissociative Identity Disorder (2005) state that health care professionals working with the client with DID must not encourage the client to create more alters or to adopt names if they have none, suggest clients ignore or get rid of alters, or play favorites with alters.

9. **Are alters real people within one person's body?** Downing (2003), a social worker and trained therapist, describes herself as a fully integrated person "formerly DID." Downing says that after she had integrated all her personalities, she was surprised she still had "all the thoughts and feelings that had been labeled as personalities." She wrote: "I came to realize that the personalities were always and only a collection of thoughts, feelings, experiences and memories that had been separated from normal awareness and from other collections of thoughts, feelings, experiences, and memories. Personalities are not real people."

The International Society for the Study of Dissociation agrees, saying: "The patient is not a collection of separate people sharing the same body. Personality and alter (alternative personality) have to do with dissociated parts of the mind influencing behavior of people with DID. Other terms preferred by some clinicians include self-state or part of the self or mind."

10. **Why do people who have DID self-mutilate? If you were Amanda's nurse, how would you need to respond to this client or any client who is thinking of hurting herself, threatening to hurt herself, or has hurt herself?** When people with DID inflict injury on themselves, they may be taking control, becoming an aggressor, and trying to lose the victim role (McAllister et al., 2001). Some people who inflict self-harm talk of it as a way to assure themselves they are alive or to assure themselves that they can feel.

You must take all threats of self-injury seriously, and before leaving the client, get the client to give assurance she will seek a staff member before hurting herself. Then notify the health care provider and share information about threats with the rest of the treatment team. Some clients will need an order for a one-to-one within eyesight intervention. Other clients can be managed with visual checks every fifteen minutes. You must keep in mind that clients can hurt or even kill themselves within a fifteen-minute framework. The person doing the checks needs to add some unexpected check times. This lets the client know that they can be checked at any time rather than thinking they have exactly fifteen minutes to hurt or kill themselves. If you delegate the checks to ancillary personnel, it is important to give them clear instructions, have the checks documented on a flow sheet, and provide close supervision to make sure these checks are done correctly.

You need to identify your feelings and attitudes about self-injury in general and Amanda's self-injury or potential self-injury. Some nurses will have strong negative reactions in response to people hurting themselves. These responses include a feeling of helplessness or despair, sympathy, anger or even rage, revenge, or a need to punish the client. Nurses may feel like ignoring the client, distancing from them, or making them wait. All of these feelings and behaviors tend to lead to the client feeling a lack of power and control. The nurse must provide a supportive presence through listening to the client, modeling calm, and getting the client to explore their feelings. The nurse can provide means for the client to vent feelings such as anger, rage, or guilt. Sometimes nurses mistakenly think a person who superficially cuts themselves will not commit suicide and that perhaps the client is only doing this to get attention. They may then withdraw attention from the client for this reason. The nurse must not let his or her personal feelings stand in the way of keeping the client safe. Actual injuries must be assessed and cared for in a timely fashion.

11. **What nursing diagnoses and treatment goals might the nurse write for this client?** Possible nursing diagnoses include: risk for violence: self-directed; high risk for self-mutilation; risk for violence: other-directed; chronic low self-esteem; and anxiety.

The long-term therapy treatment goal is often integration of the various personalities or at least some peaceful working agreement among the alters. Work is often directed toward an increased sense of connection between the personalities and eventually a state where none of the alternative personality states takes charge.

Goals on the nursing care plan would be directed to resolving the identified nursing diagnoses. Risk for violence to self or others or risk for self-mutilation would take priority and a goal might be no evidence of harm to self or no acts of aggression toward others.

12. **What are some of the nursing interventions and professional treatment approaches to DID?** Initial nursing interventions will focus on preventing the client from harming herself, by eliminating things that could be used for harm in her environment. The nurse will work to establish a trusting nurse-client relationship with a client who has never mastered trust. Interventions directed at building self-esteem will include identifying the client's strengths and helping the client use those strengths and modeling/teaching the client to make positive affirmations. The nurse can teach the client relaxation techniques to deal with anxiety.

Wakeman (2002) uses a facilitative model for doing with the client as opposed to doing for or to the client. Wakeman stresses helping the client gain a sense of self through pursuit of resources and strengths. The client is given the message that not remembering is not functional even though it is an important survival skill. Tools utilized by Wakeman and others include journaling; videotaping; keeping lists of goals, needs, and wishes; recording and replaying messages of support; and self-mapping. In self-mapping the client writes or draws a picture of how they see their selves at that point in time. This snapshot is compared with later self-mapping pictures. The client can see progress by comparing early to later self-mapping pictures. Watching a videotape of a client when one or more alters come out will often convince the nonbeliever in the DID diagnosis that this is indeed a real diagnosis. The client seeing him- or herself often gives up part or all of their denial. A popular term and tool used in treatment of DID has been "abreaction," a term used by Freud in 1892 to mean the re-living of a trauma. It involves a complete reexperience of some trauma including complete autonomic and sensory recall. Although controversial, hypnosis has been used as a way to facilitate abreaction for clients with DID. Combat veterans and other trauma survivors as well as persons with Borderline Personality Disorder and DID have been found to dissociate. All have in common the high incidence of trauma. In World War II health care professionals working with veterans found that when combat veterans were helped to abreact their trauma in a safe, therapeutic, controlled environment, their PTSD symptoms decreased. At some point in time after World War II, abreaction became a major part of the treatment of various dissociative disorders, as the wounds of trauma were viewed as similar to a boil needing to be opened in order to heal. With the recovered memory court challenges, abreaction fell out of favor; some clinicians are saying that abreaction does need to occur, but not to the exclusion of other therapies. Therapists must use judgment about timing, being careful not to rush the client. The client can be reconnected to the present through any of the senses. Nurses sometimes find a client having an abreaction. For example, the nurse discovers a clients screaming in the night and giving clues she or he can feel the weight of someone on them, smells the perpetrator, and so on. The nurse can gently talk to the client, saying something like: "Can you hear my voice?" Or the nurse can provide some music or a new scent and slowly and carefully reground the client.

Another tool used with clients with DID is designed to help the client feel the presence of a helping person when that helping person is not with them physically. The helping person provides the client with a simple handwritten message, a stuffed animal, or a ritual or rituals that can be seen or recalled for comfort. The caution here is to be aware of and consider the client's boundaries.

Small successes are seen as important because each small bit of progress can be a powerful step in recovery. Big steps can be overwhelming and traumatic. The client with DID may experience grief when faced with the reality of their forgotten experiences and a childhood that was lost.

During the course of therapy, the goal is often to facilitate the alters striking deals among themselves so the person is safe and can function. In West's description of his experiences with alters and therapy, he describes alters who did not feel welcome in his home. In order to get his alters to agree not to come out when he was romantically or sexually engaged with his wife, his wife had to agree, in a discussion with one of the alters, to welcome alters at specific other times (West, 1999). Some clients are described as having integrated all their personalities into one during extensive therapy; however, West and others point out that this may not always be possible.

On the other hand, Downing (2003) described a strong personal belief that "integration (of the alters) is a natural part of the healing process." She describes integration as "a choice to do more than just survive." While West seems comfortable not integrating his alters, Downing feels sorry for people who don't integrate.

13. What additional research is being done in the area of DID? Albach, Moorman, and Bermond (1996) studied ninety-seven adult survivors of extreme sexual abuse. The control group consisted of sixty-five women with ordinary unpleasant childhoods. The study group involved subjects who had been abused, and this group was divided into those who had received treatment and those who had not. About equal numbers of subjects (34 percent vs. 33 percent) in the treatment subgroup and the nontreatment subgroup reported having had the inability to recall abuse at some time. Only 1 percent of the control group reported an inability to recall unpleasant events. This study found that events seem to trigger later memories of abuse (e.g., discovering abuse of a daughter; suffering another trauma; confronting specific triggers, like the smell of a certain soap, when exhausted; being touched on the back; alcohol or tobacco on a male's breath; or footsteps on a stair). Verbal cues were found not to be as significant as olfactory, sensimotor, auditory, and visual cues. Calamari and Pini's (2003) research conducted with 162 female students suggests abused girls are insecurely attached and more prone to anger turned inward, with dissociation being a way to deal with anger.

References

Albach, F., P. Moorman, and B. Bermond. (1996). "Memory Recall of Childhood Sexual Abuse." *Dissociation* 9(4): 261–273.

American Psychiatric Association. (2000). *Diagnostic and Statistical Manual of Mental Disorders, 4th ed.* Text Revision. Washington, DC: American Psychiatric Association.

Calamari, E., and M. Pini. (2003). "Dissociative Experiences and Anger Proneness in Late Adolescent Females with Different Attachment Styles." *Adolescence* 38(150): 287–303.

Cook, L. (2005). "The Ultimate Deception: Childhood Sexual Abuse in the Church." *Journal of Psychosocial Nursing and Mental Health Services* 43(10): 18–24.

Downing, R. (2003). "Understanding Integration as a Natural Part of Trauma Recovery." http://mentalhealth.about.com/gi/dynamic/offsite.htm?site=http://www.issd.org/. Accessed November 6, 2004.

Holmes, L. "Abreaction: The Baby or the Bathwater." http://mentalhealth.about.com/cs/traumaptsd/a/abreact.htm. Accessed November 7, 2005.

International Society for the Study of Dissociation. http://mentalhealth.about.com/gi/dynamic/offsite.htm?site=http://www.issd.org/. Accessed November 4, 2005.

McAllister, M. (2000). "Dissociative Identity Disorder: A Literature Review." *Journal of Psychiatric and Mental Health Nursing* 7: 25–33.

McAllister, M. et al. (2001). "Dissociative Identity Disorder and the Nurse-Patient Relationship in the Acute Care Setting: An Action Research Study." *Australian and New Zealand Journal of Mental Health* 10: 20–32.

Middleton, W., and J. Butler. (1998). "Dissociative Identity Disorder: An Australian Series." *Australian and New Zealand Journal of Psychiatry* 32(6): 794–804.

Piper, A. (2004). "The Persistence of Folly: Critical Examination of Dissociative Identity Disorder. Part I: The Excesses of an Improbable Concept." *Canadian Journal of Psychiatry* 49(9): 592–600.

Silberg, J.L. (2000). "Fifteen Years of Dissociation in Maltreated Children: Where Do We Go from Here?" *Child Maltreatment* 5(2): 119–136.

Wakeman, S. (2002). "Working with the Center: Psychiatric Rehabilitation with People Who Dissociate." *Psychiatric Rehabilitation Journal* 26(2): 115–123.

West, C. (1999). *First Person Plural: My Life as a Multiple.* New York: Hyperion Press.

GENDER

Female

AGE

31

SETTING

- Physician's office

ETHNICITY

- White American

CULTURAL CONSIDERATIONS

PREEXISTING CONDITION

COEXISTING CONDITION

COMMUNICATION

DISABILITY

SOCIOECONOMIC

- Has a trust fund and is upper class without having to work

SPIRITUAL/RELIGIOUS

PHARMACOLOGIC

PSYCHOSOCIAL

LEGAL

- Need to avoid libel or slander

ETHICAL

- Refusing to treat client or alienating client so she goes to another health provider is questionable from an ethical standpoint

ALTERNATIVE THERAPY

- Getting a pet
- Volunteer work

PRIORITIZATION

DELEGATION

DIFFICULT

FACTITIOUS DISORDER

Level of difficulty: High

Overview: Requires keeping an open mind while carefully observing and assessing client's behaviors and sharing findings with team members who must be consistent in their responses to the client. The nurse must control any negative thoughts or reactions and select an appropriate professional attitude and behaviors. Knowledge of transference and countertransference is useful. Avoidance of defamation of character by libel or slander is essential.

Client Profile

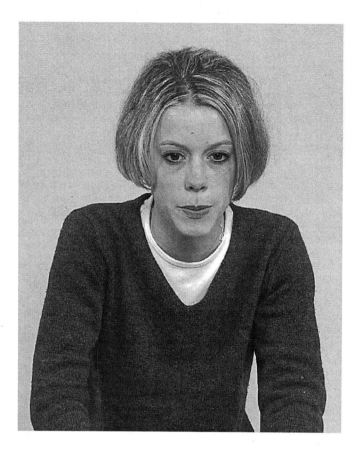

Linda is a 31-year-old single female who does not have to work as she has a trust fund left to her by a grandfather. A lawyer manages the trust fund and approves requests from Linda for money. Linda has lived in her own home, but is currently living with her parents because she says she is too ill at times to care for herself.

Linda has recently begun to frequently complain of seeing blood in her urine and having chills, fever, and bladder pain. She has been seeing a health care provider who is puzzled by her symptoms because the urinalyses are almost always normal with an occasional urine infection that responds to antibiotics. The client has a fever at each visit and looks pale and uncomfortable. On the first visit with the bladder-related symptoms, she provided a story about having extra pockets in her bladder wall that fill with urine and get infected; when they don't have urine in them, they have air, which is painful and requires hospitalization. In trying to verify this strange condition, the health care provider sought to find the name and address of the provider who identified it. The client was evasive, complaining of not remembering and providing a long involved story of earlier treatment by a urologist in a famous university hospital without supplying any real details.

Case Study

The office nurse goes to the waiting room to get Linda, weighs her, and takes her vital signs and a short history in preparation for seeing the health care provider. The nurse puts a glass thermometer in Linda's mouth and leaves the room to get a drink for the client who has complained of being thirsty. After the nurse closes the door, she remembers she forgot to remind the client to keep the thermometer under her tongue. As she opens the door, she thinks she sees the client take the thermometer from under the water faucet. The client quickly tells a story of needing to wash her hands. Linda's temperature is 101.8.

Although she cannot be sure the client had the thermometer under the faucet, the nurse mentions her suspicions to the health care provider. The provider does not say anything to the client but goes ahead with his assessment, and examination and orders a urinalysis. He tells the client he will be back after she is dressed. The doctor tells the nurse to recheck the temperature and stay in the room while it is being taken. The temperature is 98.4 on rechecking it. Neither the nurse nor the health care provider questions the client about this temperature. It is simply noted. The client is to drink at least six glasses of water a day and two glasses of cranberry juice and return in one week for further testing.

Later the health care provider mentions to the nurse in private that he suspects this client has Factitious Disorder. The provider tells the nurse he would like her to get some medical history on the client from the parents. The nurse recalls that she overheard the client tell the parents that the provider said he would have to run more tests and she was lucky to have parents to take care of her since she was so ill.

Questions and Suggested Answers

1. **What is Factitious Disorder, and how does this disorder differ from the somatoform disorders?** In the literature and in common practice, Factitious Disorder is often referred to as Munchausen's Syndrome (MS). A number of clinicians and writers prefer the term Munchausen's Syndrome, a term that preceded the name of Factitious Disorder. This syndrome was named for a famous eighteenth-century baron named Baron Karl Frederick von Munchausen, a great teller of lies. The client with Factitious Disorder feigns or causes elaborate and frequently contradictory symptoms in themselves and presents for medical attention. This person is often disappointed or angry if tests come out normal or if confronted about the possibility of feigned symptoms. The client often willingly submits to procedures that other clients would cringe about.

   The person with Factitious Disorder intentionally produces or feigns physical or psychological symptoms in order to assume the sick role. By contrast, persons with any of the somatoform disorders (Somatization Disorder, Conversion Disorder, Pain Disorder, Hypochondriasis, and Body Dysmorphic Disorder) do not consciously produce or feign symptoms, although the person with Hypochondriasis often realizes the feared disease may not be present while being unable to shake a fear of currently having the disease or getting it.

2. **What do you suppose the nurse was thinking when she opened the door and thought she saw the thermometer being held under the faucet water by the client? What emotions might this observation arouse in the nurse?** The nurse was probably wondering why the thermometer was under the water, and then it dawned on her that this could be hot water and the client could be feigning a fever. The next thought might be: "What do I need to do about this?"

   Yonge and Haase (2004) caution: "When Munchausen's or Munchausen's by Proxy is unmasked, there is a tendency for concern to be replaced by equal measures of hostility on the part of health care staff," and they remind us that these clients are deserving of compassion.

3. **Do you agree with the nurse's actions to say nothing of her suspicions about the thermometer being under the faucet to the client, but to then share her possible observation with the health care provider in private? Give a rationale for your answer.** The nurse's decision to say nothing to the client, but to report suspicions to the health care provider, is a good decision. The nurse is not sure of what she saw. The client is giving a shaky but still plausible answer for the water running. If the nurse were to confront the client, it would be the client's word against the word of the nurse. If the client was creating a higher temperature and was confronted about it, she would surely refuse to have the temperature taken again. The client could accuse the nurse of slander, storm off in a huff, and go see another health care provider who has a different and less suspicious nurse. There is the risk of legal action for slander, but there's a stronger case for legal action if the client can actually make herself sick and claim the provider and nurse missed the diagnosis due to falsely accusing her of feigning symptoms.

The nurse needs to be concerned about defamation of character, which is communication to others that is damaging to a client. Slander involves oral communication and libel involves written communication; therefore all nurses must be careful in what they say about others and in charting the nurse must be objective.

4. **If you were the nurse working with this client, how would you handle the situation if the provider asked you to recheck the client's temperature?** You would be wise to have a third person in the room with you when you recheck the temperature. Perhaps the health care provider would agree to chat with the client on a nonthreatening subject while you try to matter-of-factly recheck the temperature. Or perhaps another nurse could come in to do some task. You might offer an explanation for taking the temperature again, saying something like: "The provider is concerned that your temperature could be even higher than the reading we got, and wants me to take it now." If this seems devious, remember that there is still the possibility that this client is not feigning symptoms and that she could actually have a higher temperature than that previously recorded. You must keep an open mind and approach this situation from a problem-solving approach.

5. **Does this client have any signs and/or symptoms that match the criteria for Factitious Disorder?**

Criteria for Diagnosis of Factitious Disorder	Does This Client Match the Criteria?
Feigning of physical and/or psychological signs or symptoms, intentionally.	It would appear that the client is manipulating/changing her temperature readings. Further assessment is necessary to see if any other physical or psychological signs or symptoms are feigned intentionally.
The client's feigning of signs or symptoms is to assume the sick role.	Probably. From the overheard remark of the client to her parents, she would appear to be interested in maintaining the sick role.
Motivation other than to assume the sick role is not present (e.g., not done to get economic gain or avoid legal responsibility or improve physical well-being).	The client has a source of money, which is the estate of her grandfather. She does not appear to gain monetarily or to avoid legal responsibility or improve her well-being by feigning symptoms. Although more assessment is needed, it would appear that the only clue to motivation points to the sick role.
Subtypes of Factitious Disorder • Psychological signs and symptoms predominating • Physical signs and symptoms predominating • Combined psychological and physical signs and symptoms	This client appears to have physical signs and symptoms predominating.

(Adapted from APA, 2000)

6. **What is thought to be the cause of Factitious Disorder?** Clients with Factitious Disorder have a strong need to be nurtured. Some theorists think that the symptoms of Factitious Disorder are a type of psychological defense mechanism. Other ideas about the cause of the disorder include: having medical or surgical procedures during childhood or adolescence with a great deal more nurturance than received usually at home, anger at the medical profession or a prior medical setting employer, presence of a personality disorder, or an important relationship with a health care provider in the past.

7. **Why is the true incidence of Factitious Disorder in the general population unknown?** The true incidence, or even a close estimate, of this disorder in the general population is unknown because of several factors. The disorder may go unrecognized and unreported. Some people with this disorder present to a variety of health care facilities and may even change their names and demographic data. One man is reported to have been admitted over 850 times to 650 British hospitals and having received 42 laparotomies in a 12-year period (Papadopoulos and Bell, 1999). While he was found out, many others are not.

The incidence of the disorder within large general hospitals has been found to be approximately 1 percent of those patients on whom psychiatric consultation was requested (APA, 2000). The incidence is actually probably higher in general hospitals when you consider that a psychiatric consult was not asked for in all cases.

Papadopoulos and Bell described five cases of "patients with Munchausen Syndrome" who were neurosurgical admissions to a neurosurgical unit of a hospital. Clients presented with a variety of acute neurological complaints including head injury and hemiparesis. Although some cases of Munchausen Syndrome presenting to this unit may have been missed, the authors make a good case for neurosurgeons, who will exclude serious pathology through imaging, missing this diagnosis less often than general surgeons, who are more likely to do exploratory surgery. The incidence of patients (identified later as having Munchausen Syndrome) admitted to this unit was 0.032 percent of all admissions. These clients (with MS) all sought admission at night and 50 percent on a Friday or a Saturday. The average stay was less than twenty-four hours. None underwent surgery, but they did have a variety of costly procedures done, such as myelogram, CAT scans, MRI, lumbar punctures, and even one intubation and ventilation at the referring hospital.

8. **In what settings would a nurse encounter a client with Factitious Disorder?** In addition to encountering a client with Factitious Disorder in the health care provider's office or on a neurosurgical unit as described above, the nurse would especially find these clients in the emergency room and the admissions unit of a psychiatric hospital, although they can be in just about any health care setting. There have been cases of nursing students with Factitious Disorder (Munchausen Syndrome) reported in the literature. Yonge and Haase (2004) discuss a case of a student nurse who has Munchausen's and Munchausen's by Proxy and whose education as a nurse is delayed to "prevent the possibility of her becoming a hazard to patients." There is a case in the literature of a young adult nurse treated for septic arthritis of her knee—an infection that she produced herself (Guziec, Lazarus, and Harding, 1994). Another case presented in the literature was a woman with a history of three vaginal deliveries and six miscarriages who had previously had a hysterectomy but presented saying she was miscarrying. She later admitted to genital self-mutilation to feign the bleeding of miscarriage (Ajibona and Hartwell, 2002).

9. **If you were the nurse in this case, what additional assessments would you like to do? What nursing diagnoses would you likely find in this client or other clients with Factitious Disorder? What goals would you likely write for this client or other clients with Factitious Disorder?** If you the nurse in this case, you could try to get the client's early developmental history from the parents. You could also get a health history for the client from the client as well as from the parents. It would be helpful to learn if there is a family history of Factitious Disorder or FD by Proxy (Munchausen's by Proxy) or any other mental disorder. It would be helpful to gather some data on the family dynamics and any family crises and how crises are dealt with or how problems are solved. Working with the parents would require a release of information from the client, which could be denied. Risk for self-mutilation or suicide needs to be assessed.

Some nursing diagnoses that you might find in this client or others with FD include:

- Risk for self-mutilation
- Risk for self-directed violence
- Ineffective coping
- Loneliness
- Noncompliance
- Chronic low self-esteem
- Dysfunctional family processes

The staff in the health care provider's office may have goals that are not the goals of the client or mutually agreed upon goals. This is not an easy case, nor is any case involving a person presenting with Factitious Disorder. Some staff might be delighted if the client bolted out the door never to return, but there is an ethical issue here in not helping the client because the client will go on to use a lot of health care resources unnecessarily and will likely harm themselves. Client goals would likely include:

- Will accept mental health counseling and attend therapy sessions
- Will identify needs and share feelings
- Will identify and engage in new and appropriate ways to nurture self

10. **What interventions would you likely write for this client or another client with a similar situation?** Some interventions that might prove helpful include:

- Build a therapeutic relationship with the client. The client needs to learn to trust others. Building trust often starts with just one person. There are many things that the nurses can do and model in order to increase a client's trust. This is difficult when a nurse believes or knows the client is not telling the truth about their symptoms and may be feigning illness by self-inflicted injury or causing symptoms and cannot be trusted alone in a room with a thermometer or a urine sample or other items. Building a relationship with the client is a process most often requiring patience, planning, consistency, and time. It is essential to getting the client into therapy and/or to eventually give up seeking nurturance through feigning medical or psychological symptoms. Clients will have what is known as transference, which involves unconsciously viewing and reacting to the nurse, health care provider, therapist, or other person as someone from his past, and this causes them to distort or misperceive the behaviors of that person. The distortion and misperception can involve negative views or positive views of that person. Thus the client may be more drawn toward a staff member who unconsciously reminds him or her of someone who was kind and nurturing and repelled by someone who reminds him or her of someone who was not. A skilled therapist can work with clients with varying transference and use the transference to help the client (Feldman and Feldman, 1995). The average nurse is more comfortable with a client who seems to have a positive perception of the nurse. The nurse can also unconsciously react to the client's behavior and damage to their body or underlying issues and have intense reactions. Feldman and Feldman conclude that "recognition management of the counter transference reactions likely to emerge in work with factitious disorder patients are particularly important if the therapy is to be maximally effective." Willenberg (1994) discusses the use of countertransference in Factitious Disorder.

- One or two assigned staff to deal with client consistently. Yonge and Haase (2004) state that the nursing care plan needs to be developed in such a way as to combat pitting of one staff member against other members. It is helpful for building relationships as well as to discourage manipulation of staff for the client to see the same staff consistently. Options for assigning staff may be limited, but if not, then assign a staff member the client seems to have some positive regard for and/or a nurse who wants to accept the challenge of working with a client in whom progress may be slow. The nurse needs professional support and consultation. In many settings, including the setting of this case, the nurse will be hard pressed to find time and support for working with a client with Factitious Disorder and will of necessity need to avoid even beginning to believe he or she is the only one who can help the client. This client needs to be finessed into seeing a mental health professional. Staff nurses and health care providers are capable of finding out what would motivate a client to see a mental health professional such as a psychiatric nurse clinician, a psychologist, or social work professional trained in working with this type of problem.

- Journaling to identify feelings and needs. If the client is willing to share a journal with you or another nurse or health care provider, positive feedback can be given to encourage the client to continue when they are writing about difficult feelings and perceptions that might be judged badly by others. The person reading the journal can simply write in the margin of a strange perception, "Is there another way to think about this?" or something similar to get the client to entertain other ways of thinking.

- Encourage client to identify ways to nurture him- or herself or assign client specific self-nurturing tasks. The nurse can engage the client in a brainstorming session about ways that she can think of to nurture herself. The introduction might be something like: "Lots of our patients/clients have difficulty doing things to nurture themselves. What special things do you do to nurture yourself?" and "What other things have you thought of that you might like to try? " The health care provider might prescribe something like a weekly massage or yoga sessions.

- Encourage a pet and volunteer work to reduce focus on self and to reduce loneliness. The person with Muchausen's syndrome may be lonely and in need of attention. Finding ways for the client to get legitimate attention without endangering self or others is a challenge. Having a pet and doing volunteer work are two ways for the client to get attention in lieu of using the sick role.

11. One of your peers asks you to explain Munchausen's Syndrome by Proxy. Give a brief explanation. This syndrome is referred to as Factitious Disorder by Proxy in the DSM-IV-TR and is discussed in Appendix B under Criteria Sets and Axes Provided for Further Study. Research criteria rather than criteria for diagnosis are provided (APA, 2000). The criteria for research involve not the production or feigning of symptoms in oneself like Factitious Disorder, but rather the intentional causing or feigning of the physical or psychological signs or symptoms in someone else who is under the person's care. It usually involves a caretaker and most often the mother producing or feigning signs and/or symptoms in her child. There are famous cases, which have gone to trial, in which a nurse has induced or fabricated signs and symptoms in infants, children, and even adults under his or her care. The motivation for the perpetrator's behavior has to be to assume the sick role by proxy in order to meet the research criteria. External incentives such as economic gain must be absent, and the behavior cannot be better explained by different mental disorder or disorders.

Factitious Disorder by Proxy (Munchausen's Syndrome by Proxy) constitutes child abuse, which involves legal requirements for reporting by health care professionals, and is a serious charge against a parent. It is serious for the victim as they suffer from physical problems that are unnecessary and pathological and can be life threatening.

References

Ajibona, O.O. and R. Hartwell. (2002). "Feigned Miscarriage by Genital Self-Mutilation in a Hysterectomised Patient." *Gynaecology* 22(4): 451.

American Psychiatric Association. (2000). *Diagnostic and Statistical Manual of Mental Disorders, 4th ed.* Text Revision. Washington, DC: American Psychiatric Association.

Feldman, M.D. and J.M. Feldman. (1995). "Tangled in the Web: Countertransference in the Therapy of Factitious Disorders." *International Journal of Psychiatry in Medicine* 25(4): 389–399.

Guziec, J., A. Lazarus, and J.J. Harding. (1994). "Case of a 29-Year-Old Nurse with Factitious Disorder: The Utility of Psychiatric Intervention on a General Medical Floor." *General Hospital Psychiatry* 16(1): 47–53.

Papadopoulos, M.C. and B.A. Bell. (1999). "Factitious Neurosurgical Emergencies: Report of Five Cases." *British Journal of Neurosurgery* 13(6): 591–593.

Willenberg, H. (1994). "Countertransference in Factitious Disorder." *Psychotherapy Psychosomatics* 62(1–2): 129–134.

Yonge, O. and M. Haase. (2004). "Munchausen Syndrome and Munchausen Syndrome by Proxy in a Student Nurse." *Nurse Educator* 29(4): 166–169.

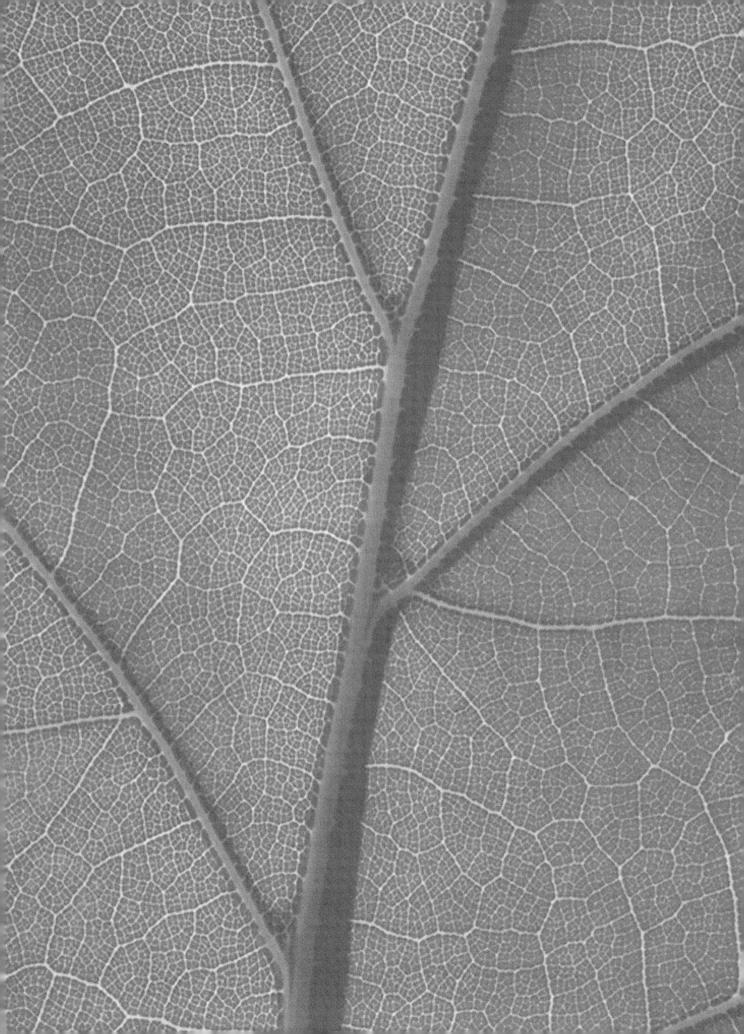

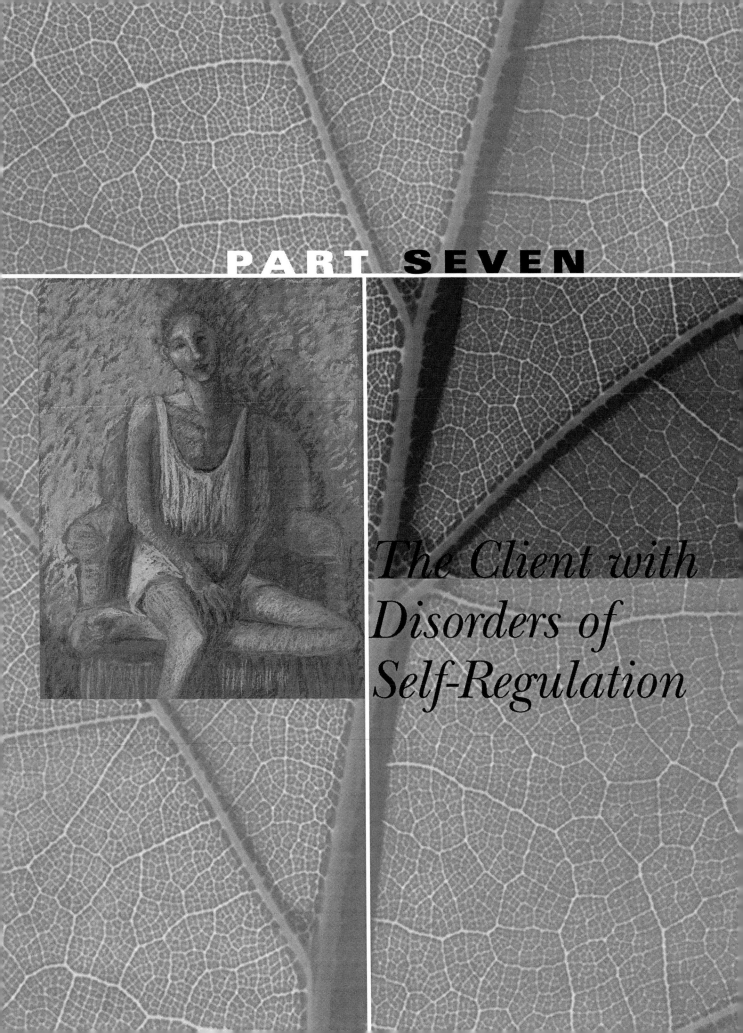

PART SEVEN

The Client with Disorders of Self-Regulation

Sabine

GENDER

Female

AGE

26

SETTING

- Eating disorders unit of a private psychiatric hospital

ETHNICITY

- White American

CULTURAL CONSIDERATIONS

PREEXISTING CONDITION

COEXISTING CONDITIONS

- Nicotine abuse
- Alcohol abuse
- Depressed mood

COMMUNICATION

DISABILITY

SOCIOECONOMIC

- Upper middle class

SPIRITUAL/RELIGIOUS

- Connecting with a higher power to deal with abuse of food and alcohol and as a means of dealing with anxiety

PHARMACOLOGIC

- Buproprion hydrochloride (Wellbutrin, Zyban)

PSYCHOSOCIAL

- Socialization impaired by need to hide eating behavior

LEGAL

ETHICAL

ALTERNATIVE THERAPY

- Twelve-step program of AA for alcohol abuse and abuse of food
- Hypnosis for smoking

PRIORITIZATION

DELEGATION

BULIMIA NERVOSA, PURGING TYPE

Level of difficulty: Moderate

Overview: Requires knowledge of the signs and symptoms and behaviors associated with Bulimia Nervosa in order to identify clients who may have this disorder early on. Critical thinking is necessary to identify therapeutic approaches to clients with Bulimia Nervosa and to help them change harmful behaviors associated with binging and purging. Knowledge of the disorder is necessary in order to educate clients about the disorder.

Client Profile

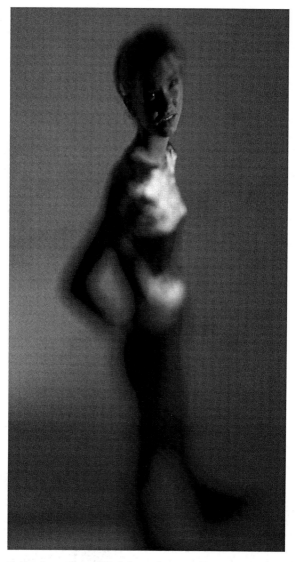

Sabine has a distorted body image because of her eating disorder.

Sabine is a 26-year-old single woman who grew up in an urban upper-middle-class family in a western state. Her parents both worked and gave her whatever she wanted except their time, so she soothed herself with food. Sabine was a cheerleader in junior high school but failed to make the team in high school due to being over-weight. Currently she is living alone in an apartment complex. She has a master's degree from a major university and earns over $100,000 a year managing a software development team. Sabine wants an attractive figure and will do almost anything not to be overweight like she was as a teenager. For the past four months, four or five times a week, she has been stopping at night at the grocery store on the way home from work and buying foods she has been denying herself in her previous dieting phase—donuts, cookies, potato chips, and ice cream bars—which she eats as fast as she can in the car on the way home. When she gets home she goes to the bathroom and makes herself vomit. She feels guilty after the binging and vows she won't do it again, but within a few days she finds herself binging again. She also eats excessively at all-you-can-eat buffets, then goes home and takes an excessive amount of laxatives and prune juice. Sabine feels guilty about her binging and purging, abuses alcohol to make herself forget, then feels guilty about drinking too much, and eats some more. She smokes from one to two packages of cigarettes a day. Sometimes she feels "depressed."

Sabine began to have abdominal discomfort and pain in the middle of her chest (esophageal area). She went to see a nurse practitioner, who noticed that she had enlarged parotid glands and eroded teeth enamel. When questioned about her eating habits, Sabine admitted to binging and purging. The nurse practitioner convinced Sabine to get treatment at an inpatient eating disorder program. Sabine went home, called work to arrange time off, drank a few drinks, packed a couple of suitcases, and called a taxi to take her to the eating disorders unit.

Case Study

Sabine is admitted to the eating disorders unit. During the initial assessment by the primary nurse, Sabine describes bowel irregularities and says she will need the laxatives she brought with her. The nurse advises Sabine that all the laxatives she has will have to be turned in and any she takes will have to be ordered by the doctor and dispensed by the nurse. Sabine becomes very upset and says: "I will talk to the doctor about this. I will just leave if I can't have my laxatives that I need."

The nurse reviews Sabine's chart and the CBC report, and during the initial assessment notices the client's affect is somewhat blunted. The nurse notices the client's enlarged parotid glands and the erosion of dental enamel. The nurse looks at Sabine's hands and asks: "Are you left-handed or right-handed?" Sabine answers: "Left-handed."

The nurse finds that Sabine weighs 142 pounds and is 5 foot 5 inches tall. Sabine sees herself in the mirror and says: "I look like a beer barrel." A psychiatrist, who examines Sabine, makes a diagnosis of Bulimia Nervosa (BN). He orders individual and group therapy, a twelve-step program, and buproprion hydrochloride (Wellbutrin). She asks for hypnosis to help with smoking cessation, and the psychiatrist orders it. After a few days, Sabine is offering to help on the unit.

Questions and Suggested Answers

1. **What signs did the nurse practitioner and the nurse find that would lead any health care professional to suspect an eating disorder? What signs and symptoms suggest Sabine has Bulimia Nervosa and not Anorexia Nervosa? How do these eating disorders differ and how are they similar?** The nurse practitioner and the admitting nurse saw the teeth with enamel erosion and the parotid gland enlargement, signs found in clients who have self-induced vomiting. The acid of the vomitus erodes the enamel of the teeth over time. Dentists are often the first to suspect an eating disorder when they see a client with these signs.

   Sabine has complaints of esophagitis, abdominal discomfort, and bowel irregularity, which are common complaints in Bulimia Nervosa. People with Anorexia avoid food, especially high-calorie food, whereas the client with Bulimia eats these foods and purges. Sabine is not underweight for her height, and she would likely be at least 15 percent underweight if she had Anorexia Nervosa. In Bulimia Nervosa the client may or may not have menstrual irregularities, and this symptom is not part of the criteria for the diagnosis; however, in Anorexia Nervosa, the client must have missed at least three menstrual cycles.

   In both Anorexia and Bulimia there are two subtypes: purging and nonpurging. For a diagnosis of Bulimia Nervosa, the client must not only binge but also have inappropriate compensatory behaviors two or more times a week on average for three months. In the nonpurging type these compensatory mechanisms can be fasting or excessive exercise but not self-induced vomiting or misuse of enemas, laxatives, or diuretics, which, if used, would constitute purging. The "nonpurging type" of Bulimia Nervosa means only that the client has not used purging behaviors during this episode of Bulimia Nervosa, but may have used them in a previous episode.

2. **The psychiatrist gave Sabine a diagnosis of Bulimia Nervosa, Purging Type. What criteria does she have to meet to receive this diagnosis? Does she appear to meet these criteria?**

Criteria for Bulimia Nervosa	Do Client's Signs and Symptoms Match?
Has repeated binge eating (i.e., eating within a short amount of time more food than most people would eat in the same amount of time under similar conditions) with a feeling of loss of control over eating during this time.	Yes, Sabine is buying large amounts of high-calorie foods and eating them in the car on the way home as quickly as she can or binging in buffet restaurants and then making herself vomit when she gets home.
Repeated use of inappropriate methods to avoid weight gain, such as but not limited to: overuse/misuse of laxatives, diuretics, enemas, exercise, and periodic fasting.	Yes, she uses large amount of laxative and prunes and prune juice and has taken large amounts of laxatives to the treatment facility in her suitcase.
Average of biweekly or more frequent binge eating episodes and inappropriate compensation over a three-month period.	Yes, for past four months, four or five times a week Sabine has binged and purged and used laxatives to excess.
Body shape and weight must exert an undue influence on the person's self-evaluation.	Sabine was a cheerleader, and she does not want to lose her shape. She thinks of herself as a beer barrel at weight 142.
Binging and compensatory behaviors must not occur only during episodes of Anorexia Nervosa.	No evidence of Anorexia Nervosa.
Criteria for Purging Type	
Has induced vomiting and/or misused laxatives, diuretics, or enemas, on a regular basis, during this current episode.	Yes, has induced vomiting and misused laxatives on a regular basis in last four months.

(Adapted from APA, 2000)

It is important to realize that a person can begin a binge in one setting and continue in another (e.g., begin in a restaurant and continue at home or eat in more than one restaurant during a binge). Sometimes clients with Bulimia Nervosa try to hide the problem by eating in more than one setting so others are less aware of their total consumption during a short period of time. Snacking small amounts throughout the day or eating excessively at a holiday meal or a celebration are not considered binging.

3. **Why was the nurse interested in knowing whether the client was left-handed or right-handed? When the nurse reviews the lab tests, which tests are likely to be abnormal in this client because of purging by self-induced vomiting?** The nurse no doubt saw Russell's sign when looking at the client's hands. Russell's sign is a callus or scarring on the back of the client's hand due to trauma caused by the teeth when inducing self to vomit.

Lab tests likely to be abnormal because of purging and resultant dehydration include hypokalemia (low potassium) and metabolic acidosis. The client can also have low sodium, low chlorides, and/or low potassium levels due to self-induced vomiting. Zepf (2004) points out that hypokalemia in healthy young women is indicative of Bulimia Nervosa but is not a screening test. Most young women with BN who purge do not present with electrolyte abnormalities. Clients who abuse laxatives may have low magnesium and low phosphate levels. The client may have hypernatremia or hyponatremia from drinking too little or too much fluid to control weight (Ressel, 2003).

4. **What two screening questions could the nurse practitioner have used to screen this client for Bulimia? What other screening(s) might the nurse have done?** Frisch and Frisch (2006) point out that although clients with Bulimia can be very evasive about their binging and purging, they do respond well to direct clinical questioning. These authors suggest two screening questions: 1. Are you satisfied with your eating patterns? and 2. Do you ever eat in secret? Frisch and Frisch note that a study by Freund, Graham, Lesky, and Moskowitz found that 100 percent of people with Bulimia would answer "no" when asked the first question and "yes"

when asked the second question. It was found in this study that only 10 percent of clients without Bulimia answered the same way as clients with Bulimia.

The nurse could screen for depression and alcoholism, which are often seen in clients with eating disorders. Alcohol is a depressant drug and could cause depressed mood. On the other hand, some clients self-medicate their depression with alcohol. Sometimes depression precedes the eating disorder and may be one of several factors triggering binge eating and purging. Depression can follow the eating disorder as a complication.

5. **What possible reasons could the nurse practitioner have had for referring the client to an inpatient eating disorders clinic rather than an outpatient program?** This client is likely to find many reasons not to attend outpatient meetings. The client has more opportunities to binge and purge on an outpatient basis. Extensive education and therapy can be done in less time on an inpatient basis. The inpatient unit may be the safest place for the client to deal with any underlying depression and issues associated with depressed mood. Inpatient treatment allows the nursing staff to gather data and closely observe the client for any suicidal ideation as well as improvement in mood that brings increased energy needed for carrying out suicidal ideation. Some clients with eating disorders do have suicidal ideation and do commit suicide ("Eating Disorder Behaviors Linked to Suicide Risks," 2004).

If the client had a severe decrease in potassium and metabolic acidosis, she would benefit from hospitalization to improve her electrolyte and metabolic state. Typically clients with these problems receive 40 to 80 mEq of supplemental potassium until their potassium level is normal, and sometimes clients receive IV saline to turn off the rennin angiotensin aldosterone system to allow normalization of the potassium level (Cumella, 2003).

6. **What items might Sabine have brought with her to the hospital that would need to be inventoried and locked up? Can the nurse delegate these tasks to ancillary staff? How can the nurse deal with Sabine's threat to leave if she is not allowed to keep her laxatives?** The nurse can delegate the inventory, and the locking up, of all items with which Sabine could harm herself (e.g., razors, scissors, and mirrors) to ancillary staff who have been trained to do this. The staff needs to check the client's belongings for laxatives, enemas, medications, and other means to purge such as prune juice and write these items on an inventory list and secure them from the client. The nurse retains responsibility for this delegated task and must make certain it is done correctly.

Sabine can leave against medical advice (AMA) if she chooses to do so in response to being denied her laxatives and other purging items. The nurse needs to stay calm and matter-of-fact and stress that the staff want Sabine to stay in the program so they can help her. The nurse can let her know that the rules on laxatives and other purging materials apply to other clients too and that she or he knows it is difficult for the client. Empathy and respect are important.

7. **Sabine offers to help the nurse's with little tasks and in general tries to please the nurses on the unit. Is this common behavior of someone with Bulimia Nervosa, and what must you and other nurses keep in mind when this occurs?** Working to please the nurses and others is a common behavior in clients with BN. The client with BN may attempt to manipulate the nurse(s) (Dichter, Cohen, and Connolly, 2002) and expect nurses to relax the rules for him or her. Although nurses need to be aware that clients may attempt to manipulate, they must keep an open mind about an individual client's behavior and give positive verbal reinforcement when it changes in a positive direction. Manipulation opportunities are reduced or eliminated when nurses are consistent in holding all clients to unit rules and adhering to the treatment plan.

8. **You are teaching a class on the eating disorders unit. Sabine wants to know if males ever suffer from Bulimia Nervosa. She has observed that all the clients on the unit are female. Peers ask about the usual onset of Bulimia and the cause of Bulimia. How would you answer these questions?** The onset of BN is usually between the ages of 15 and 24. Figures on the incidence of Bulimia Nervosa may be skewed due to the ability of people with this disorder to hide it well. An estimate of the prevalence in females is 1–3 percent with the prevalence in males being about a tenth of that found in females (APA, 2000). Clinic and population studies have found

90 percent of those with the disorder to be female. Dichter, Cohen, and Connolly (2002) point out that this disorder is most common in White American women but there has been an increase in eating disorders in minority populations and areas of the world that previously did not experience these problems.

The American Academy of Pediatrics (Ressel, 2003) has stated that 1–5 percent of adolescent females in the United States meet the criteria for Bulimia Nervosa and that there are numerous mild cases not meeting criteria for diagnosis but having physical and psychological consequences.

Eating disorders in males may occur after dieting due to teasing about weight, a desire to be more lean for participating in a particular sport, or a desire to be more attractive to potential significant others. Eating disorders may be increasing among men involved in particular sports such as track and wrestling and in homosexual males (Cumella, 2003).

The cause of Bulimia Nervosa is unknown at this time. Some genetic studies are being conducted. A Japanese study reported by H. Koizumi and others from Chiba University Japan found significant differences in brain-derived neurotrophic factor (BDNF) 198G/A when comparing levels in 198 subjects with eating disorders and 222 normal controls ("Neurotrophic Factor 196G/A Polymorphism May Trigger Eating Disorder," 2004).

Some theorists suggest that Bulimia Nervosa is a culture-bound syndrome and that Anorexia Nervosa (AN) is not culture-bound (Keel et al., 2003) whereas other theorists think AN is also culture-bound. Keel and his colleagues argue that for a person to binge and purge, there must be an abundance of food available and a strong desire to not be overweight, both factors influenced and/or controlled by culture.

Cooper, Wells, and Todd (2004) describe a cognitive theory of causation of Bulimia Nervosa as well as a cognitive model of treatment. They suggest some event, such as a negative statement about the client by someone else or a sight of him- or herself in the mirror, triggers negative self-appraisals and a belief of being unacceptable in some way. The negative self-appraisals bring negative emotions (e.g., anxiety, depression, or guilt) that are managed by eating. Eating distracts the person from the negative emotions and decreases the intensity of the emotions. The client has conflicted thoughts as a result of positive beliefs about eating along with negative beliefs about the consequences of eating. The conflict is resolved by permissive thoughts and/or thoughts of no control or both, and the person then binges, continuing the cycle of binging and purging.

9. **Clients with Bulimia who are in the education class about the disorder, learn about medical problems arising from binging and purging. What medical problems associated with Bulimia Nervosa do these clients, nurses, and other health care professionals need to be aware of?** In severe cases of Bulimia Nervosa (and Anorexia Nervosa also) lower mineral density in the bones of the whole body and especially the lumbar spine can develop. It is important to be aware of the need for bone marrow density (BMD) screening and replacement calcium ("Study Recommends BMD (bone mineral density) Assessment in Severe Bulimia and Anorexia Nervosa Cases," 2004) Other health problems that can occur with Bulimia Nervosa include abdominal pain, esophagitis with possible scarring and stricture, gastroesophageal reflux disorder (GERD), gastritis, perforation of the esophagus, pancreatitis, and oropharyngeal problems such as dental caries, swollen salivary glands, and chronic sore throat. The esophagus can perforate or rupture, which can be fatal. The client may develop cardiovascular problems including palpitations and arrhythmias due to the metabolic abnormalities, which come from self-induced vomiting (e.g., low potassium and chloride levels and alkalosis). Electrolyte imbalance can lead to fatal cardiac arrthymias. The client may also have metabolic abnormalities from laxative abuse (e.g., low magnesium and phosphate levels.) Clients with Bulimia Nervosa may have fertility problems and irregular menses.

10. **When assisting in gathering data on this client, what information would you especially be interested in gathering?** You need to take the vital signs no less than once a day. Clients almost always have bradycardia due to either exercising excessively or as a result of starvation (Frisch and Frisch, 2006). While the staff needs to know the baseline weight and possibly a biweekly weight, the team may or may not want the client to be focusing on this weight. Sometimes clients are weighed backward on the scale to prevent their knowing their weight. Weights are always done at the same time of day to provide a more accurate comparison. It is

important to have an accurate measure of what the client is eating at meals and during the twenty-four-hour period as well as an intake and output. The client's elimination is also an important part of data gathering. The nurse will do a brief assessment of all body systems daily and will include an assessment of mood and affect. Data will be gathered on past patterns of eating. The pattern generally is fasting, binging and purging, and making efforts to keep others from knowing. It is helpful to know these patterns and what thoughts and moods precede and follow the binge. This will be useful in identifying any triggers for binging and ways to reduce these triggers.

The nurse will need to assess the client's self-esteem and body image. A simple way to gather data on the client's body image is to ask the client what they say to themselves when they look in the mirror. Another way is to have the client draw a picture of themselves and describe it. A third method is to ask the client what they like best about their body and what they would change if they could and why they would change it.

The nurse will assess the whole person and in doing so will include a spiritual assessment to identify spiritual strengths and needs.

11. **What nursing diagnoses would Sabine likely have that are related to her diagnosis of Bulimia Nervosa? What goals would you likely write for this client?** Likely diagnoses for Sabine include:

- Ineffective individual coping
- Anxiety
- Powerlessness
- Altered nutrition: more than body requirements
- Disturbed body image
- Chronic low self-esteem

Goals could include:

- Will describe the problem-solving process
- Will have no evidence of binging or purging
- Will eat food slowly, taking at least thirty minutes to consume prescribed diet
- Will identify three things liked about own body and three things about self
- Will state feels more in control and less anxious

12. **What interventions would you need to write and implement for this client? What nonpharmaceutical interventions are commonly used with clients who have Bulimia Nervosa? Are medications used to treat Bulimia Nervosa? What are the likely reasons for the health care provider ordering buproprion hydrochloride (Wellbutrin, Zyban)?** An important intervention is to build trust and rapport with the client by means such as promising only what can honestly be delivered and being honest, empathetic, and respectful.

The nurse and treatment staff can help clients build self-esteem and a healthy body image by encouraging clients to identify and talk about their strengths. In group and individual one-to-one, clients can be asked to give positive affirmations, such as "I am a good mother or father" or "I am good at math." People with low self-esteem are prone to say they cannot think of one good attribute that they have. The nurse can help clients use their talents to get positive feedback from others. Nurses can help clients improve their body image by encouraging grooming and giving positive feedback to clients. The nurse is like a mirror. The client can see himself or herself in a more positive way through the nurse.

The nurse can encourage the client to identify feelings. Sometimes people soothe bad feelings such as loneliness or inadequacy with food binges and then experience guilt over eating too much. Helping the client to find appropriate healthy ways to deal with feelings is an important intervention.

After assessing the client's knowledge of Bulimia Nervosa, the nurse can reinforce correct knowledge and beliefs and give the client additional information they are lacking. Accurate knowledge about the disorder tends to help the client feel and be more in control. Nutritional education is also important.

The nurse can encourage the client to journal about or talk about significant interpersonal relationships and to find healthy ways to relate to others as well as encourage the client to go to scheduled family, individual, and group therapy. On the inpatient unit the nurse may get the client to go to sessions by simply saying it is time to go or by offering to walk with the client to the session. The twelve-step program of AA is used not only in the treatment of alcohol abuse but is used with clients with eating disorders also. This twelve-step program can help this client with both problems.

Mantle (2003, 42) discusses how hypnosis can be used in the treatment of eating disorders to help the client "develop feelings of control and mastery over their thoughts and behaviors." Sabine asked for hypnosis for smoking cessation, but it will be helpful for cessation of binging and purging too.

Structured cognitive behavioral therapy is often used with clients who have Bulimia Nervosa. Cooper, Wells, and Todd (2004) found four types of thoughts preceding binge eating: positive beliefs about eating, negative thoughts regarding weight and shape especially related to acceptance by self and acceptance by others, permissive thoughts, and "no control" thoughts. In the cognitive behavioral therapy, these four key types of thoughts need to be changed.

The selective serotonin reuptake inhibitor (SSRI) fluoxetine (Serotonin) has been approved by the U.S. Food and Drug Administration for the treatment of Bulimia Nervosa (Zepf, 2004). The psychiatrist in this case prescribed buproprion hydrochloride (Wellbutrin, Zyban) probably because it is not only helpful in treating depression, but it is used to help clients quit smoking.

References

American Psychiatric Association. (2000). *Diagnostic and Statistical Manual of Mental Disorders, 4th ed.* Text Revision. Washington, DC: American Psychiatric Association.

Cooper, M.J., A. Wells, and G. Todd. (2004). "A Cognitive Model of Bulimia Nervosa." *British Journal of Clinical Psychology* 43(1): 1–16.

Cumella, E.J. (2003). "Examining Eating Disorders in Males: An Obsession With Bulging Biceps and a Sculpted Six Pack Can Lead to Serious, But Treatable, Problems." *Behavioral Health Management* 23(4): 38–42.

Dichter, J.R., J. Cohen, and P.M. Connolly. (2002). "Bulimia Nervosa: Knowledge, Awareness, and Skill Levels Among Advanced Practice Nurses." *Journal of the American Academy of Nurse Practitioners* 14(6): 269–276.

"Eating Disorders Linked to Suicide Risks." (2004). *Woman's Health Weekly*, June 3, 63–64.

Frisch, N.C. and L.E. Frisch. (2006). *Psychiatric Mental Health Nursing, 3rd ed.* Albany, NY: Thomson Delmar Learning.

Keel, K.P. et al. (2003). "Are Eating Disorders Culture-Bound Syndromes? Implications for Conceptualizing Their Etiology." *Psychological Bulletin* 129(5): 747–769.

Mantle, F. (2003). "Eating Disorders: The Role of Hypnosis." *Pediatric Nursing* 15(7): 42–44.

"Neurotrophic Factor 196G/A Polymorphism May Trigger Eating Disorder," (2004). *Womens Health Weekly,* July 8, 82.

Ressel, G.W. (2003). "AAP Releases Policy Statements on Identifying and Treating Eating Disorders." *American Family Physician* 67(10): 2224–2226.

"Study Recommends BMD Assessment in Severe Bulimia and Anorexia Nervosa Cases." (2004). *Women's Health Weekly,* June 3, 72.

Zepf, B. (2004). "Metabolic Abnormalities in Bulimia Nervosa." *American Family Physician* 69(6): 1530–1531.

GENDER

Female

AGE

21

SETTING

- General hospital

ETHNICITY

- East Asian American mother and White American father (deceased)

CULTURAL CONSIDERATIONS

- Eastern value of honesty conflicts with need to hide and lie about hair pulling

PREEXISTING CONDITION

COEXISTING CONDITION

- Depressed mood

COMMUNICATION

DISABILITY

SOCIOECONOMIC

- Low-income college student with scholarship and part-time job with little or no help from family

SPIRITUAL/RELIGIOUS

PHARMACOLOGIC

- Fluoxetine (Prozac)

PSYCHOSOCIAL

- Prior sexual abuse
- Isolates herself to pull hair

LEGAL

- Adult client reveals sexual abuse as a child

ETHICAL

ALTERNATIVE THERAPY

- Marjoram leaves
- Aromatherapy
- Acupuncture
- Hypnosis

PRIORITIZATION

DELEGATION

MODERATE

IMPULSE CONTROL DISORDERS: NOT ELSEWHERE CLASSIFIED TRICHOTILLOMANIA

Level of difficulty: Moderate

Overview: Requires knowledge of impulse control disorders, understanding of the client's background and personal situation, empathy and rapport with the client, and understanding of the impact of traditional and alternative medications and therapies.

Client Profile

Deidre is a 21-year-old student at a large university, on scholarship and part-time work with little financial help from her family. When she was 7, her mother went into the psychiatric hospital for depression. Her father had been killed in an accident when she was a toddler so a grandfather cared for Deidre and her brother. The grandfather sexually abused her, and by the time her mother came home Deidre literally was pulling her hair out. She would pull first one hair and then another from the top of her head and then eat the hair. Deidre also pulled out eyelashes at times and began to pull out pubic hair, thinking no one would see that area and she could better hide her hair pulling. She did not tell her mother about the sexual abuse because her grandfather said her mother would either go away again or die if she found out. Deidre isolates herself, choosing not to date or go places with other girls. She tries hard not to pull her hair out and may go several days without pulling, but always begins again. Her habit is to carefully choose a hair, twirl the hair, pull it in such a way as to remove the hair bulb with the hair, rub the hair between her fingers, and then eat it.

Case Study

Deidre has been eating marjoram leaves and doing aromatherapy in an effort to stop eating hair. She experiences a loss of appetite, weight loss, weakness, diarrhea, nausea and vomiting, increased white blood cells, and fever. She has resisted going to see a health care provider, but finally allows her mother to take her to the provider's office. The provider notices Deidre has a strange pattern of baldness on her head. He asks her if she pulls her hair, but she denies it. Deidre is admitted to the hospital for observation prior to possible exploratory laparoscopy. The primary nurse assigned to Deidre does a head-to-toe assessment and makes a note of the bald spot at the top of Deidre's head. Later the nurse forgets to knock before entering Deidre's room, and just as she is getting ready to apologize for not knocking, she sees Deidre, with her eyes closed, put what looks like a hair in her mouth and swallow it. During the hospitalization, Deidre undergoes an exploratory laparoscopy. The surgeon finds a trichobezoar. When the surgeon confronts Deidre about the trichobezoar, the mother becomes angry with Deidre for insisting on the first visit to the health care provider and thereafter that she was not eating her hair. Deidre's mother demands that Deidre stop eating hair and stop lying immediately.

The health care provider diagnoses Deidre with Trichotillomania, suggests acupuncture and hypnosis, and prescribes fluoxetine (Prozac).

Questions and Suggested Answers

1. **Why do you suppose Deidre denied pulling her hair when the health care provider asked her? Is it common for people who pull their hair out to deny it?** Deidre is possibly ashamed of her hair pulling, and does not want anyone to find out. People who pull their hair out often believe they are the only ones to pull their hair out and that no one else could possibly understand their doing this. In addition, people who pull out their own hair are both the perpetrator and the victim, which creates a sense of shame as well as the fear that others will view them in the same way as self-mutilators.

   The literature and Internet is full of stories of people with Trichotillomania who denied pulling their own hair when taken to a pediatrician by their parents and who denied it a second time when taken to a dermatologist when the parents, angry at the pediatrician for suggesting such a thing, took their child to see another specialist. Some children make up stories to explain the hair loss (e.g., ringworm or a skin disease), while others pile their hair on their head over the bald spot or wear a hat all the time. Some sufferers get a wig, and they may then pull hair from the wig, as their compulsion to pull out hair is intense at times.

2. **What is Trichotillomania, and what are the essential features of Trichotillomania? Describe some common behaviors carried out by individuals with Trichotillomania.** Trich is from the Greek for hair, tillo is from the

Greek for to pull, and mania is for the morbid impulse to pull. This name for pulling out one's own hair was first suggested in 1889 by Hallopeau, who was caring for a young man who pulled out all his body hair.

To meet the diagnostic criteria for Trichotillomania, a person must:

- Pull out his or her own hair on a recurrent basis and the hair loss must be noticeable by others. Hair can be pulled from any part of the body on which hair grows. The common sites for pulling hair out are scalp, eyebrows, and eyelashes.
- The person must feel an increasing sense of tension just prior to pulling the hair out or when trying to resist pulling the hair out.
- The person must feel pleasure, gratification, or relief when pulling the hair out.
- This behavior must not be accounted for by some other mental disorder or medical condition such as a dermatological problem.
- The behavior must cause clinically significant distress or impairment in important areas of the person's functioning such as social or work. (Adapted from APA, 2000)

There are people who meet all of the criteria except one: they deny experiencing tension prior to pulling their hair out. There are researchers and authors who suggest this criterion be removed.

Common behaviors of people with Trichotillomania include studying a hair root, twirling it off, pulling the strand between the teeth like dental floss, grinding it between the teeth, or engaging in trichophagia (eating hairs), but they usually do not do this in front of others. According to one study, 50 percent of all hair pullers had an oral component with one in ten describing swallowing of the hair (Keuthen, Stein, and Christenson, 2001). People who pull their own hair often have other nervous behaviors such as biting their nails and cuticles, picking scabs or picking their nose or lips, rocking, and head banging (Keuthen, Stein, and Christenson, 2001).

A person with Trichotillomania may have an urge to pull hairs from other people and do it casually. They may also pull hair from pets, dolls, and fibrous materials such as in carpets or sweaters.

3. **You have entered the client's room without knocking. You are pretty sure that the client is unaware that you entered the room and saw her eating a hair. What will you do now? If you confront the client and she says: "You must be mistaken. I would never think of doing such a thing," what do you say or do?** You have several options, such as backing out without saying anything, confronting the client in some way, or pretending you saw nothing and apologizing for not knocking. One response that would seem appropriate would be to model honesty. You could say gently: "Deidre, I am so sorry that I entered your room without knocking. You deserve your privacy, and I apologize for forgetting to knock. I saw you swallow what looked a hair. I can understand your doing this. I want you to talk with me so I can help you." If the client denies eating a hair, you can plant the idea in her mind that it is all right to change her mind and admit the behavior later. You could say something like: "Perhaps you didn't, but I would understand your denying it if you did. Most people who pull their hair don't want anyone to know it, but once they admit it and get help, it gets better for them. If you change your mind, I will help you."

4. **Is there a relationship between Trichotillomania and self-esteem and/or body image?** A study at the Massachusetts General Hospital Obsessive-Compulsive and Trichotillomania Clinics had sixty-two women with Trichotillomania complete a survey, which posed questions about their hair pulling and their feelings about themselves. It turned out that the more time a person spent pulling their hair, the lower their self-esteem, although the severity or amount of hair loss was not related to the level of self-esteem. The study also found that high levels of anxiety and depression in subjects were associated with low self-esteem. Subjects also reported a high rate of dissatisfaction with aspects of their appearance unrelated to hair pulling and the greater the dissatisfaction the lower the self-esteem. The researchers pointed out that this study suggests the treatment not focus solely on hair pulling but on issues of self-esteem, depression, anxiety, and dissatisfaction with appearance or body image (Soriano and O'Sullivan, 2005).

5. **What is a trichobezoar? Is the response of the mother, to the news that Deidre has a trichobezoar, helpful or not? How will you respond to the client and her mother in regard to what the mother has said to the**

client? A trichobezoar is a hair ball. Trichobezoars can grow large enough to fill the entire area of the stomach before they are discovered. Cases of trichobezoars have occurred in which the small intestine was filled as well as the stomach. Trichobezoars are relatively rare in the United States. Keuthen, Stein, and Christenson (2001) wrote that they saw three hundred cases of Trichotillomania and only one of them had a trichobezoar. A study of children with Trichotillomania in India is said to have found over 38 percent with trichophytobezoars, which are hair balls consisting of hair and vegetable matter. The nurse needs to develop a working relationship with the mother and find out if she or any of her family in India experienced Trichotillomania.

The mother chastising the client for lying and talking about being disappointed in her may arise out of an Eastern value of honesty and not causing the family to experience shame because of your actions. The mother's remarks no doubt lower the client's probably already low self-esteem.

Although the mother's response is not a helpful response, it is a fairly common response or reaction of significant others of hair pullers. Telling the person to just stop is particularly common and not helpful because trichotillomania is a compulsive disorder, not a choice. It is a challenge to the nurse to model a more empathetic approach to the client and to find additional ways to get the mother to use a more empathetic approach.

After developing some rapport with the mother, you can speak with her alone and enlist her help in working with Deidre. Talk with her about the need to be supportive and how to be supportive. Educate her about Trichotillomania and give her some suggestions of what to read, such as *Help for Hair Pullers: Understanding and Coping With Trichotillomania* (Keuthen, Stein, and Christenson, 2001) and/or *The Hair Pulling Problem; A Complete Guide to Trichotillomania* (Penzel, 2003).

You can also work with Deidre alone. Encourage Deidre to talk about her feelings and about the hair pulling. Listen to her. Work on a nursing care plan with her input.

6. **Deidre's mother asks you, "What causes Trichotillomania? and "What are the complications of Trichotillomania?" What is your response?** What little is known about the cause of Trichotillomania includes the idea that the hair pulling often begins with a stressful event (e.g., a loss, the first menstrual period, or sexual abuse); however, it does not always begin with a stressful event. Some people with this diagnosis describe beginning to pull their hair out on a dare from a peer and continuing this behavior for years, while others describe pulling hairs out to make things more perfect (e.g., pulling whiskers from a cat because they stick out too far). Some of the people with Trichotillomania have a perfectionist tendency (Keuthen, Stein, and Christenson, 2001), while others claim the hair pulling started with no explanation.

Some researchers think Trichotillomania may be genetic with more than one gene involved. Some theories suggest a link with neurotransmitters. It may be a genetic predisposition that is activated by stress and other factors.

You will want to educate the client and her mother that one complication is trichobezoars like the one the client had removed surgically. A bezoar can lead to anemia, abdominal pain, hematemesis, nausea and vomiting, bowel obstruction, and even perforation and death in rare cases. In addition to bezoars and the obvious alopecia, there can be infection and scarring. The hair growth may be slowed or stopped, and there can be changes in hair color or texture. There can be damage to the teeth as well.

7. **What happens when people with Trichotillomania try to just stop pulling their hair as Deidre's mother suggests?** While some people on the Internet sites about Trichotillomania claim to have resolved their hair pulling by prayer and turning it over to God, most sufferers of this disorder seem to try hard to stop and struggle for years until they get into some treatment that works for them, and even then they often have periodic relapses. Sufferers of Trichotillomania describe going to great lengths to stop pulling their hair and/or eating it. They discuss using various methods such as wearing a ski mask over the head and face and/or tying their hands together, and making deals and contracts with themselves as well as threatening themselves to keep from pulling out their hair. Failure to stop pulling and/or eating hairs is often blamed on the extreme need to release tension.

8. **The client asks you if you think munching marjoram leaves and some aromatherapy will calm her enough to stop the impulses to pull out her hair. What will you tell her? What type of treatment has been found to work for people with Trichotillomania? Discuss acupuncture and hypnosis as treatments for Trichotillomania.**
The Internet offers many herbal, aromatherapy, and homeopathy cures for Trichotillomania. The website www.trichotillomania.co.uk/treatment/index.htm lists aromatherapy oils that are "great for scalp pullers" including ladies PMS mix #4 and unisex fragrance. There is herbal homeopathy for Trichotillomania such as belladonna cuprium, lillium tigrinum, arsenicum, Lachesis, and more. There is aloe vera for itching scalp, chamomile tea, Kava Kava, and marjoram leaves for munching to calm the self and to "help lash and scalp pullers to remain calm and stay centered and pull free." However, Penzel (2003) lists these herbal cures as among things that don't work. You could refer the client to Penzel's book, which provides a great deal of information about what does not work, what may work, and what does work, for treating Trichotillomania. You might tell her that chewing marjoram leaves may do no harm and may help if she strongly believes it will, but she will need to check with her doctor to see if there is any interaction between marjoram leaves and other medication she is taking. Even if her doctor approves of chewing marjoram leaves, this will not be the whole answer to stopping hair pulling.

Self-monitoring has been found to be helpful to clients, and it also provides a good assessment database. Keuthen, Stein, and Christenson (2001) and Penzel (2003) both provide information on self-monitoring in which the client writes about every episode of hair pulling and describes it in detail, graphs the number of hair pulled on a chart, and counts every hair pulled. There is often a decrease in the occurrence of a negative behavior when a person records its occurrence. Some people decrease the behavior to avoid seeing the physical evidence. The hair puller also can rate the severity of hair pulling using the Massachusetts General Hospital Hair Pulling Scale, which has seven questions that measure not only the severity of hair pulling but rate the frequency of urges, intensity of urges, and ability to control urges. Triggers such as situations, particular times, specific rooms, and activities are also noted by the client. There are also forms for noting hair pulling feelings and thoughts. When the client fills out these assessment forms, clues are given as to how to reduce the hair pulling (e.g., if hair pulling mainly occurs when watching TV, the person could reduce the amount of time watching TV and could use something for tactile contact like a piece of satin on a blanket).

According to Penzel (2003), treatments that work for some but not others include hypnosis and biofeedback. An article by Mark Lehrer (2005), director of the Biofeedback Clinic Santa Monica, discusses biofeedback for people with Trichotillomania. Lehrer claims this method helps by teaching the client a new way to release and reduce tension. The goal is to reduce muscle tension in the face, forehead, and neck and provide a healthier focus on these areas.

Treatments that have been found to work in many cases include Habit Reversal Training, which was developed by Drs. Azrin and Nunn and their colleagues, and Cognitive Behavioral Therapy (CBT).

Habit Reversal Training as designed by Azrin and described by Prenzel (2003) involves monitoring behaviors for a given period of time, for example, one week. This includes all urges to pull; occurrences of pulling including a description of when and where; emotions prior to pulling and feelings just after; and identifying response precursors such as what is being done with the arms and hands just before starting to pull (e.g., touching or stroking hair. The response detection procedure involves experiencing and describing muscles used when pulling and in a series of actions with pauses of ten seconds between each action the client describes and experiences the movements he or she uses to get ready to and to pull the hair. Response training involves choosing a behavior that prevents pulling such as clenching a ball. The person practices clenching the ball for three minutes and releasing one minute and repeats this five times; identifying habit prone situations such as talking on phone or reading; relaxation training such as deep breathing exercises or body relaxation exercises to use when the urge to pull occurs; and positive attention, which is a form of overcorrection. If pulling occurs, the client can practice positive attention, such as brushing or repairing eye makeup.

Penzel (2003) provides a self-help program in his book and it incorporates Habit Reversal Training steps and additional work as well. It includes destigmatizing self, building strengthening and awareness of the disorder, behavior analysis, self relaxation training, diaphragmatic breathing training, stimulus control, motivation building, weekly review and self evaluation, and maintenance and relapse prevention.

9. **What teaching will you do on fluoxetine (Prozac)? What response will you give to the client sharing her fear she cannot afford the Prozac?** You will advise the client that fluoxetine is an antidepressant—a selective serotonin reuptake inhibitor, which makes more serotonin, a neurotransmitter, available to the brain. It has been found to be helpful in impulse control in studies of people with Trichotillomania. It takes about four weeks or longer for full therapeutic effects. If the client is a night sleeper, you will advise her to take the medication early in the morning and avoid taking the medication in the afternoon since it can cause some nervousness and insomnia. Advise the client that she needs to talk with the psychiatrist first before stopping this drug, changing the dose that she takes, or before taking any other prescription, OTC drugs, or herbal preparations. You could tell the client that fluoxetine has helped many people with their depressed moods and their Trichotillomania, but that if for some reason after four to six weeks, it is not helping her, she needs to talk with her doctor about another SSRI or another type of medication rather than stopping medication completely.

You could share with the client that the drug companies producing the various SSRIs have assistance programs for clients who can't afford the medication. She can ask her health care provider about this. The provider can call the Pharmaceutical Research and Manufacturing Association for information on the various assistance programs of the drug companies. The client can also access Internet information about financial assistance in obtaining SSRIs.

10. **What is your response to the client's revelation that she was sexually abused when she was 7 years old and she wants to keep it a secret?** You need to advise the client that this kind of information must be shared with at least her health care provider and psychiatrist as it is a critical piece of information in helping her deal with her depression and her Trichotillomania. Advise her also that you must share this information with your supervisor. Her psychiatrist will probably advise her to deal with her sexual abuse in therapy either concurrently or prior to dealing with her Trichotillomania in therapy. Talking with your supervisor will help you determine if this information needs to be shared with the rest of the treatment team and what, if anything, is to be charted.

Had the grandfather not been dead, you would also have to comply with any state laws regarding the reporting of sexual abuse. All the states have laws about reporting child sexual abuse, which involves sexual abuse of anyone under age 18. The states differ in their statutes of limitations for the time frame in which the sexual abuse can be reported and prosecuted. In many states the statute of limitations (i.e., a designated time limitation for reporting and prosecution) begins when the abused is at the age of maturity (usually 18). In some states the time runs out when the adult is 28, whereas in others it is a certain number of years after the person realizes they were harmed.

11. **What do you think is the primary nurse's role in caring for this client?** The primary nurse is a client advocate, educator, and role model. Other staff members may not understand the complexities of Trichotillomania and be critical of the client's behavior. The nurse must not join in this criticism but instead describe the client's behavior objectively and paint the client as a worthwhile individual. The role of the nurse is to educate not only the client about the disorder and its treatment but the staff as well. The nurse can suggest sources of information for the client. The nurse can teach and model relaxation techniques. Encouragement to seek further treatment is within the role of the nurse. The staff or primary nurse is not going to do the therapy for sexual abuse or Trichotillomania with the client, but can support and encourage the idea of the client getting help with her sexual abuse issues and point the client to information that describes current treatments and the degree of success various treatments have had.

12. **Based on the information you have, what nursing diagnoses, goals, and interventions would be appropriate for this client?** Nursing diagnoses you could write include but are not limited to:

- Pain
- Chronic low self-esteem

- Ineffective denial
- Anxiety
- Hopelessness
- Deficient knowledge regarding Trichotillomania related to unfamiliarity with information resources
- Risk for loneliness

Some likely goals include but are not limited to:

- Will be free from pain
- Surgical site will evidence healing and no signs of infection
- Will be able to give positive affirmations
- Will state is motivated to get treatment for depression, sexual abuse, and hair pulling
- Will develop personal goals associated with depression, sexual abuse, and hair pulling (e.g., Will join a Trichotillomania support group)
- Will be able to feel comfortable with self
- Will be able to have some control over behavior
- Will have a plan to deal with any relapses
- Will develop a plan to stop isolating and develop social friends

Interventions that hold promise for being helpful include:

- Provide pain medication promptly as ordered
- Instruct client to call for pain medication when pain is 4 to 5 on a scale of 1 to 10
- Instruct client on signs of infection and to report these signs promptly
- Provide time for client to talk about feelings and concerns and to ask questions
- Model and teach positive affirmations
- Educate client and family about Trichotillomania and provide resources for their further self-education
- Instill hope that client can be helped to overcome hair-pulling impulses
- Discuss tendency of people with Trichotillomania to isolate and have client talk about ways she may have isolated
- Provide client with resources to read about other people with Trichotillomania and how they dealt with relapses while in treatment e.g. the Trichotillomania Learning Center Website http://www.trich.org/about_ttm (Soriano and Sullivan, December, 2005).
- Ask client for her ideas on how to begin to interact socially with other people
- Encourage client to begin journaling

References

American Psychiatric Association. (2000). *Diagnostic and Statistical Manual of Mental Disorders, 4th ed.* Text Revision. Washington, DC: American Psychiatric Association.

Keuthen, N.J., D.J. Stein, and G.A. Christenson. (2001). *Help for Hair Pullers: Understanding and Coping With Trichotillomania.* Oakland, CA: New Harbinger.

Lehrer, M. (2005). "Biofeedback: Its Use and Application." Available at www.trich.org/about_ttm/alttherapies.asp. Accessed December 7, 2005.

Penzel, F. (2003). *The Hair Pulling Problem: A Complete Guide to Trichotillomania.* New York: Oxford Press.

Soriano, J.L. and R. O'Sullivan. (2005). "Trichotillomania and Self-Esteem." Available at www.trich.org/about_ttm. Accessed June 14, 2006.

GENDER	**PSYCHOSOCIAL**
Male	■ Isolation due to stigma and fear of being found out
AGE	■ Stress on marital relationship due to past and current sexual contact with children
25	**LEGAL**
SETTING	■ Reporting requirements in regard to a child telling about sexual activity with an adult
■ Pediatric unit then local jail	■ Acting on sexual urges with children is a crime and punishable by law
ETHNICITY	**ETHICAL**
■ White American	■ Do Pedophiles deserve treatment and compassion or just punishment such as incarceration, probation, lifelong tracking, and ostracism?
CULTURAL CONSIDERATIONS	
■ Small town, large family	**ALTERNATIVE THERAPY**
PREEXISTING CONDITION	**PRIORITIZATION**
COEXISTING CONDITION	■ Safety of the child
COMMUNICATION	■ Safety of other children (future victims)
DISABILITY	■ Need for psychological and medical help for child as victim as well as for child's family
SOCIOECONOMIC	■ Psychological and other treatments for the client as perpetrator
■ lower middle class	■ The perpetrator needs to be kept safe from hurting others and safe from suicide attempts
SPIRITUAL/RELIGIOUS	**DELEGATION**
PHARMACOLOGIC	

PEDOPHILIA

Level of difficulty: High

Overview: Requires the ultimate in professionalism to help a person who has Pedophilia learn to control their sexual urges and to live in society without being sexually involved with children. Involves reporting to a state agency any information provided by children who have been the subject of sexual acts or personal knowledge of sexual activities between a child and an adult. Requires ability to assess for suicidal ideation and to "anchor" a person who has suicidal potential.

Client Profile

Edgar, a 25-year-old married male with a stepdaughter and a natural daughter, grew up the youngest child in a large family. The family lived in a small town where everyone knew everyone, but there were secrets in Edgar's family. Edgar's father drank a lot and talked about sex a lot, and something did not seem right when he was around small children. A couple of his grown children would not trust him alone with their children.

When Edgar graduated from high school, he moved into his married sister's home. In the car one day, her 6-year-old son said something that caused her to suspect sexual activities between her brother and her son. She had no proof, but she asked Edgar to leave. Edgar immediately moved in with his brother's family. He shared a room with the brother's 5-year-old boy. Edgar's brother had no idea of what had transpired in the sister's home. Not too long after Edgar moved in, his brother was playing with his son and the son asked if he wanted to play "tiger bellies" like Uncle. When he was asked what that was, the boy's father was shocked to hear it involved some genital stimulation. Edgar admitted to his brother that he had experienced fantasies and sexual urges about sex with children since he was 16 years old. Edgar was asked to leave and told by his brother to get counseling. Edgar did not go to counseling, but instead found himself another place to stay and a well-paying job. Within a couple of months, he married an attractive woman who had a 3-year-old daughter and a year later they had another child.

Case Study

Edgar's 5-year-old daughter, Mindy, is in the hospital for treatment associated with her diabetes. The hospital is in the closest city to the small town where the family lives. Edgar is going to stay all night on the cot in the child's room while his wife stays at home with the other daughter. The night nurse makes rounds and finds Mindy sleeping on the cot with Edgar. The night nurse did not think too much about this as children often feel insecure in the hospital and want their parents close by. The next day Mindy says to her primary nurse: "Don't touch me down there. Only my daddy can touch me there. Oops, I am not to tell anyone. Don't tell anyone, please."

Edgar finds himself in jail waiting to see the judge in regard to child sexual abuse charges. His wife has threatened divorce. He has begged her not to divorce him. He has agreed to go into treatment, yet he is afraid he will be sent to prison and lose his wife, his job, and all respect from any source due to the stigma attached to sexual preference of children and child molestation. The nurse working at the jail makes rounds. The nurse is to do a brief check on this new inmate.

Questions and Suggested Answers

1. **What actions had to taken in response to Mindy's revelation that her daddy is the only one who can touch her "down there" (her genitals) in a certain way?** The child's statement had to be reported to, and investigated by, the proper state authorities, which in many states is the Department of Child and Family Services. The nurse was legally required to report this information and was also obligated to share this information with her supervisor and with the child's pediatrician. The pediatrician then has the option to talk with the mother and with the father separately or leave this up to the proper authorities. Most states have a hotline telephone number for reporting suspected cases of child abuse and/or neglect. Some states have the option for school nurses and nurses in pediatric clinics to do the reporting on a secure Internet line.

2. **Does Edgar's behavior match the diagnostic criteria for Pedophilia? Does a person who meets these criteria have to experience distress in some area of functioning to have the diagnosis of Pedophilia? Do most Pedophiles abuse only children in their family or belonging to friends or neighbors?**

Criteria for Diagnosis of Pedophilia	Does Client Behavior Match These Criteria?
For a time period of at least six months, the client has reoccurring, intensely sexually arousing fantasies, urges of a sexual nature, or has some type of sexual activity with a prepubescent child or children.	It would appear that the client has experienced reoccurring sexual fantasies and had some sexual activity with children around five to six years old for over six months, but this needs to be verified.
Sexual urges have been acted on or there is marked distress or interpersonal difficulty caused by sexual urges or fantasies.	Yes, sexual urges have been acted on with nephews and his own female child.
Person is age 16 or older and five years or more older than the child or children who are subjects of the sexual urges, fantasies, or behavior.	Yes, Edger is over 16 and more than five years older than the children who are subjects of his sexual urges, fantasies, or behavior.

This client's behavior appears to match most or all criteria for Pedophilia. The client does not have to experience distress in some area of their life to have a diagnosis of Pedophilia, unlike some of the other diagnoses in the Diagnostic and Statistical Manual of Mental Disorders (APA, 2000). Many with this diagnosis are said to not experience distress.

Some clients with Pedophilia are attracted to only males and some to only females. This client is attracted to males and females and perhaps adults as well as children. The phrase "Exclusive Type" is used if the person is attracted only to children and the phrase "Nonexclusive Type" if the person is attracted to both children and adults. Murray (2000) states that some Pedophiles and child molesters actually prefer sex with adults, but select children since they are vulnerable and available.

Some people with Pedophilia seem to limit their behavior to children within their household, including their own children or stepchildren or other relatives, while others with this disorder are sexually aroused by any child and may or may not act on their urges (APA, 2000). Some Pedophiles have hundreds of children they act out sexually with during their lifetime while "most pedophiles tend to be either a direct relative of the child or a friend of the family with the sexual abuse occurring within the child's own home" (Rosenberg, 2002). There are reported cases of people abducting children or taking in foster children for sexual purposes or, like our client, marrying someone with children (APA, 2000); however, Rosenberg states that "less than 3 percent of all reported sexual abuse cases are perpetrated by strangers who kidnap and sexually assault the child."

3. **Are some Pedophiles attracted only to children of a certain age? Do most pedophiles begin to have sexual urges, fantasies, or activity with children in adolescence like Edgar? What justification do people with Pedophilia use when they have sexual activity with a child or children?** People with Pedophilia often report they are attracted to children of a certain age group. The adult who is attracted to female children tends to prefer 8- to 10-year-olds, while those attracted to males often prefer boys older than 10. Some, like the father in this case, prefer 5- to 6- or 7-year-olds or even younger children.

   According to accounts by people with Pedophilia and observations by people who work with Pedophiles, the behavior most often starts when the person is an adolescent or young adult in the early 20s (Rosenberg, 2004; APA, 2000).

   Themes used by adults who have sexual activities with children include: "He or she wanted it" or "It was educational" or "He or she was being sexually provocative." These comments can be thought of as "thinking errors" since they basically consist of blaming or minimizing.

4. **Is it unusual that this client is married, has sex with his wife, and has a second child? Are all Pedophiles male like the client in this case?** According to Rosenberg (2002) the Pedophile has little, if any, interest in sex with adult men or women, but many Pedophiles get close to or marry adults of the opposite gender to gain access to children. There is a type of Pedophilia in which the Pedophile is sexually attracted to adults as well as children (APA, 2000).

People often think that all Pedophiles are males, but there are also female Pedophiles. Periodically we read in the news of women being involved in child pornography and of young female teachers seemingly unable to resist having sex with younger underage male students. Perhaps some of these female teachers who had sex with young male students are Pedophiles: fantasizing and having urges about sex with children and then acting on these urges.

5. **What are the current beliefs about the cause(s) of Pedophilia? Are all child abusers Pedophiles?** The cause of Pedophilia is not known. Dr. Berlin, a noted Pedophilia expert associated with Harvard University, believes that this disorder is a "lifelong sexual orientation just as hetero and homosexuality" are and points out that "patients can be terrified by the discovery of pedophilic cravings." (Edwards, 2004). In an article in the *Harvard Mental Health Letter* (Rosenberg, 2004), it is suggested that this tendency is established genetically before birth or early in life. The idea of inherited biological abnormalities is strengthened by the reported cases of men who developed Pedophilia and other atypical sexual urges in midlife as a result of developing brain tumors in the area of the brain that regulates judgment and impulse control.

Another popular theory is that people with Pedophilia are compensating for feeling a lack of power and lack of control in relationships with adults by engaging in sexual activities with children—activities where the adult Pedophile can have control. Yet another theory is that people who are Pedophiles were abused as children and they simply continue the cycle of abuse by abusing children. This theory is weakened by the fact that not all Pedophiles were abused as children. The *Harvard Mental Health Letter* (Rosenberg, 2004) points out that not all child abusers are Pedophiles and describes a recent study in which only "about 12 percent of 200 convicted child molesters were sexually abused as children."

Child abuse can be physical and not sexual. Not all people labeled as child abusers, even if the abuse is sexual, can meet the DSM (APA, 2000) criteria for Pedophilia. Rosenberg (2002) points out that a child molester "can sexually offend for other reasons (than the urges of a pedophile) and his or her sexual interest in children is usually secondary or tertiary to such interests in adults."

6. **What did you think or feel when you read that Edgar had sexual activity with two of his nephews and then his stepdaughter?** Perhaps this information made you angry or made you feel nauseated. Perhaps you felt badly and were concerned for the abused children and their families. Perhaps you identified with the victims and bad memories came to mind because you had been abused yourself. Perhaps you could identify with Edgar and his predicament because you have this problem or someone in your family does. Whatever your feelings, it is good to recognize them and admit that it is all right to feel these feelings, then you must sort these feelings and thoughts out and decide if you can put them aside and work with Edgar in a professional and therapeutic manner. You may want to do this or you may want to stay as far away from the Edgars of this world as you can. It is best to keep an open mind about the possibility that the person with Pedophilia needs treatment, and it needs to somehow be provided as a means of protecting children. Punishment rarely if ever changes this person, who, even if incarcerated, will be released into the community at some time.

7. **Edgar was advised by his brother to go into counseling for his unacceptable behavior with children. Were you surprised that he didn't go to counseling? Why or why not?** When people with Pedophilia get treatment, it is usually because they are coerced by the legal system mandating it or because they think it will get them a lesser sentence or perhaps occasionally to avoid a divorce if they are married. A number of authors (Rosenberg, 2002; APA, 2000) point out that rarely does a person with Pedophilia seek treatment. People with pedophilia are afraid that if they do, their secret is out and this may cause them repercussions such as incarceration, probation, signs in their yard identifying them, hate acts by others, or any number of other legal and social problems.

8. **If you were the nurse working in the jail, what would you ask Edgar and/or tell him when you go to do a brief check on him?** As the nurse working in the jail, you need most to assess this client for suicide ideation and for depression. Periodically in your local newspaper, perhaps you have seen an article saying that a person, who committed a crime with some social stigma attached to it, has committed suicide in jail. People with pedophilia come from all social strata, some without work and some from professional and high level jobs.

Regardless of social standing, a person can become depressed and hopeless when facing charges of crimes against children—crimes with great social stigma. You need to quickly build some rapport with this client by introducing yourself by name and stating that you are the nurse and that you would like to talk briefly with the client to see how you might help him. You might ask how he is feeling and then spend a few minutes listening. Before you leave, however, you must ask: "Have you thought about hurting yourself or killing yourself?" Whether this client denies having thoughts of suicide or not, you can then ask: "What would keep you from killing yourself? (What anchors you to this world?)" This technique of "anchoring" the client is a well-known and often used technique of therapists working with depressed clients who are potentially suicidal. Many times it is the person's children and thoughts of his or her children being without a father (or mother) that keep the client from killing him- or herself. In this case, this anchor may not work. The client may say something like: "When I am dead, people will be sorry they treated me so badly." A response by the nurse or other professional of: "What if they are not? What if you are lying there in the coffin, no mourners as they are all out partying and you have died for nothing?" Response by client may be: "Oh well, I will be out of my pain." The nurse might counter with: "How do you know? Perhaps you will be in more pain." At some point you can suggest that killing yourself is always an option but a one-time option that you cannot take back and perhaps it would be better to wait and see how things turn out. You can also say something like: "I want you to promise me you will not kill yourself, and I want a written contract with you." Getting a written contract for no suicide does work. Another necessary action on your part is to let the psychiatrist on call and the jail personnel know that this client is at risk for suicide.

9. **Will Edgar go to prison and/or to treatment, and will he have to register as a sexual offender?** What happens to Edgar will depend on what happens in his court hearing(s). He may go to prison where he may or may not get treatment, which varies from facility to facility and may or may not be effective. Or he may be on parole mandated to treatment.

There are states that mandate imprisonment then probation with outpatient treatment while some provide treatment during incarceration then supervision and monitoring by a parole officer. Some states (fifteen in 2004) permit civil commitment after a prison term. In 1996 federal law was passed requiring states to require sexually dangerous offenders to register with local police and public notice of their location be made available.

California has recently enacted what is referred to as Megan's law, which was effective January 1, 2005. This law requires the registration every 30 days of people who have been convicted of any one of 107 different sex crimes or crimes equal to them or if the court mandates such registration. People who were convicted as long ago as July 1, 1944, are required to register with the police (www.calsexoffenders.net/pages/769214/index.htm).

10. **Can Pedophilia be treated, and if so, what kinds of medications, therapy, and other treatments are being used today to treat Pedophiles?** Medications used to treat Pedophilia are principally the antiandrogens because they have been shown in controlled studies to lessen sexual fantasies, urges, and behavior. These drugs decrease the amount of available male hormones and include medroxyprogesterone (Provera) and leuprolide acetate (LPA, Luperon). These medications are given orally or intramuscularly for slow release. Some treatment regimens include selective serotonin reuptake inhibitors (SSRIs) given concurrently with antiandrogens to reduce anxiety, depression, and any obsessive-compulsive symptoms (Rosenberg, 2004).

Treatment of pedophilia is difficult, and professionals doing this need to have specialized training. Rosenberg (2002) describes therapists using polygraphs and penile plethysmographs in a thorough psychosexual evaluation before developing a treatment plan. Some of the treatments that have been utilized include aversive conditioning techniques, individual and group therapy, twelve-step programs, or treating Pedophilia as a post-traumatic stress disorder.

Recently, the focus in a number of programs has been on changing beliefs and attitudes as a means of increasing self-control. This is accomplished by methods such as imaginal desensitization, covert sensitization, cognitive restructuring, externalization, and victim empathy training (Rosenberg, 2004). Aversion therapy has been used in treatment of alcoholism and overeating and essentially involves imaging the behavior that is objectionable while seeing or smelling something very unpleasant in order to associate the undesirable behavior with the unpleasantness such as maggots crawling or an ammonia or feces smell. In imaginal desensitization the client is to talk about sexual situations while being taught to relax and deal with the discomfort and suppress sexual urges. Covert sensitization involves training to think beyond the sexual behavior to bad consequences of it. Cognitive restructuring usually involves having the client discuss his rationalizations in group and having peers challenge them and identify the thinking errors. In externalization the client discovers how his actions look and feel to a child. Victim empathy may take the form of reading writings or watching videotapes done by those who have been abused. In some facilities perpetrators and victims do role reversals in psychodrama led by someone highly trained in the techniques of psychodrama.

A treatment regimen for a Pedophile with a low intelligence quotient, who had grown up in institutional care, is described by Dowrack and Ward (1997). Therapists were able to change his behavior through self-modeling videos. He was scripted to behave at a superior level while being videotaped. For example, he would be videotaped saying that he was thinking of sex with a child and then saying he was going to stop and call the appropriate person or do the appropriate thing. He then was shown his own video many times. At first no behavior changed, but within ten days of seeing his self-modeling videos, he improved and followed through with appropriate behavior. This self-modeling technique has also been used to teach assertiveness.

11. **Where will nurses encounter and care for people with Pedophilia in addition to pediatric units and the jail, and what will their role be?** Some advanced practice nurse clinicians prepared at the graduate level may get training to work with people with Pedophilia. Staff nurses may be assisting in gathering data and writing treatment plans as part of a multidisciplinary treatment team in prisons, private psychiatric hospitals, outpatient programs, or community mental health centers and may be working with these folks in helping them resolve medical problems in a variety of settings. It is important that nurses have some understanding of Pedophilia so they can be therapeutic and professional in their work with this group.

References

American Psychiatric Association. (2000). *Diagnostic and Statistical Manual of Mental Disorders, 4th ed.* Text Revision. Washington, DC: American Psychiatric Association.

Dowrack, P. W. and K.M. Ward. (1997). "Video Feedforward in the Support of a Man with Intellectual Disability and Inappropriate Sexual Behavior." *Journal of Intellectual and Developmental Disability* 22(3): 147–161.

Edwards, D.T. (2004). "Mental Health's Cold Shoulder Treatment of Pedophilia." *Behavioral Health Management* 24(3): 32–36.

Murray, J.B. (2000). "Psychological Profile of Pedophiles and Child Molesters." *Journal of Psychology* 134(2): 211–225.

Rosenberg, M. (2002). "Treatment Considerations for Pedophilia." *Behavioral Health Management* 22(4): 38–42.

———. (2004). "Pedophilia." *Harvard Mental Health Letter* 20(7): 1–5.

www.calsexoffenders.net/pages/769214/index.htm. Accessed November 26, 2004.

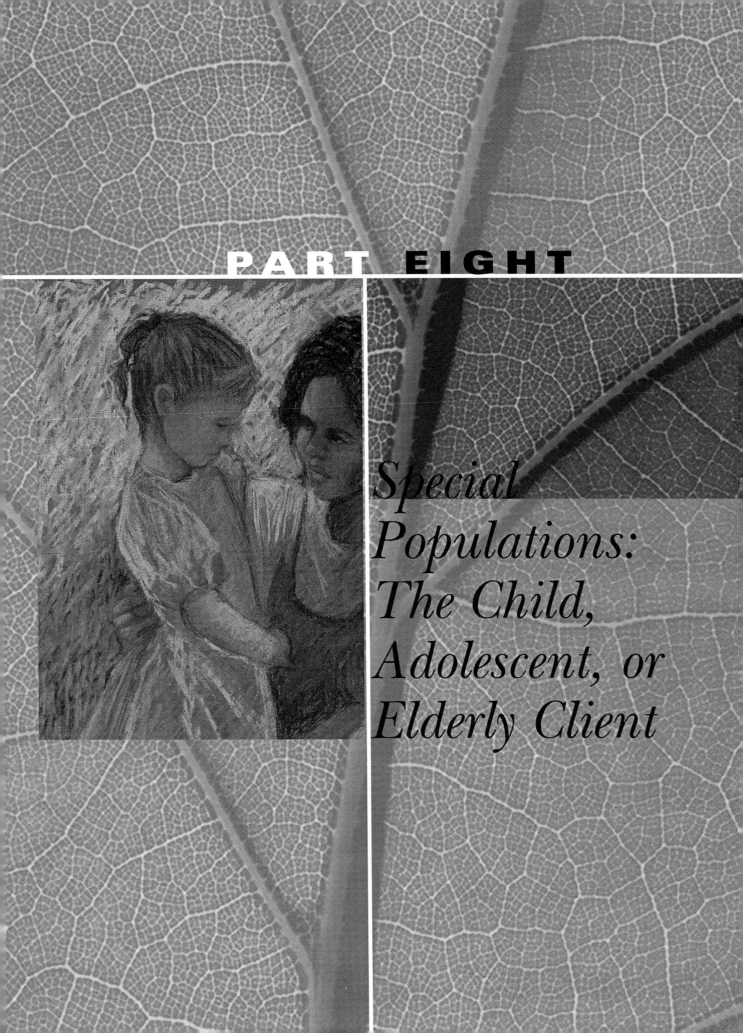

PART EIGHT

Special Populations: The Child, Adolescent, or Elderly Client

Len

GENDER

Male

AGE

13

SETTING

- Residential treatment facility for adolescents

ETHNICITY

- White American

CULTURAL CONSIDERATIONS

PREEXISTING CONDITIONS

COEXISTING CONDITIONS

COMMUNICATION

DISABILITY

SOCIOECONOMIC

- Parents divorced; mother is low income and father is middle income

SPIRITUAL/RELIGIOUS

PHARMACOLOGIC

PSYCHOSOCIAL

- Priority is being seen as tough by male acquaintances
- Difficulty establishing peer relationships

LEGAL

- History of sneaking out past legal curfew and drinking with older boys
- Found in neighbor's house uninvited; neighbor could press charges if Len leaves treatment early
- History of tardiness and skipping school

ETHICAL

ALTERNATIVE THERAPY

PRIORITIZATION

DELEGATION

MODERATE

OPPOSITIONAL DEFIANT DISORDER

Level of difficulty: Moderate

Overview: Requires working collaboratively as part of a multidisciplinary team, including client and client's family, to change the behavior of the client (a child) who has difficulty with authority figures. The nurse must be able to set limits consistently and help the client's family to recognize the need for, and to set, consistent limits for the child.

Client Profile

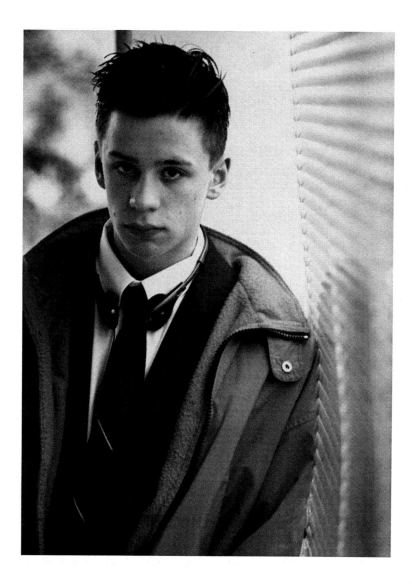

Len is a 13-year-old boy whose parents are divorced. Len's father is remarried and has two children by his second wife. The father is a truck driver and home only periodically. Len's mother tries to compete with his father in giving Len and his younger brother Nathan (Nate) material things. The mother recently bought Len some outrageously expensive tennis shoes that he demanded she buy. The mother doesn't work and has been buying things for Len and his brother on her brother's credit card. She is running up a large credit card debt on her brother's account and refuses to let him look at the bills that come in the mail. The boys and their uncle live with their mother, who is not good at setting limits. Their uncle and their father are also poor at setting limits.

Len has been in and out of trouble at school for the past year. He curses in class and is argumentative with teachers and the vice principal of his middle school. His mother takes Len's side in any disagreement between Len and authority figures. Len tells her that these adults are unfairly picking on him or they are stupid, and his mother believes him or at least she seems to when she goes to the school to "straighten the school people out." Recently a neighbor returned home to find Len in his house with some bizarre story of why he was there. The neighbor called the police who took Len into custody. The neighbor dropped charges when he learned that a deal had been worked out for the school system and Len's father's insurance to pay for Len going into residential psychiatric treatment.

Case Study

Len is admitted to a unit for adolescent boys at a residential treatment center by the nurse on duty. The nurse shows Len and his mother around the unit and gives both of them a copy of the unit rules. The nurse goes over the rules and has Len sign a statement that he has read, understands, and will abide by the rules. Consequences of breaking various rules are on the document. The unit is on a level system in which residents are promoted to a higher level and granted more privileges as they comply with rules and treatment. The nurse notices Len crossing his fingers, rolling his eyes, and then winking at his mother before signing the document.

Len and his mother are introduced to a nurse clinical specialist in child and adolescent mental health (certified by the American Nurses Association and prepared at the master's level in nursing) who will be Len's case manager, individual therapist, and the family therapist. Case managers in this facility can be nurse clinical specialists, master's prepared social workers or psychologists, or licensed professional counselors. The treatment plan is managed by the case manager but is developed, implemented, and evaluated by the treatment team members, from various disciplines, at formal meetings at designated time intervals.

Mother says to the nurse clinical specialist and the unit nurse: "I hope you will fix him so I can take him home soon. How soon can I visit?"

During the next few days, Len tests the staff by refusing to comply with unit rules, such as refusing to get out of bed and refusing to complete hygiene tasks without several prompts and using cuss words. Len loses his temper with peers and staff. Peers accuse him of hiding their belongings and playing pranks on them, which he denies and blames on someone else.

At a meeting of the staff in which Len's case is discussed, treatment team members from the various disciplines offer input about Len's behavior since admission. The psychiatrist suggests a diagnosis of Oppositional Defiant Disorder. Len and his mother meet with the treatment team. Len is given his diagnosis, and it is explained to him. His input and his mother's input are sought in regard to treatment goals and interventions. Len's response to the team is: "I am not oppositional and I am not defiant. You are all wrong and stupid."

Questions and Suggested Answers

1. **If you were the nurse admitting Len to the unit, how would you respond to Len when he crosses his fingers, rolls his eyes, and winks at his mother before signing the rules agreement form? Give a rationale for your response.** You would use the therapeutic communication tool of "observation," saying something like: "I noticed that you had your fingers crossed, were rolling your eyes, and you winked at your mother." Len may deny doing this. If he does, do not get into an argument with him. You are simply making an observation, not interpreting it or being accusatory. Len loves arguing with authority figures, and if you ask his mother for verification that Len made these gestures, she may lie and say "no." She is in the habit of doing what she thinks protects her son. You don't have a trusting relationship with the mother yet, and the mother has not yet been taught the importance of changing her behavior and how to do it. You can respond simply to Len's denial with a serious expression: "This agreement is firm. You have signed this agreement to abide by the rules and you will be held to it." You are giving Len "the bottom line."

   It is important that Len have limits firmly set. He has few if any limits set at home. When looking for limits, children escalate their behavior, exhibiting more and more socially unacceptable and/or objectionable behaviors until they find the limits.

2. **How could you as a staff nurse develop some rapport with Len? How would you develop rapport and a trusting relationship with the client's family?** Staff nurses often spend one on one time with a resident. Whether you are assigned to do this or not, you can take time to play a game or encourage the client to talk about

something nonthreatening, such as his hobbies or interests as a step in building rapport. You must be careful not to promise Len more than you can deliver or anything that is not therapeutic. Clients with Oppositional Defiant Disorder are good at manipulating people into promising those things. You are aware that Len has been very good at getting material things from his parents. The most valuable thing you can give this child is your time and help in learning to stay within set limits while still getting attention or having fun. Discuss ideas to give him anything other than time and attention with your supervisor.

To develop rapport with Len's mother and other family members, you need to watch your verbal and nonverbal language with the family so that both aspects of communication are congruent and that you are conveying a noncritical helping attitude. Empathy also helps. If mother is talking about being lonely with her son away, the nurse can empathize: "Yes, I realize this is hard for you, but you are such a good parent to help him get treatment." During visits you can have the client take his family on a tour of some of the facility and you can go along. Informal time with the family is helpful in relationship building. When the family comes to visit, make certain that you introduce yourself and offer to answer questions. Give positive reinforcement to the child for complying with limits. This positive reinforcement encourages the child and helps the family view you as not just an enforcer of rules but one who can recognize when the child is doing the right thing. You can also model behavior you want the family to have.

3. **You are assigned to have a one on one with this client and he says he has nothing to say and you cannot make him talk. How would you react to this?** If the client refuses to talk or interact with you, it is important to avoid a control battle. Say something like: "It's up to you. I have some time for you now." Or, "Perhaps you will feel like talking a little later. I have some time at 12:30 and some time at 2 o'clock. Let me know if you want one of those times to talk or just play some cards." Most clients who feel they have lost control are looking for some area they can control. Talking or not talking is an area the client can control. Choosing a time to talk also provides a feeling of control.

4. **The health care provider asks you and the rest of the staff to identify behaviors in this client that match the diagnosis of Oppositional Defiant behavior. Does the client have behaviors that match the criteria for this disorder?**

Criteria for Oppositional Defiant Disorder	Does Client Match Behavior?
For six months or more has had a pattern of being negativistic, hostile, and defiant with four or more of following behaviors:	Yes, for about a year he has had this pattern and has had several of the behaviors listed as criteria.
• Loses temper frequently	Yes
• Frequently argues with adults	Yes, he was argumentative with teachers and vice principal and with unit staff.
• Frequently defies or is noncompliant with adult's requests or rules	Yes, he has needed several prompts on the unit to comply with requests and was noncompliant in school.
• Frequently deliberately annoys others	Yes, peers complain that he annoys them.
• Projects blame for his/her mistakes or misbehavior on others	Yes
• Frequently behaves in "touchy" manner or seems easily annoyed by others	Yes
• Frequently is angry and resentful	Yes
• Displays spiteful or vindictive behavior often	Not evidenced. To be evaluated.
For items above the behavior must be more often than typically seen in those of comparable age and developmental stage.	Yes

(Continued)

Criteria for Oppositional Defiant Disorder	Does Client Match Behavior?
There must be significant impairment in an important area of functioning which is caused by the disturbance in behavior.	Impairment in social area and school work
Behaviors are not seen only in the course of psychotic or mood disorders.	Yes
The client must not meet criteria for conduct disorder (if he/she does, that is the diagnosis) or if he/she is 18 years of age or older, criteria is not met for antisocial personality disorder (if he/she does, then that is the diagnosis).	Does not meet criteria for conduct disorder which involves more aggressive acts and he is not 18 years of age or older.

(Adapted from APA, 2000)

5. **What if you as a staff nurse decide you don't like some of the interventions that the team has implemented and you would like to try something different? Can you do this?** One of the most important aspects of treatment in residential treatment centers is staff consistency in everything said to the client and in all treatment interventions. You cannot change the consequences or rewards, and you cannot interpret the rules differently than other staff members. If you don't like an intervention, you need to bring this up at a team meeting and state your rationale for why you would like to change it and how you would like to change it. If you are not consistent with the rest of the staff in applying interventions, you may be mimicking the inconsistency the client sees between the rules of his father and those of his mother: an inconsistency that reinforces the client's behavior of testing limits.

6. **One of the staff asks you: "What causes Oppositional Defiant Disorder?" What would you reply?** The cause is unknown. This disorder has been found to occur more often in families with:

   - At least one parent with a history of one or more of several disorders such as Mood Disorder, Oppositional Defiant Disorder, Conduct Disorder, Attention-Deficit/Hyperactivity Disorder, Antisocial Disorder, or a Substance-Related Disorder; or
   - In families with serious marital discord (APA, 2000).

   Markward and Bride (2001) state that there is a good bit of evidence suggesting that "family problems are responsible for the behaviors that typify those of children with ODD," with poor discipline a possible cause of Oppositional Defiant Disorder. These authors also state: "Although this (family problems and poor discipline) may be the most acceptable explanation, some evidence supports the notion that genetic factors play a role in ODD."

7. **What nursing diagnoses would you write for this client? What goals would you write for this client?** Note: The multidisciplinary care plan does not have nursing diagnoses, but you can write a nursing care plan that is consistent with the multidisciplinary plan.

   Nursing diagnoses could include:

   - Ineffective coping
   - Noncompliance

   Goals could include:

   - Will comply with 100 percent of unit rules without argument
   - Will accept responsibility for actions and have no instances of blaming others

- Will identify two socially acceptable ways to deal with anger
- Will have no instances of angry outbursts

8. **Would you expect this child to be on medication to treat Oppositional Defiant Disorder? What interventions do you think would work with this client?** Maughn and associates ("New Study Explores Comorbidity Conduct Disorder and Oppositional Defiant Disorder: Trends and Treatment," 2004, 4), state that "for ODD the pharmacological treatment should not be considered except in cases where aggression is a significant problem." Since this client does not have significant aggression, medication would not be expected to be part of the treatment. Maughn and colleagues describe interventions for disruptive behavior as including parent training, classroom intervention, family therapy, social skills therapy and cognitive behavior therapy (CBT). They point out that parent training and school intervention can be used to target oppositionality wheras social skills programs and/or CBT are effective in reducing aggression/impulsivity.

   Nursing interventions would probably include some or all of the following interventions:

- When client's behavior is unacceptable or when he does not comply with unit rules, advise the client that his behavior is unacceptable, stressing that he is acceptable but his behavior is not. Basically convey this message: "I like you, but I did not like a particular behavior from you."
- Correct unacceptable behaviors when they occur and not later when the child cannot recall the behavior or cannot recall it clearly.
- Have client sign a statement of what is expected of him and repeat it back to you or ask questions of client to ensure understanding.
- Provide the client a list of unacceptable behaviors on one side of a 3 × 5 card and acceptable behaviors on the other. Client can keep this in his pocket to remind himself, and staff can ask him to look at the card when he engages in unacceptable behavior and denies doing anything wrong.
- Post not only consequences for breaking rules, but also the rewards for following them.
- Blaming is a thinking error. Teach peers and client about thinking error of blaming. Peers can call each other on acts of blaming
- Model acceptable behavior for client (e.g., taking responsibility, following rules, thinking through decisions).
- Give positive reinforcement for following rules and any movement toward positive change.
- Have client and peers role play or do a play about behaviors that cause people to like you.
- Do role playing in which the client is himself and you are the vice principal, and then reverse roles with the idea of learning to communicate without arguing and to communicate effectively.
- Identify client's talents and strengths and encourage client to build on these.
- The client also will receive individual and family therapy and may be scheduled for classes such as social skills class or self-esteem building class.

9. **The client talks with his mother on the phone and convinces his mother that he is better and asks her to come get him. He has not been discharged. How would you convince the mother that her son is not ready to be discharged?** You will certainly let the mother know that this idea of discharge comes as a surprise and that the team has not recommended discharge yet. You could ask the mother to think about what her son's behavior was like when the decision was made to admit him. Ask her to consider the possibility that he is not ready to go and will revert back to his old behaviors, but with a little more time, a new pattern of behavior might be more set. You might use the analogy of a cake not quite baked. The health care provider may ask you to talk with mother about a discharge against medical advice (AMA); however, the school system may refuse to pay for treatment if the child is removed AMA. Some third-party payments are denied when the client leaves AMA.

10. **Is there a link between Oppositional Defiant Disorder and Conduct Disorder and is there a link between ODD and ADHD?** An article in the *Brown University Child and Adolescent Newsletter* ("New Study Explores Comorbidity Conduct Disorder and Oppositional Defiant Disorder: Trends and Treatment," 2004, 1) states that "experts estimate that about 50% of children with ADHD are comorbid for ODD and/or CD, while

almost all children under 12 years of age with these disruptive behaviors meet the criteria for ADHD." According to Maughn cited in that same *Brown University Child and Adolescent Newsletter* (2004), not all children with Oppositional Defiant Disorder go on to develop Conduct Disorder and some children develop Conduct Disorder without having met the criteria for ODD, but there seems to be a strong overlap between ODD and CD.

References

American Psychiatric Association. (2000). *Diagnostic and Statistical Manual of Mental Disorders, 4th ed.* Text Revision. Washington, DC: American Psychiatric Association.

Markward, M.T. and B. Bride. (2001). "Oppositional Defiant Disorder and the Need for Family Centered Practice in Schools." *Children and Schools* 23(2): 73–83.

"New Study Explores Comorbidity Conduct Disorder and Oppositional Defiant Disorder: Trends and Treatment." (2004). *Brown University Child and Adolescent Behavior Letter* 20(5): 1–4.

Brandon

GENDER

Male

AGE

14

SETTING

- Pediatric unit of hospital

ETHNICITY

- White American

CULTURAL CONSIDERATIONS

PREEXISTING CONDITION

COEXISTING CONDITIONS

- Seizure disorder and mild mental retardation

COMMUNICATION

DISABILITY

- Impaired social interaction

SOCIOECONOMIC

- Middle to upper-middle income family

SPIRITUAL/RELIGIOUS

PHARMACOLOGIC

- Carbamazepine (Tegretol)
- Vicodin

PSYCHOSOCIAL

- Withdraws from others
- Limited speech
- Poor social skills
- Dependent on parents for help with activities of daily living

LEGAL

- Need for informed consent to gather information from health care providers and others outside the hospital system

ETHICAL

ALTERNATIVE THERAPY

PRIORITIZATION

DELEGATION

AUTISTIC DISORDER

Level of difficulty: High

Overview: Requires using the usual caregiver as a resource in planning and implementing care for a child who has Autistic Disorder and does not relate well to people. Requires prioritization of clients and determination of tasks to be delegated.

DIFFICULT

Client Profile

Brandon is a 14-year-old boy who was diagnosed with Autistic Disorder just before his third birthday. His older sister Anne also has Autistic Disorder. Three other siblings do not have the disorder. As a toddler Brandon would go off by himself and when people tried to get near him, he would make flapping motions and strike out at them. He has always been sensitive to clothing touching him, refusing to wear any rough feeling or new clothing. When seasons change his mother has to hide Brandon's old clothes or he would insist on wearing winter clothing in summer and summer clothes in winter. Brandon loves to put pebbles or marbles in a container then take them out and put them back one by one. He plays with a piece of string, a rubber band, or a small stick for hours. Brandon did not have very many words or sounds until he was enrolled in an early childhood education program prior to going to preschool. The speech therapist and teachers' aides worked very hard with him until he had sufficient vocabulary to make some of his needs known and to communicate in simple words and to give a hug to people who are familiar to him. He can use a message board if someone holds his elbow in a certain way. He exhibits echolalia. Brandon does not make eye contact with others, and sometimes people say he looks like he is in his own world. The teachers and mother get his attention by holding his face up or pinching his arm and using behavior modification rewarding techniques for his doing or saying what they are asking of him. Brandon sometimes rocks his body in a stereotypical fashion. He gets very upset when things are moved around in his room, his home, or in the classroom. Brandon plays tee-ball in a special league for kids with special needs, and he is very proud of his tee-ball uniform. He collects baseball cards and has them in a certain order. If they are out of order, he works hard to get them back in order. He often uses headphones and listens to music.

Brandon is a big boy for his age, nearly 6 feet tall, 200-plus pounds, and muscular. He is difficult to handle when he is upset. His mother is a petite women, and she has gotten a few bruises when interacting with Brandon and has had to stop the car sometimes when Brandon was pulling her hair or throwing things in the car. Brandon's father helps with Brandon when he is home, but the father travels with his job and is often away from home for several days.

Case Study

Brandon was practicing playing ball at home in the yard. His sister threw the ball in the street, and Brandon ran after it with his mother close behind yelling at him to stop. Brandon was hit by a car and taken by ambulance to the emergency room where he had a seizure and was moved to ICU for observation and treatment with Valium and an anticonvulsant. After about twenty-four hours he was moved to the pediatric unit of the hospital and admitted for further observation. He has a fractured radius, and his arm is scheduled to be casted in the morning. The pediatric nurse assigned to care for Brandon and admit him to the pediatric unit observes that he is clearly upset as he makes all kinds of sounds and is flapping his arms. Brandon won't let anyone come near him. This is problematic as the health care provider wants Brandon's forearm in a splint wrapped with an ace bandage, the lower arm elevated in a sling, and an ice pack applied. The provider also orders carbamazepine (Tegretol) two times a day, Vicodin for pain as necessary, and bed rest.

Brandon's mother is near hysterical and crying. She tells the pediatric nurse that the ambulance personnel did not want her to ride in the ambulance with Brandon, although she advised the ambulance personnel that they would soon wish she were with Brandon. She relates that the same thing happened in ICU at the hospital. The ICU nurse did not want to have Brandon's mother stay with him in ICU without documentation she was the legal guardian. Within minutes of asking the mother to leave ICU, the ICU nurse assigned to Brandon came to get the mother to help her with Brandon. The mother did have to telephone Brandon's father and ask him to fax proof she is a legal guardian.

The pediatric nurse assigned to Brandon has been listening to Brandon's mother tell her story, but realizes that there are three other assigned clients as well as Brandon. The nurse is to give two pediatric clients their

9 A.M. medicines that are ordered and do a specific gravity on the urine of the third client. It is now 8:55 A.M. A preoperative medication must be given to a burn client at 9 A.M. prior to going to a whirlpool treatment. Brandon still needs his forearm wrapped and elevated in a sling with an ice pack. He gets upset and strikes out at the nurse (but misses) when the nurse tries to give him a hospital gown and asks him to put it on.

Questions and Suggested Answers

1. **What is going on with the mother that she is near hysterical and crying, and what would be a good response if you were the nurse in this case?** You don't know what is going on with mother so you need to keep an open mind. The mother is possibly blaming herself for Brandon getting hit by a car and/or worried about whether he has internal injuries or not. She could be concerned that she won't be allowed to stay with Brandon and he will get extremely upset being cared for by strangers. It sounds like she has had a very difficult day with Brandon getting hurt, suffering a seizure, being told by EMS they don't need her to ride in the ambulance when she knows that they do, and being told in ICU that they have to have proof she is a legal guardian. Put yourself in the mother's place and think about how you would feel. At any rate, a good response would be for you to use a kind voice and empathetic words and let the mother know that you are going to work with her and help her care for Brandon. Let her know that she is part of the team. Tell her you think it will help Brandon if you leave for a few minutes and give him a chance to calm down and get used to the room. Let her know when you will be back to talk with her about Brandon's needs and how to approach him. Tell her how to call for you if she needs you sooner.

2. **Assuming you were the nurse in this case and looking at the clients assigned to you and their needs, what would be your first and second priorities? What sort of things would make Brandon's care a first priority to you? Could you delegate some of the tasks that you have to do, and if so, what and under what circumstances?** The premedication for whirlpool is a top priority. Whirlpool for burns is painful so the client needs the premedication given on time. The 9 A.M. meds can be given one half hour on either side of 9 A.M., and you need to pass these before attending to Brandon. Putting Brandon's splint on and wrapping Brandon's forearm can wait a few minutes until he calms down and you begin to get some relationship going with Brandon. It may help him to relax if he has a few minutes alone with his mother. The procedure of getting Brandon's splint on and wrapped will go easier if you have urgent tasks done, are patient, and let the mother do as much as possible. If she can be instructed to do the entire procedure, it will be less traumatic to Brandon.

Brandon is not the first priority given the information you have. If Brandon has another seizure or seizures or does something else where he could hurt others or hurt himself, he could become your first priority. If Brandon becomes a first priority, you can ask a fellow licensed nurse to give the pain medication to the client getting premedicated for whirlpool. Brandon's problem will probably resolve in time to give the routine medications within one half hour after they are due to be given, and if not, you can call the supervising nurse for help. What you can't do easily is delegate Brandon's care. No one can run in and do something quickly for him and not upset him. A steady stream of different nurses will be upsetting to him.

3. **What is Autistic Disorder (AD), and does Brandon have behaviors that meet the criteria for AD? Do all children with AD have the same symptoms as Brandon?** The American Psychiatric Association (2002) uses the term Autistic Disorder in describing criteria for what clinicians and researchers more commonly call Autistic Syndrome or Autism. Children with Autistic Disorder (Autism, Autistic Syndrome) have impairment in social interaction and communication and a greatly decreased number of activities and things they are interested in. A review of the current literature reveals that clinicians are using the term "Autism Spectrum Disorders" and looking at the similarity between high-functioning people with autism and an IQ higher than 79 and people with Asperger's Syndrome.

The criteria for Autistic Disorder is somewhat lengthy as described below.

Criteria for Autistic Disorder	Does Client Match Criteria?
The client must have at least two behaviors from category 1 and at least one behavior from categories 2 and 3 for a total of six or more behaviors.	
Category 1: Impairment in social interaction as shown by at least two of the following:	
• Impairment in using nonverbal behaviors (e.g., facial expression, body posture, eye to eye gaze, and gestures normally used to regulate social interaction).	Client has lack of eye contact.
• No peer relationships appropriate to developmental level.	Client does not have peer relationships appropriate for a 14-year-old.
• Does not spontaneously seek others to share enjoyment, interests, or attachments with others (does not point out, bring or show objects of interest to others).	Client matches.
• Does not have social or emotional give and take.	Client matches.
Category 2: Has impairments in communication demonstrated in at least one of the following ways:	
• Delayed, or lack of, development of spoken language and no attempt to compensate with other means of communication like mime or gestures.	Yes, client has this impairment. With lots of hard work by speech therapists, he has gained some words and can use a message board. He did not initiate gestures on his own.
• If adequate speech present, there is marked impairment in starting or keeping a conversation going with others.	Yes, client matches. He rarely initiates a conversation, and he does not attempt to keep it going.
• Stereotypical and repetitive or idiosyncratic use of language.	Yes, client matches. He has echolalia. He repeats words over and over.
• Does not have varied or "spontaneous make-believe play or social imitative play appropriate to developmental level."	Yes, client does not have much variety in play, and he does not imitate others or do make-believe play.
Category 3: Behavioral patterns are restricted, repetitive, and stereotypical. Must have one or more of the following:	
• Extreme preoccupation with at least one stereotyped restrictive area of interest that is abnormal in intensity or focus.	Yes, client has played with rocks or marbles or a string or stick for hours at a time.
• Seemingly inflexible sticking to "specific nonfunctional routines or rituals."	Yes, has a certain order for his baseball cards and must handle them a certain way or he is upset. He does have routines, some of which are nonfunctional.
• Stereotypical motor mannerisms that are repeated over and over such as flapping of the fingers, hand, or arm or twisting or complex motor movements involving the entire body.	Yes, the client does have flapping motions.

(Continued)

Criteria for Autistic Disorder	Does Client Match Criteria?
• Preoccupation with object parts rather than whole objects.	Unknown, needs assessment.
Prior to age 3, the child must have delays or abnormal functioning in one or more of three areas: 1. Social interaction, 2. Social communication language, 3. Symbolic or imaginative play.	Yes, he matches this as he was displaying these delays and abnormal functioning in these areas before age three.
Behavior is not associated with Rett's Disorder or Childhood Disintegrative Disorder.	As far as is known, this is true.

(Adapted from APA, 2000)

Brandon's lack of eye contact is consistent with a diagnosis of Autistic Disorder. Pierce et al. (2001) point out that "autism may be one of the only disorders where affected individuals spend reduced amounts of time engaged in face processing from birth."

All children with Autism do not have the same symptoms as Brandon. After you work with a number of children with Autistic Disorder, you will find that the symptoms vary a great deal. The intelligence quotient (IQ) of children with Autism varies greatly. Some of these children have mild mental retardation, some have severe forms of mental retardation, and others do not have mental retardation at all. Some will learn to communicate verbally, and others will have great difficulty learning even a few words. Some will work a part-time job in high school, such as sacking groceries in a large supermarket right along with peers who have no disabilities. Some will work after leaving the educational system, which is obligated by law to educate them up through the school year in which they celebrate their twenty-first birthday. Gross (2004) describes a variety of children with Autism and their strengths and limitations. It is clear from the article that they all present a challenge to their families in everyday activities such as getting a haircut or going to a restaurant or shopping.

4. **How would you approach getting Brandon to wear the hospital gown and stay in bed? How would you get Brandon's splint on his arm and get it wrapped and put ice on it?** Seek the mother's advice on how to accomplish this task. It may be that he won't wear a hospital gown. If the gown is a colorful print and is soft, it will probably be easier to get him to wear than if the gown is white and scratchy. You may have to just let him wear his pajama bottoms or his underwear only. With children who are Autistic, the phrase "choose your battles wisely" is appropriate. Brandon's mother may have to hide his clothes while he is asleep or send them home in order to get him to give up wanting his clothing.

To put Brandon's splint on his arm, get it wrapped, and put an ice pack on it, you will need to be patient, make a few short visits with Brandon, and follow his mother's advice on how to build a relationship with Brandon. You need to again enlist the help of the mother and see if she alone, with your instructions, can get the splint on, wrapped, and the ice in place or if the two of you need to work together on this task. If nothing works, you will need to call the health care provider and advise him or her of the problem(s).

5. **How would you figure out when Brandon is in pain and in need of a pain pill?** Use your observational powers to see if Brandon is grimacing, rubbing his arm, or making some other motion that gives you a clue he is in pain. You can check with his mother who can probably tell when Brandon is in pain. You could give him pain medicine on a regular basis (congruent with the health care provider's order) to prevent pain from escalating.

This client can also be taught a sign for pain or to communicate pain on the message board, although asking an Autistic child if they are in pain often brings a nonvalid response. The child may say "yes" when you ask them if they have pain. Five minutes later if you ask the same question, they may say "no."

6. **Brandon needs to urinate, and his mother wants to take him to the bathroom. She insists he will be upset if he urinates in the bed, and he won't understand the urinal. Brandon is on bed rest. How would you handle this situation?** You may end up letting his mother get Brandon to the bathroom and calling the health care provider

to see if you can get an order to cover bed rest except to get up for bathroom. Parents of Autistic children will frequently say: "I do what I have to do." Mothers describe having to go into the men's bathroom to get their son with Autistic Disorder to come out. Parents of Autistic children often find that other people don't understand this need and they feel criticized frequently, but they assure you that what they do is necessary.

7. **Brandon's parents ask you several questions including: "What are the current theories about the cause of Autism?" "What is the prevalence/incidence of Autism, and is it more prevalent in one gender compared to the other or not?" "What is the usual onset of Autistic Disorder?" and "What disorders or medical problems are commonly associated with Autism?" What would you include in your answer?** Kalb (2005) points out that although we have known about Autism for more than sixty years, we still don't know what causes it. Theories of causation range from a virus to toxic metals and a deficiency of glutathione to a genetic cause.

Baylor College of Medicine researchers led by Yong-hui Jiang have proposed that the majority of cases of Autism "can be explained by a complex model for genetic malfunction that may or may not include an altered DNA sequence." These researchers have suggested that "epigenetic and genetic factors (both de novo and inherited) cause autism through dysregulation of two or more principal genes, one of which maps within (specific) chromosomes" (Roser, 2004).

Wakefield, a British researcher, conducted research with three collaborators that "identifies a new inflammatory intestinal disease in some children who appear normal but regress into autism, it suggests the intestinal disease is viral." ("Scientist Links Gut to Autism in Children," 2004). Dr. Timothy Buie, a pediatrician and nationally recognized autism expert, specializing in gastrointestinal disorders at Massachusetts General Hospital for Children, has been studying bowel diseases and autism (Roser, 2004).

Kleffman (2004) talks about some work at the University of Arkansas for Medical Sciences in which researchers found "some children with autism have a weakened ability to protect themselves for toxic metals in their bodies." The children were said to have a deficiency of glutathione, which is used by the body to detoxify and excrete heavy metals like lead and mercury. The study had twenty subjects with Autism, eight of whom were given folinic acid, which is a form of folic acid and vitamin B-12. After taking these supplements, their glutathione levels improved. Dr. Mumper of the University of Virginia Medical School is quoted as saying she has given similar supplements to children with Autism and seen a marked improvement in some of them.

It has been reported that researchers are going to "apply new genome searching technologies to available samples and information from 463 families including 979 individuals with autism to find any genetic factors contributing to autism." ("Brain Inflammation Found in Autism," 2004). Dr. Chakravarti, the principal investigator of this project and director of McKusick-Nathan's Institute of Genetic Medicine at Johns Hopkins, is cited as saying: "We are looking for combinations of genetic mutations and extra or missing gene copies that are much less common, even in the affected group, than more scientists are used to thinking about."

Prevalence reported in the literature ranges from 2 to 29 cases per 10,000 population. It has been reported that Autism is estimated to affect 2 to 5 of every 1,000 children, and it is 4 times more likely to occur in males compared to females ("Hunt for Autism Genes to Be Led by Hopkins Researchers," 2004). Kalb (2005) states that there has been a tenfold increase in Austism Spectrum Disorder in the last twenty years and now 1 in 166 children will receive a diagnosis of ASD.

The onset of the disorder has to occur before age three in order to meet the criteria for diagnosis of this disorder.

As many as 25 percent of clients with Autism will have seizures, especially in adolescence. Some clients with Autism have delayed hand dominance. Mental retardation is frequently found in clients with Autistic Disorder.

8. **Discuss any assessments you need to do. What nursing diagnoses and goals would you write for Brandon, and what interventions would you include in the plan of care?** Brandon is not a reliable historian. While nurses are used to getting information from the client as the expert on himself or herself, in this case the history will have to be obtained from the parents and the health care professionals who have worked with Brandon. Release of information forms must be signed by the parents in order to get information from providers other than those currently caring for the client in the hospital. The provider may provide an extensive history

and physical document, and the nurse may not need to probe any further than talking with the parents and reading the chart.

The nurse will want to determine Brandon's usual schedule, likes and dislikes, strengths and limitations, special needs, allergies, and usual medications taken. The parent's knowledge about the disorder and sources of support and help need to be assessed.

Likely diagnoses could include the following:

- Risk for injury
- Impaired verbal communication
- Pain related to fracture
- Anxiety
- Noncompliance
- Self-care deficit
- Impaired social interaction
- Relocation Stress Syndrome: could encompass such characteristics as anxiety, fear, anger, frustration, dependency, insecurity, and involuntary temporary move
- Mother may be at risk for caregiver role strain

Possible goals could include:

- Will be free of injury during hospital stay
- Will demonstrate communication in some manner with nurse assigned to care for him
- Will communicate by some means that pain is absent or minimal
- Mother will report few or no incidences of agitated behavior evidenced by arm or hand flapping
- Will demonstrate compliance with essential aspects of care
- Will interact with at least one person other than mother
- Will adapt to hospitalization
- Mother will report finding at least one source of respite care

Interventions may include the following:

- Provide pain relief on a regular basis and within the allowable amount prescribed
- Encourage parents to bring familiar objects/items from home that will calm Brandon, such as his MP3 player and headphones
- Post Brandon's preferred daily schedule in a visible place in his room
- Encourage staff to adhere to Brandon's preferred schedule and educate them as to the reason(s) for doing this
- Provide play activities that are ability appropriate and age appropriate when possible
- Provide teaching as needed to family about medications, respite care, information on or where to find information on Autism Spectrum Disorders, and how to help siblings of children with Autistic Disorder. Some families will know much more about Autism, having researched it fully. Some may have accessed many specialists in treating this diagnosis. Staff must be careful not to talk down to the family. It may be helpful to refer the family to support groups and to suggest books such as one by Sandra Harris and Beth Glasberg entitled *Siblings of Children with Autism: A Guide for Families* (Harris and Glasberg, 2003)
- Work with mother to insure she has adequate respite care and support
- Use concrete language, not abstract language

9. **What would you need to know, and want to make sure the mother knows, about carbamazepine (Tegretol)?**
Carbamazepine (Tegretol) is an anticonvulsant used to prevent clonic-tonic, mixed, and complex partial seizures. Off-label uses include treatment of bipolar disorder and management of pain in trigeminal neuralgia. This drug is metabolized by the liver, so it must be used cautiously if client has any hepatic or cardiac problems. Adverse reactions and side effects reported are varied and include: drowsiness, vertigo, blurred vision, corneal opacities, pneumonitis, hypotension, hypertension, hepatitis, urinary hesitancy and retention,

photosensitivity and skin rashes and hives, syndrome of inappropriate antidiuretic hormone, blood dyscrasias, chills, fever, and swollen lymph nodes. It is given orally in tablet, suspension, and extended release forms.

Before this client is discharged on carbamazepine (Tegretal), you will want to teach the family to give the carbamazepine as ordered. Doses should not be doubled if a dose is missed. The family needs to be instructed to call the health care provide if more than one dose is missed, the client has fever, sore throat, ulcers in the mouth, chills, rash, bruising or easy bleeding, pale stools or dark urine, abdominal pain, or jaundice. You can instruct the family to have Brandon use sunscreen and protective clothing to prevent reactions when in the sunlight. The family needs to know that follow-up lab testing and eye examinations periodically are important. The family needs to be instructed on the importance of consistent good oral hygiene practices for Brandon.

10. **What research is being done in the field of Pervasive Developmental Disorders including Autism and Asperger's Disorder/Syndrome? Is there research into families in which than one child has an Autism Spectrum Disorder?** In 2005 the National Institutes of Health spent more than 99 million dollars on Autism research with new research on how to find clues to the disorder in babies as young as six months (Kalb, 2005). In addition, the Yale Developmental Disabilities Clinic has some of the most renowned experts in the area of Pervasive Developmental Disorders including Autism, Asperger's Syndrome, and other disorders, and performs extensive research on Autism Spectrum Disorders. Another research project reported by McAlonan et al. (2005) involved mapping the brain in seventeen "stringently diagnosed children with autism and 17 age-matched controls and all 34 had IQs of 80 or better." The researchers were able to map the brain of all subjects for regional grey and white matter and to compare differences. Significant findings in children with autism included the following: a reduction in grey matter volume, an increase in CSF volume, "localized grey matter reductions within fronto-straital and parietal networks," reduction of white matter in the cerebellum. The controls who did not have a diagnosis of Autism were found to have "significantly more numerous and more positive grey matter volumetric correlations" than those with Autism. The researchers used similar "diagnostic criteria and image analysis methods in otherwise healthy populations with an autistic spectrum disorder from different countries, cultures and age groups," and reported a number of consistent findings. The researchers suggest "abnormalities in the anatomy and connectivity of limbic–striated 'social' brain systems which may contribute to the brain metabolic differences and behavioral phenotype in autism." (McAlonan et al., 2005, 268).

Pierce et al. (2001) conducted research work involving adults with Autism, comparing them to so-called normals in terms of brain activity in carrying out tasks. They point out that babies with Autism do not process the human face or have difficulty processing it with several areas of the brain involved in this difficulty. These researchers view eye contact as the core of most social interactions. Pierce et al. have pointed out that Autism may be one of the only disorders in which those with the disorder spend less time engaged in face processing. In their research, these researchers found that Autistic individuals seem to have reduced or no activation in four areas of the brain studied. On the other hand, only in the amygdala in Autistic patients were anatomical differences found when compared with control subjects. It also appears that, when compared with normal subjects, those with Autistic Disorder perceive faces utilizing different neural systems. Each person with Autism uses a unique neural circuitry to perceive faces. "Such a pattern of individual-specific, scattered activation seen in autistic patients in contrast to the highly consistent FG activation seen in normals, suggests that experiential factors do indeed play a role in the normal development of the FFA."

The National Institutes of Health is funding a study, with Susan Folstein as the principal investigator, to identify Autistic susceptibility genes for the purpose of improving diagnosis and treatment. There is no travel or expense to be in the study, and it appears the team travels to the family to do the study. This study can involve two siblings or an uncle/aunt and nephew or niece pair (http://ladders.org/currentar.php, January 29, 2005). Brandon's family could be given this website address so they could become knowledgeable about these studies, which could be of interest and help to them.

References

American Psychiatric Association. (2000). *Diagnostic and Statistical Manual of Mental Disorders, 4th ed.* Text Revision. Washington, DC: American Psychiatric Association.

"Brain Inflammation Found in Autism." (2004). *Pain and Central Nervous System Week*, November 29, 20–22.

Gross, J. (2004). "For Families of Autistic, the Fight for the Ordinary." *New York Times*, October 22, 1.

Harris, S.L. and B. Glasberg. (2003). *Siblings of Children with Autism: A Guide for Families.* Bethesda, MD: Woodbine House.

"Hunt for Autism Genes to Be Led by Hopkins Researchers." (2004). *Pain and Central Nervous System Week*, November 1, 23.

Kalb, C. (2005). "When Does Autism Start?" *Newsweek,* February 28: 45–52.

Kleffman, S. (2004). "Study Links Autism, Toxic Metals." *Austin American Statesman*, December 14, 14.

McAlonan, G.M. et al. (2005). "Mapping the Brain in Autism: A Voxel-Based MRI Study of Volumetric Differences in Intercorrelations in Autism." *Brain* 128(2): 268–276.

Pierce, K., R.A. Müller, J. Ambrose, G. Allen, and E. Courchesne. (2001). "Face Processing Occurs Outside the Fusiform 'Face Area' in Autism: Evidence from Functional MRI." *Brain* 124(10): 20–22.

Roser, M.A. (2004). "New Genetic Hypothesis Offered for the Cause of Autism." *Pain and Central Nervous System Week*, September 20, 21.

"Scientist Links Gut to Autism in Children." (2004). *Austin American Statesman*, November 1, B1 and B3.

GENDER

Female

AGE

8

SETTING

- School nurse's office

ETHNICITY

- White American

CULTURAL CONSIDERATIONS

- American culture values independence

PREEXISTING CONDITION

COEXISTING CONDITION

COMMUNICATION

DISABILITY

SOCIOECONOMIC

SPIRITUAL/RELIGIOUS

PHARMACOLOGIC

PSYCHOSOCIAL

- No close relationships with peers due to fear something will happen to mother if not near mother

LEGAL

- School attendance

ETHICAL

- Forcing child to work through anxiety and go to school versus homeschooling and not distressing child

ALTERNATIVE THERAPY

PRIORITIZATION

DELEGATION

MODERATE

SEPARATION ANXIETY DISORDER

Level of difficulty: Moderate

Overview: Requires awareness of behaviors associated with Separation Anxiety Disorder in order to identify children at risk for this disorder. The nurse must work cooperatively with the parent, teacher and others, as well as the child, to plan and utilize interventions to resolve issues associated with separation anxiety.

Client Profile

Christine is an 8-year-old female who becomes very anxious when separated from her mother. She refuses to go to school or to stay there. Christine clings to her mother and cries and begs her not to leave her in the morning when she takes Christine to school. Christine has not made friends with peers. Christine recently tried to stay overnight at the house of a girl who wants to be her friend. Within an hour of arriving at the girl's home, she began describing fears that something bad was going to happen to her mother, so she was permitted to call home several times. Each time she learned that everything was fine. She did not eat much at dinner, complaining she was allergic to everything or did not like it. At bedtime, she began to cry because she had forgotten her pillow from home and she wanted her mother to bring it or to go home and get it. About 2 A.M., when she called home again, her mother came to get her. Christine's mother describes her as like a shadow, saying that Christine won't let her out of her sight at home. Most nights she comes and gets into the parents' bed because she is fearful of not being close to mother. She hears a siren in the dark and thinks the ambulance is coming for her mother.

Case Study

Christine comes to the school nurse's office complaining of a stomachache and wanting her mother to come and get her and take her home. When the nurse calls the home, no one answers the phone. The school nurse offers to call the father at work and have him come and take her home. Christine says, "No, I don't want my father to come for me." Christine seems very upset until she recalls her mother was going to the dentist. The school nurse is aware that Christine has been falling behind her class in schoolwork due to having her mother come and get her and take her home from school two or three times a week. Christine asks the school nurse: "Would you please call the dentist's office to see if my mother is there and if she is all right? Could you ask her to come get me and take me home when she is finished at the dentist's office?" The nurse makes the call and then asks Christine if there has been a time in which her mother was sick or a time in which she worried about mom.

When the mother arrives at the school, she tells Christine that she can't keep taking her out of school and that she must learn to stay in school. When the nurse says: "It sounds like you are concerned that Christine stay in school," the mother replies: "Why wouldn't I be with the school truancy officer calling and coming to the house? Besides that she won't pass this grade if her attendance does not get better."

The mother asks the school nurse if she thinks Christine could have school phobia and wants to know if she should homeschool Christine.

When the nurse asks Christine's mother whether there was a time when she was sick and Christine worried about her, the mother shares that two years ago when Christine's sister was born, she was in labor for an extended time and then had to have a caesarian section. The sister was premature and had to remain in the hospital for a month. The mother had a number of complications, almost died, and also was in the hospital for three weeks. The nurse asks how long Christine has been like a shadow to her and worried about her. The mother answers that it has been about two years, although it has been worse since summer vacation ended six weeks ago.

Questions and Suggested Answers

1. **What could you do instead of calling the mother to come get Christine? What would you do if you could not reach the mother?** While it is all right to call the mother, it would be good to try some distraction to get Christine's mind off her mother and focused on something else. Sometimes nurses and/or teachers distract a child by giving them a hard task that takes concentration, and they ignore any references to the mother. If distraction does not work and the child is extremely distressed and the mother is not answering the phone, you could call the father even though the child is insisting on the mother.

2. **Christine's mother has asked if Christine could have school phobia. How would you answer, and what is your rationale?** It is unlikely that Christine has school phobia. Her main worry does not seem to be school but rather a fear of something happening to her mother and not wanting her mother out of her sight. You

could point out gently that you do not diagnose. You could also help the mother recognize that Christine seems not so much afraid of school as she is afraid of being separated from her mother. You could answer the mother's question with a question such as: "Do you think Christine is more afraid of being away from you than she is afraid of school?" Getting people to come up with their own insights into the problem is more effective than telling them what you think.

3. **Could Christine have Separation Anxiety Disorder? Does her behavior match any of the criteria for Separation Anxiety Disorder?** It is more likely that Christine has Separation Anxiety Disorder than school phobia.

Criteria for Separation Anxiety Disorder	Does Client Match Criteria?
Excessive anxiety, which is not developmentally appropriate, about being separated from other people to whom the person is attached, with at least three of the following eight behaviors:	Yes
Reoccurring and excessive distress when away from home or major attachment persons happens or is anticipated.	Yes, Christine's wanting her mother to come get her at school repeatedly and when she tried to stay overnight with a peer exemplifies this.
Ongoing excessive worry about loss of or harm coming to major attachment significant others.	Yes, Christine described worrying about something bad happening to her mother and called home several times to check on her when trying to overnight away from home.
Worries excessively and persistently that a significant attachment figure will fall victim to an untoward event such as getting kidnapped or lost.	Needs further assessment.
Being reluctant or refusing to be away from attachment figure(s) to go to school or anywhere else due to being afraid of separation.	Yes, her mother describes Christine as like a shadow to her.
Persistent excessive fear or reluctance to stay alone or without attachment figures in the home or without significant adults elsewhere.	Needs further assessment.
Persistent refusal or reluctance to go to bed or fall asleep without proximity to a major attachment figure or to sleep somewhere away from home.	Yes, Christine goes to her parents' bed at night and had difficulty trying to sleep away from home.
Reoccurring nightmares around the theme of being separated.	Needs assessment.
Periodic repeated complaints of physical symptoms when anticipating separation or when separated from attachment figures.	Yes.
The problem must last at least four weeks.	Yes, the mother shares the problem has lasted about two years and has been worse since summer vacation ended six weeks ago.
There must be clinically significant distress or impairment in important areas of functioning such as school, social, or work.	Yes, the client is leaving school two to three days a week and unable to defocus on mother long enough to make friends.
The behavior does not occur only during the course of some other disorder or is not better accounted for by another disorder.	As far as is known, there is no other disorder.

If the disorder is diagnosed before six years of age, it is called "early onset" (Adapted from APA, 2000).

4. Why does the nurse ask Christine and then her mother if there was a time when the mother was sick and Christine was worried about her mother? The nurse is assessing to see if there is a reason why Christine might be so fearful something will happen to mother. The question produces a logical reason for why Christine has become so attached to mother: there was a recent time when her mother almost died, and at the time she was in the hospital, separated from Christine. Assessment will sometimes, but not always, produce a logical explanation for Separation Anxiety Disorder. In some cases of Separation Anxiety Disorder the history reveals no discrete event where the major attachment figure was in danger.

5. What causes Separation Anxiety Disorder? What is the usual course of Separation Anxiety Disorder? It may have been more than the life stressor or stressors. The child may have been more vulnerable to this disorder through biological differences or learned behavior. It has been found that Separation Anxiety Disorder is found more often in first-degree biological relatives of someone with the disorder compared to the general population. The disorder is also found more frequently in children whose mothers have Panic Disorder. It is said to occur more frequently in close-knit families. The exact role of biology and environmental factors has yet to be discovered.

The onset of Separation Anxiety Disorder can occur anytime from preschool to sometime before age 18. It is most common in children between the ages of 7 and 9 (www.adaa.org). It may occur after a life stress such as moving to another neighborhood or country, changing schools, a pet or family member dying, or someone in the family being ill. The majority of children with this disorder respond to treatment; however, it is typical to have exacerbations and remissions. Exacerbations may occur under stress, such as hospitalization, in which it is natural for a child to want their parents; however, the child with Separation Anxiety will tend to demonstrate more distress than other children. In some cases the anxiety about separation and avoiding situations of separation goes on for years (APA, 2000). The client may have trouble getting married and/or moving away from home.

6. Christine's mother asks: "Are there many other children who have difficulty separating from their mothers at school age?" How would you answer her? You would probably let mother know that this problem is common. Various sources point to about 4 percent of children and adolescents experiencing separation anxiety (APA, 2000; Frisch and Frisch, 2006).

7. At what developmental stage (according to Erickson) is Christine, what are the tasks of this stage, and is she mastering these tasks? Christine's mother asks the school nurse if she should homeschool Christine. What would you say to her if you were the school nurse? Christine is in the stage of industry versus inferiority (age 6 to 11). This is a stage to master social and cognitive skills, develop skills outside of the family in the wider culture, and develop peer relationships. Christine is trying in some ways, as evidenced by trying to stay overnight with a girl who wants to be her friend, but she is failing because she cannot separate from her mother.

Homeschooling is not a question that the school nurse can answer with yes or no. The school provides a practice ground for Christine to learn to separate and to feel a sense of mastery of independence and trust that her mother will return for her. If the mother allows Christine to stay within her sight at all times, the problem will likely not resolve or will not resolve for a long time. This idea might be better accepted by the mother if it were in the form of a question, such as: "Do you suppose that Christine would learn to separate from you better if, for now, we worked on it using the present school situation rather than her being with you all day at home?" Homeschooling is a big commitment on the part of a parent or parents. The nurse can provide the mother with some resources for finding out more about homeschooling and how home schooling parents provide peer socialization opportunities so the parents can make their decision about continuing in public school or home schooling.

8. What treatments have been found to be successful in reducing separation anxiety from major attachment figures? Behavior modification and cognitive behavioral therapy have been found to be effective in reducing separation anxiety from major attachment figures. Gosschalk (2004) says that school psychologists like behavioral interventions best in working with children who have Separation Anxiety Disorder. Gosschalk describes the case of a 5-year-old girl who is treated successfully for school refusal. The girl was "shadowing" her mother at home, getting into her mother's bed at night, and having long, drawn-out separations from her mother at school and asking for her mother frequently during the day or crying for her mother. The successful treatment approach in this case included: education about the disorder for the parents, teaching the parents and child deep breathing exercises and progressive muscle relaxation, as well as providing a session on how to separate at the classroom door, saying such things as "Have a good day." The teacher was taught to take the child's hand at the door and walk her away from her mother while praising her. At home the mother would leave the room but was where she could hear the child. She gradually increased the time she could be outside the child's view (but could still hear her) using a timer and a reward system.

In another case involving the treatment of a 6-year-old boy with a diagnosis of Separation Anxiety Disorder, Dia (2001) describes successful treatment using a four-phase cognitive behavioral therapy. In the first phase the boy and his parents were taught about anxiety and about cognitive behavioral therapy. The parents were given reading materials and informed about the Anxiety Disorders Association of America. The boy was told some stories to help him learn to label his feelings and to understand that he was to conquer his fear by gradual exposure. Phase II involved creating a collaborative relationship with the therapist so they could set the pace of therapy together and formulate some strategies, used to help with the child cope with anxiety, such as distraction, coping self-statements, and contingency management techniques. The latter involved use of plastic poker chips that the child could earn for risk taking and doing well during the session. Prizes and treats could be bought with the chips. Coping statements were such words as "I can be brave." The treatment began with goals designed to provide success and gradually progressed to longer periods away from parents. In Phase III the situations used were those provoking more anxiety, such as parents taking a walk rather than being outside the door. The child used his positive self-coping statements and then was given pleasurable activities and was also taught distractions such as counting backward from ten then saying "blast off" and taking a deep breath. Another distraction was generating words beginning with a, then b, then c, and so on. In this phase the family was taught to be cotherapists at home and to practice skills at home. The father had engaged in aversive parent-child interactions. He had yelled and teased when the boy became anxious. The father was educated to change his belief that the child could do better if only he wanted to do so and to help him deal with his anxiety in more productive ways. In phase IV, the strategies were reviewed and the child informed that his success was due to his use of the coping strategies as this increases a sense of self-efficacy.

9. **From the information you have about Christine, what nursing diagnoses would you write for her? What are common nursing diagnoses for clients with Separation Anxiety Disorder? What are some reasonable goals for Christine?** Common nursing diagnoses for Separation Anxiety Disorder, which Christine would seem to have, include:

- Fear
- Anxiety
- Impaired social interaction
- Ineffective individual coping

Some goals could be:

- Will report using relaxation techniques such as deep breathing and self-talk to reduce anxiety and fear at school, at night, and in other situations when mother is not close by; in addition to reducing fear and anxiety, it is appropriate to try to make the separation at school go more smoothly and to increase the amount of time the client stays in school until a long-term goal of staying in school 100 percent of the time is met
- Will reduce time it takes to separate from mother at the classroom door or the school entrance
- Will increase the amount of time that passes before mother is called during school day
- Will stay in school 100 percent of the time

10. **What interventions do you think would work for this client, and how could you go about getting the mother and teacher(s) invested in initiating these interventions? How would you evaluate success of interventions?**

Interventions successful in resolving Separation Anxiety Disorder will need to focus on increasing the child's sense of safety and trust in not only the mother's return but a sense of safety and trust in other individuals in her life such as the father, the nurse, and the teacher as well as a sense of safety in the environment. It is helpful to emphasize that the work with the child is a team effort and the parents, as well as the school personnel who interact with the child, are an important part of the team. The nurse needs to build trust and rapport with the child, the mother, the teacher, the truancy officer, and the school psychologist and anyone else who is involved in working with the child.

It will be helpful for the nurse to do some education about Separation Anxiety Disorder. She can provide some materials as well as information about websites and local resources, if any, to the mother. The nurse can keep the psychologist informed and get information and help or at least feedback from the school psychologist.

The nurse can explain to the parents that small children first learn that objects out of sight are not gone when parents play games like hide and seek. The mother can still do some of this. It may still be helpful to play hide and seek or a game using walkie-talkies.

The nurse could teach the mother and Christine some simple relaxation techniques. The mother can role model and encourage the use of these techniques by Christine. Deep breathing exercises and progressive muscle relaxation techniques are well within the expertise of the nurse to teach.

The nurse can work with the mother to set up a simple behavior modification program at home. The mother could start by timing how long Christine can be away from her side at home and gradually increase that time. If stickers such as stars are something Christine would work for, the mother can reward Christine for meeting goals with stars on a chart that she can exchange for a small treat or small privilege.

It would be good for the mother to take Christine to school close to the time the bell rings the start of class as this gives her less time to get anxious. The mother can explain that the goodbyes are going to be different and get Christine to help script the goodbyes. A play can be written about a girl saying goodbye to her mom, and Christine and her mom can practice their lines.

The teacher can be taught relaxation exercises so she can work with Christine to relax before she gets too anxious. Teacher can also give Christine a star or some reward for each hour of staying in class and staying focused on task. This can be gradually increased to a reward for staying in class all morning. It may be helpful to give Christine a task such as taking the roll.

The interventions are designed to help the client meet the goals. Evaluation involves looking at goals and deciding if the client met these goals completely or partially. Goals can be increased or decreased and interventions changed to better help the client meet the revised goals. If goals are met, interventions were successful.

References

American Psychiatric Association. (2000). *Diagnostic and Statistical Manual of Mental Disorders, 4th ed.* Text Revision. Washington, DC: American Psychiatric Association.

Dia, D. (2001). "Cognitive-Behavioral Therapy with a Six-Year-Old Boy with Separation Anxiety Disorder: A Case Study." *Health and Social Work* 26(2): 125–129.

Frisch, N.C. and L.E. Frisch. (2006). *Psychiatric Mental Health Nursing, 3rd ed.* Albany, NY: Thomson Delmar Learning.

Gosschalk, P.O. (2004). "Behavioral Treatment of Acute Onset School Refusal in a 5-Year-Old Girl with Separation Anxiety Disorder." *Education and Treatment of Children* 27(2): 150–160.

www.adaa.org. Accessed December 4, 2005.

GENDER	SOCIOECONOMIC
Female	■ Middle class

GENDER

Female

AGE

7

SETTING

■ School nurse's office

ETHNICITY

■ Asian American (Myanmar, formerly called Burma)

CULTURAL CONSIDERATIONS

■ Military culture and Asian (Myanmar)

PREEXISTING CONDITION

COEXISTING CONDITION

■ Possible Social Phobia

COMMUNICATION

DISABILITY

SOCIOECONOMIC

■ Middle class

SPIRITUAL/RELIGIOUS

PHARMACOLOGIC

PSYCHOSOCIAL

■ Shy and selective mute

LEGAL

ETHICAL

ALTERNATIVE THERAPY

PRIORITIZATION

DELEGATION

MODERATE

SELECTIVE MUTISM

Level of difficulty: Moderate

Overview: Requires enlisting the cooperation of the client's family, teacher, and peers to work together to help the client feel safe and motivated to talk out loud in a variety of settings and to a variety of people.

Client Profile

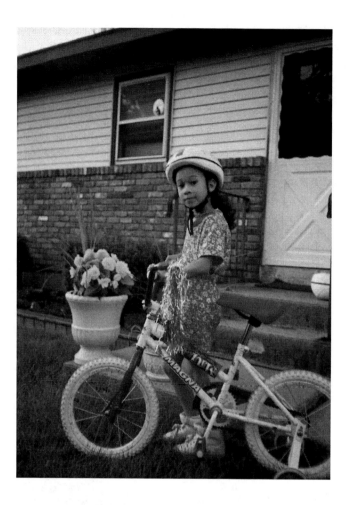

Phyu (pronounced Pee You) is 7 years old and lives with her mother and stepfather and an older sister. Her biological father lives in Myanmar (formerly Burma). Phyu's stepfather is a career military officer and currently on duty away from the family. The mother is from Myanmar. Phyu's mother and stepfather met in Bangkok where her mother had a job and the stepfather was on leave from the service. Phyu has moved frequently with her family, living first in Myanmar until her mother remarried, then on two different military bases in Asian countries. Recently the family moved to a small town in the Northwest near Phyu's stepfather's relatives while her stepfather was away on active duty.

Phyu has always been shy around distant relatives, strangers, and in strange situations. At 5 years old, she was talking to her sister in both English and the Myanmar language, but would not talk to anyone else. The parents and teacher did not worry about it the first month of school because they thought she was just shy and would start talking as soon as she got used to being in a different country and being at school. After the second month of not talking at school, the parents took Phyu to a pediatrician who diagnosed Phyu as having Selective Mutism. The parents thought Phyu would grow out of this problem, but it has persisted and now she is in the second grade and still does not talk in school.

Case Study

An older sister has brought Phyu to the school nurse's office. Phyu looks serious and somewhat sad. When the nurse asks her a question, Phyu plays with her hair, looks at the floor, and says nothing. The older sister talks for

Phyu, saying that Phyu came to school this morning even though she was not feeling well and that she is now feeling worse and wants to go home. The school nurse starts to talk to Phyu, and her sister says: "She doesn't talk." The school nurse takes Phyu's temperature, and it is normal. Talking through the sister to Phyu, the school nurse learns that Phyu does not hurt anywhere but is "feeling bad." The school nurse asks Phyu and her sister to remain in the office and goes to talk briefly with the teacher. The teacher explains that the children in Phyu's class were going to be doing oral presentations, and a peer had teased her about her inability to talk in class and said: "I bet you won't give your report because the cat has got your tongue." Phyu was diagnosed with Selective Mutism when she was 5 years old, the teacher explains to the school nurse. The teacher says: "I would really appreciate it if you would work with me to find ways to help Phyu succeed at school. Perhaps you could get her mother involved in working with us. So far I have not had any luck getting the mother to participate in anything at school or to talk with me about Phyu on the phone."

Questions and Suggested Answers

1. **If you were the school nurse, how would you respond to Phyu's request to go home?** There are several options for responding to this student's request to go home. You could call her mother and ask her to come for Phyu and do nothing more. The student would gain temporary relief of anxiety and do little to solve the problem of how to succeed in school. It might reinforce the idea of going home whenever she is anxious.

   After sending Phyu home, you could go several steps further. You could go to the classroom and have a discussion with Phyu's classmates in which you and the teacher enlist their help in working with Phyu to overcome whatever fears or thoughts are keeping her from talking.

   Another option would be to call the mother and ask her to come in and talk with you about how best to help Phyu. Together you can decide whether or not to take her home this time or how to help her be more comfortable in class the rest of the day. What you do not want to do is to take Phyu back to class to be present for a discussion of what happened in regard to the teasing and how the class needs to stop doing this teasing. The rationale for this is that children with Selective Mutism do not want to be the center of attention. They tend to withdraw more when they feel others are judging them. You can get an idea of how a child with Selective Mutism would react to being the subject of discussion in a classroom by reading the comments by adults who were selectively mute as children on a chat line sponsored by the Selective Mutism Group Childhood Anxiety Network (www.selectivemutism.org).

2. **You are the nurse in this case, and you decide to call the mother to come in and talk with you and the teacher. What action will you take if Phyu's mother offers a number of excuses for not coming to school to meet with you? What could be going on with the mother if she refuses to come to school for a discussion?** You first need to find out how capable the mother is in speaking English. You may have to have the client's sister interpret. People in Myanmar speak 111 languages; however, the majority of the people there speak Myanmar language (www.myanmars.net).

   There are a number of possible reasons for the mother not agreeing to come to school to meet with you. It is quite common for a close relative (such as the mother) of a child with Selective Mutism to have an anxiety disorder. Coming into the school to meet with the nurse and teacher, or even just the nurse, may be threatening to the mother.

   If the mother speaks English, you can consider offering to meet with her in her home or a location of her choice if at all possible. You could also talk with her by phone in a supportive, helpful way and suggest sources of support and information about Selective Mutism. Before suggesting the Internet as a source of information, you need to ask if she has access to the Internet. There are some people who do not use computers for a variety of reasons, including avoiding contact with others.

3. **What is Selective Mutism? Which of the diagnostic criteria of Selective Mutism does Phyu meet?** Selective Mutism is a diagnosis given to a person who consistently, over the time frame of more than a month, does not talk in one or more situations but talks in other situations. This term "Selective Mutism" is most frequently used with children and adolescents who do not talk at school, although some children may talk at school but

not in other situations where talking would be expected. For example, a child might elect to be silent with most family members and speak only with and through a sibling, a cousin, or mother or grandmother and not to others in the family.

Some researchers and theorists in the mental health field question whether Selective Mutism is a disorder or not. Some theorists have suggested that Selective Mutism is a symptom of Social Phobia. About 90 percent of the children with Selective Mutism can meet the diagnostic criteria for Social Phobia, according to Dr. Elisa Shipon-Blum, executive director of Selective Mutism Group Childhood Anxiety Network (www.selectivemutism.org, 2004a). Some clinicians have suggested that Selective Mutism might not only be a symptom of Social Phobia but perhaps a symptom of some other disorder closely related to Asperger's Syndrome. Other nonpopular theories include Selective Mutism as a symptom of Dissociative Disorder or a symptom that could develop into Schizophrenia (Kumpulainen, Rasanen, Raaska, and Somppi, 1998).

Phyu meets a number of the criteria for Selective Mutism.

Diagnostic Criteria for Selective Mutism	Does the Client Meet These Criteria?
Child does not talk in select places or social situations where it is expected the child will speak (e.g., at school or at home or to specific people), even though speaking in other situations.	Yes, does not talk in class or outside the close primary family.
The child's not talking interferes with school or occupational achievement or social communication.	Yes, not talking interferes with Phyu performing at school and having friends.
Not talking has lasted at least a month and not just the first month of school.	Not talking in selective situations has lasted at least two years.
Not speaking is not due to lack of knowledge of or comfort with the language required in the situation.	This client knows how to speak English and is comfortable talking English according to her sister.
The problem is not better explained by presence of a Communication Disorder such as stuttering and does not happen only during course of a Pervasive Developmental Disorder, Schizophrenia, or other Psychotic Disorder.	As far as is known the client does not have a communication disorder or a Pervasive Developmental Disorder, Schizophrenia, or a Psychotic Disorder.

(Adapted from APA, 2000)

4. **When one of Phyu's teachers asks: "What causes Selective Mutism?" and "How common is Selective Mutism?" what will you tell him or her?** The most popular current belief is that most of the children who develop Selective Mutism have inherited a genetic predisposition to anxiety. It is believed that these children have inherited severely inhibited temperaments and are extremely shy and timid. A current theory is that children with Selective Mutism have a decreased threshold of excitability in the amygdala and when confronted with something they fear, the amygdala sets off a series of reactions.

Perhaps some children with a genetic predisposition to Selective Mutism have their mutism triggered by stressful experiences. In a study by Kumpulainen, Rasanen, Raaska, and Somppi (1998), teachers reported that sixteen of thirty-nine children with Selective Mutism had experienced a stressful situation in their lives, and some experienced it just before becoming mute. Stressful situations included death of a significant person in their lives, alcoholism in their family, or changing schools.

Older theories include the psychodynamic theory in which Selective Mutism is seen as a result of unresolved conflict; for example, when a child who is orally or anally fixated wants to punish their parents, they choose not to speak in certain situations. Under this theory, the desire to punish the parents may come from such experiences as having been punished or abused, or from having to harbor a family secret. Mutism is thus a coping mechanism under this theory. The child copes with anger and/or anxiety by not speaking.

A variety of sources state that this disorder is found in less than 1 percent of children and that it is fairly rare (APA, 2000; Krysanski, 2003), although talking with school nurses and teachers, you will find that most of them have a current relationship with a child who has Selective Mutism or can recall having worked with a child with this disorder in the recent past. There are researchers and clinicians who think the disorder is more prevalent for children of early school years. Hultquist (1995) in a review of the literature on Selective Mutism found support for somewhat higher rates after age 5. One epidemiological study, Hultquist, pointed to agree with the rate cited above but only up until age 5. After age 5, the rate found was 7.2 percent per 1,000. A prevalence rate of 2 percent in second graders was found in a study by Kumpulainen, Rasanen, Raaska, and Somppi (1998). These researchers sent information explaining symptoms of Selective Mutism to teachers in one county and asking if they had any children with these symptoms. When a teacher responded "yes," a follow-up questionnaire was sent to this teacher. There were 2,010 children covered by the original questionnaire, and 39 were found that could meet the criteria for diagnosis of Selective Mutism.

5. **Does this client fit the usual pattern for age of onset of Selective Mutism? Is Selective Mutism found equally in boys and girls or not? What other disorders are frequently diagnosed concurrently with Selective Mutism?** Phyu does fit the usual pattern for age of onset of Selective Mutism, which most often begins before age 5, but frequently is not realized until the child starts school. Some children demonstrate the symptoms of this disorder in later school years.

   All reports found in the literature on Selective Mutism say that more girls have this disorder compared to boys. The ratio reported most often is five to one (although some studies have found two to one) (Stein, Rapin, and Yapko, 2001).

   Common concurrent diagnoses for children diagnosed as having Selective Mutism include Social Phobia, Avoidant Disorder, and Simple Phobia (Stegbauer and Roberts, 2002). Enuresis and Encopresis have also been reported in greater than expected percentages of children with Selective Mutism, and some researchers have found high rates of obsessive-compulsive features and/or depression (Krysanski, 2003).

6. **What are children with Selective Mutism like?** Children and adolescents with Selective Mutism are typically described as shy to the extreme. When attention is brought to them, they will do things to indicate their anxiety and lack of desire to be the focus of attention. Some children respond to attention by giving a blank stare while others turn their heads, look away or look down, try to hide, play with their hair, or suck their fingers. They are described as having a severely inhibited nature and being very sensitive. Intelligent, curious, perceptive are other terms often used to describe this child or adolescent. They are often viewed as artistic and talented. In a study of thirty-nine second-grade children who were selectively mute, Kumpulainen, Rasanen, Raaska, and Somppi (1998) found the children being described with the following characteristics in the following percentages: shy 63 percent, withdrawn 63 percent, serious 58 percent, expressionless 34 percent, cheerful 34 percent, hyperkinetic 13 percent, and aggressive 13 percent.

7. **What role do you think culture might play in this case?** The stepfather's military culture required frequent family moves. Each time a move was made to another military base, Phyu was required to enter a new class of peers, which was somewhat threatening. It may have been easier to be accepted by military dependents who also moved frequently and were multicultural. In the Northwest nonmilitary culture, the client probably joined a group of students who had been friends for some time and making friends in this group may have been even more difficult than in the military schools.

   The Myanmar culture has as a key concept "cetana," which has to do with goodwill, good intentions, and benevolence practiced in everyday life as well as religion. The culture encourages respect. Moving from the Myanmar culture to the totally different culture of the United States could be stressful.

8. **What additional data would you like to gather on this child? What tentative nursing diagnoses would you likely write for this client? Working with Phyu's teachers and hopefully Phyu and her mother, what goals would be reasonable for Phyu?** You probably would like to have a comprehensive assessment on this child, but this may not be possible at this time. You might be able to get the mother to sign a release of information form so you could talk with the pediatrician who diagnosed the Selective Mutism and get whatever

developmental history you could from him. As you build a trusting relationship with the mother, she might be willing to answer some questions. If she too has difficulty dealing with social situations and talking with people, you might get more information from her initially by giving her a questionnaire to answer. Phyu, through her sister, may be able to tell you about her interests. The teacher may also be aware of Phyu's interests and talents as well as limitations. You will want to assess to find out if Phyu does have peers that she talks to in school and/or out of school.

You would most likely write nursing diagnoses of anxiety and fear. Depending on assessment findings, other diagnosis could include but not be limited to: defensive coping, chronically low self-esteem, and powerlessness. You might be tempted to use impaired verbal communication, but fear and anxiety are more appropriate in the case of Selective Mutism.

Goals would include some or all of the following goals:

- Will identify and report using at least one means of reducing anxiety
- Will report being less anxious in class
- Will identify at least one strength

9. **What approach/interventions would you suggest to Phyu's mother, family, and teachers?** You would advise the family and teachers to avoid pressuring the child to speak. You could explain that the focus needs to be on providing a climate, techniques, and a process for gradually talking over time, but that pressure is counterproductive as it only increases the anxiety. It is also helpful to let the child know that you understand that they are afraid to speak and you and others will help them through their difficulties. A major point to get across is that punishment for not talking is counterproductive as well as inappropriate and should never be used.

Ideas for increasing comfort with the teacher and classroom that you could suggest include having the child arrive at school early before other children are there so the child can work quietly for a few minutes or help the teacher with some tasks while developing a comfort level with the teacher and classroom. If the teacher cannot or will not do this, you might ask the mother if the child could come early to help you do some small tasks. Believing that at least one person is caring, whether it is the teacher or the nurse or both, is an important step in helping Phyu reduce her anxiety enough to talk in school.

As you build a trusting relationship with the mother, you can explore with the mother the possibility of her taking Phyu to a mental health professional (e.g., a psychiatric nurse clinician, a psychologist, or psychiatrist) with experience in treating children with selective Mutism. Stegbauer and Roberts (2002) say that parents need to select a mental health professional who is willing to work with the school personnel as well as the mother to set up a "home and school program that rewards communication and socialization and discourages behaviors that increase anxiety such as punishment for nonverbal behavior, insistence on speech, or pressuring a child to speak." If the mother cannot access a mental health professional to help in developing a cognitive-behavioral program or is not willing to pursue professional help for Phyu, your school district may have a mental health professional who can assist with developing a program for Phyu.

10. **Why do you suppose some parents whose children have Selective Mutism don't want to get professional help for their children? Why do experts urge early diagnosis and treatment for children with Selective Mutism rather than waiting it out to see if it disappears?** The reasons probably vary greatly. One reason could be that the parents themselves may have some social anxiety and the child's behavior does not seem too unreasonable, especially when thinking that the child might outgrow the problem. Children seem to manage in school without speaking to teachers. Some children manage for years. In the study by Kumpulainen, Rasanen, Raaska, and Somppi (1998), teachers responded that while about half the parents had a normal open relationship with them, some of the parents were not interested in their child's schoolwork and some had no contact at all with the teacher. Two parents were even hostile and blamed the school for the child not speaking. The teachers in this study indicated that the children managed all right. With parents wanting to wait or not indicating any interest in therapy and with teachers thinking the child is managing all right, coupled with the expense and time involved in therapy as well as fears about therapy and medication somewhat generated by the media, it is understandable when parents demonstrate resistance to getting therapy for their children.

If left untreated, the anxiety associated with Selective Mutism can get much worse over time. The child can develop depression and become socially isolated and withdraw. Self-esteem can become very poor, and the child can have increasing lack of self-confidence. There is a great risk of underachievement in school and later in the workplace. Some students will self-medicate with alcohol and drugs. Some children will have suicidal thoughts. Postings on the chat line on the Selective Mutism Group Childhood Anxiety Network's webpage (www.selectivemutism.org) reveal that most people there are reporting miserable experiences as children having Selective Mutism and many have current difficulty in the work world. Early treatment of their disorder would have greatly helped many of these people.

Some people on the Selective Mutism chat line do report having experienced very caring and helpful school staff during their school years, people that made all the difference in their lives. If this client's mother won't get professional help for her, you as the nurse working with the teachers can hopefully help this child avoid, or reduce, the problems listed above.

11. **In a conversation with the mother, she asks: "Is medication ever used to treat Selective Mutism, and if so, what medications?" How would you respond? What are the treatment approaches in addition to or instead of medication that are currently being used with children and adolescents?** Medications have and are being used to treat Selective Mutism. Phyu's mother might be willing to look at the Selective Mutism Group Childhood Anxiety Network webpage (www.selectivemutism.org, 2004b) to read what Dr. Elisa Shipon-Blum says about medication and Selective Mutism. She states that "studies clearly indicate that the best approach to therapy [for Selective Mutism] is a combination of behavioral techniques and medication." In addition, she states that since most parents are hesitant or opposed to giving medication, often behavioral approaches alone are used for awhile and if the child does not respond, then medication is used. Medications used to treat Selective Mutism are those that have been successful in treating anxiety disorders and include serotonin selective reuptake inhibitors such as Prozac, Paxil, Celexa, Luvox, and Zoloft. Other medications which are used successfully include: Effexor XR, Serzone, Buspar, and Remeron. Medication lowers anxiety to a point that behavioral techniques can work more easily and successfully, according to Shipon-Blum.

The primary nondrug treatment for Selective Mutism is behavior modification using positive reinforcement and desensitization. The first step is to find ways to lower the child's anxiety and only when this is accomplished and the child is ready is positive reinforcement for speaking introduced. In some cases a token system has been used with children who are selectively mute.

Self-modeling is a technique described by Krysanski (2003). This technique involves the child viewing repeated and spaced edited videotapes of themselves. The videotapes show only appropriate behaviors. In some instances a child has been videotaped talking to someone they normally talk to and then the film is edited to replace this person with a person they do not talk with usually, such as the teacher. This method is designed to help the child feel more comfortable about talking to someone without fear that something awful will happen as a result. Krysanski points out that some children with Selective Mutism are treatment resistant, and when working with these children, self-modeling becomes more of a challenge.

Play therapy is another technique/approach used in treating Selective Mutism. Play therapy needs to be done by someone trained and certified as a Play Therapist. Play therapy utilizes such items as dollhouses and small models of people, anatomically correct dolls, sand trays, and water as well as games. These "props" and various techniques help the Play Therapist identify the level and source of fears and to identify other issues such as control or lack of control, abuse and neglect, jealousy, anger, and more.

Cognitive Behavioral Therapy is also used with children and adolescents who have Selective Mutism. Cognitive Behavioral Therapy helps children and adolescents change their fear-based and fear-reinforcing thoughts into positive thoughts.

Family therapy is yet another treatment approach in Selective Mutism. The family members can learn to adjust interactive and/or parenting styles to best help the child with Selective Mutism reduce anxiety and stress, identify their feelings, and build their confidence in themselves.

Planting suggestions is another technique. Diane Yapko (Stein, Rapin, and Yapko, 2001) points out that clinicians can use language in a suggestive and influential manner. She suggests saying something like: "I wonder which day it will be when Peter chooses to talk at school" or I wonder which friend Peter will choose to talk with first." Yapko says this method lets the child know that they have choices and some control. Yapko cautions the clinician not to discuss the child's condition with parents in front of the child but to either send the child to do something else or phone the parents later. It is important to remember that just because a child does not talk doesn't mean that they cannot hear.

References

American Psychiatric Association. (2000). *Diagnostic and Statistical Manual of Mental Disorders, 4th ed.* Text Revision. Washington, DC: American Psychiatric Association.

Hultquist, A.M. (1995). "Selective Mutism: Causes and Interventions." *Journal of Emotional and Behavioral Disorders* 3(2): 100–107.

Krysanski, V.L. (2003). "A Brief Review of Selective Mutism Literature." *Journal of Psychology* 137(1): 29–40.

Kumpulainen, K., E. Rasanen, H. Raaska, and V. Somppi. (1998). "Selective Mutism Among Second-Graders in Elementary School." *European Child and Adolescent Psychiatry* 7(1): 24–29.

Shipon-Blaum, E. (2004a). "Understanding Selective Mutism: A Guide to Helping Our Teachers Understand." Available at www. selectivemutism.org/pdf/teachers.pdf.

_____. (2004b). "When the Words Just Won't Come Out: Understanding Selective Mutism." Available at www.selectivemutism. org/pdf/words.pdf.

Stegbauer, C. and S.J. Roberts. (2002). "Identifying Mutism's Etiology in a Child." *Nurse Practitioner* 27(10): 44–47.

Stein, M.T., I. Rapin, and D. Yapko, E. (2001). "Selective Mutism Part 2." *Pediatrics* 107(4): 926–930.

www.myanmars.net. Accessed June 17, 2006.

GENDER

Male

AGE

5

SETTING

- Children's medical unit

ETHNICITY

- Asian American: parents born in Thailand and grandparents born in India

CULTURAL CONSIDERATIONS

- Culture of Thailand, including Buddhist religion and culture

PREEXISTING CONDITION

COEXISTING CONDITION

- Chronic constipation

COMMUNICATION

DISABILITY

SOCIOECONOMIC

- Parents recently finished graduate school; father has full-time work and mother has a part-time job

SPIRITUAL/RELIGIOUS

- Buddhist

PHARMACOLOGIC

PSYCHOSOCIAL

- Move from apartment to a house when child was age 2
- Followed by brief separation from parents

LEGAL

- Confidentiality issue

ETHICAL

ALTERNATIVE THERAPY

- Reflexology

PRIORITIZATION

DELEGATION

MODERATE

ENCOPRESIS

Level of difficulty: Moderate

Overview: Requires critical thinking/problem solving to develop rapport with a 5-year-old client and get him to voluntarily give up defecating in his underwear and to use the toilet for this purpose. Requires supporting not only the client but his parents, who are frustrated, angry, and embarrassed at times.

Client Profile

Theera is a 5-year-old boy who was born in the United States to parents from Thailand. His parents came to this country to attend graduate school, and that is where they met, married, and had Theera. When Theera was about 2 years old, they purchased a new home and moved from the apartment where they had lived all of Theera's life to a quiet suburban home. Soon after this family move, Theera's parents left on a business trip associated with the father's work and Theera was left in the care of extended family. Later, the mother's sister and her son, who is two years older than Theera, moved in with the family so she could attend college and help take care of Theera. At this time Theera was refusing to defecate in the commode in the bathroom, saying he would not do this until he went to school. He has had periods of passing small amounts of hard stool, usually about three times a week. Theera's mother has eagerly awaited the start of school, expecting he would defecate in the toilet; however, this has not happened. Once Theera began school, he started soiling his underwear and hiding it in various places in the school. The teacher began to discover the hidden underwear a little over three months ago and finally figured out it belonged to Theera when the mother, tiring of buying underwear because he never seemed to have any clean, decided to put labels in the underwear.

Case Study

Theera is admitted to the children's medical unit for a medical evaluation, which has revealed that although he has problems with constipation, the problem is not due to a medical condition. The primary nurse assigned to care for him reads Theera's psychosocial evaluation and learns the information in the profile above. In talking with the mother the nurse learns that the parents have been embarrassed that Theera still is not toilet trained. His room at home has been so odorous at times from hidden soiled underwear that they were embarrassed to have guests, and the cousin made fun of Theera being a baby. The father has been angry with the mother at times for not being able to make Theera use the toilet and "babying" him too much.

The mother shares that she has tried bribing Theera with promises of toys and that his father has tried spanking him to get him to use the toilet, all without success.

During a team meeting to do treatment planning for Theera, the nurse practitioner on the team says that she is building a somewhat conspiratorial relationship with Theera in which she has offered to help Theera hide his underwear. She has told Theera that he is not hiding them well enough and perhaps he could use her help to hide them better.

The nurse practitioner also shares reading about a social worker who has had good luck working with children with Encopresis to get them to not let the "poop" be the boss, much in the way children learn not to let bullies get the best of them. Some of the team members tell the primary nurse that they think these ideas are crazy and what this child needs is laxatives, suppositories, and/or enemas followed with bowel training as well as limit setting.

Questions and Suggested Answers

1. **What are some common feelings nurses might have when working with a child who soils his underwear and hides it in inappropriate places like under his bed or in the dresser drawers? What are some responses that parents might have to a child with Encopresis?** Nurses can experience a variety of feelings when assigned to work with a child with Encopresis. These feelings include but are not limited to: disgust; anger at the situation, parents, or child; discomfort associated with the thought of picking up soiled underwear; feeling the child is a "brat" or is "misunderstood" or "controlling," or just being stubborn.

   Parents may feel shame or anger or a variety of responses. Blaming the child's stubbornness for Encopresis was reported as having increased as a parental attitude over recent years in a study by Fishman, Nurko, Rappaport, and Schonwald (2003) that looked at referrals to an Encopresis clinic over a twenty-year period.

After learning more about Encopresis, nurses, parents, and others may be able to give up the idea that stubbornness causes this problem. Another response nurses can have to working with the child with Encopresis is to feel challenged or intrigued with this problem to solve and this interesting child to work with. Whatever nurses feel, they have to stop and deal with these thoughts and feelings and try to adopt the most professional therapeutic attitude that they can in order to help this client and his family.

2. **What rationale could the nurse practitioner have had for offering to help Theera hide his underwear?** The offer by the nurse practitioner to help hide soiled underwear would seem to be directed toward building a therapeutic relationship between the child and the nurse practitioner. It may help the child feel he is supported. Strange as it may seem, in some cases where Encopresis arises out of psychological issues, just this alliance and support from an adult will cause the child to begin to use the toilet rather than defecating in inappropriate places. The nurse practitioner can at some point in time transfer this alliance or share it with another nurse, perhaps yourself if you are the primary nurse for this child. The nurse practitioner will not want to be the only one with a trusting relationship with the child but will want to help the child deal with trust versus mistrust and enlarge the number of trusted persons.

3. **What are the criteria for a diagnosis of Encopresis, and do you think Theera meets these criteria?** To be diagnosed with Encopresis, a child must have had repeated incidences of defecating in inappropriate places, such as clothing or the floor or a furniture drawer, whether it is voluntary or not. The client with Encopresis must have at least one time of defecating in an inappropriate place per month for at least three months. The client must be at least 4 years old or be mentally developed at this chronological age. The inappropriate defecation cannot be due only to the physiological effects of a substance such as laxatives or a medical disorder/condition "except through a mechanism involving constipation" (APA, 2000, 118).

Encopresis can be with or without constipation associated with overflow incontinence, though the literature describes most cases of Encopresis as being associated with constipation and pain on defecation.

Fecal incontinence that is associated with a general medical condition such as chronic diarrhea, spina bifida, or anal stenosis will not be given a diagnosis of Encopresis.

Theera would appear to meet the criteria for Encopresis as he is over 4 years old and has repeated incidences of defecating in inappropriate places and has done this at several times a week/month for all his life.

Some children with Encopresis have not been toilet trained (primary Encopresis), and some are trained and then begin to pass stool in inappropriate places (secondary Encopresis). Another term used is functional Encopresis, which indicates that there is not a medical condition involved.

4. **You are teaching an in-service education on Encopresis for your peers. How would you respond to questions regarding the cause and incidence of Encopresis and how Encopresis relates to constipation and soiling?** Constipation is a symptom defined as "a stool frequency of fewer than three times a week and a change in consistency" with stools typically small, hard, and dry. In its mildest form it is simply a delay or problem in passing stools over a period of two or more weeks. Soiling is the passage of stool by involuntary means, occurring when the external anal sphincter relaxes following a long period of contraction causing muscle fatigue (Mason et al., 2004).

Painful defecation with resultant resistance to passing the stool may play a role in causation of some cases of Encopresis. Mason et al. (2004) found an incidence of 63 percent of children with Encopresis having a history of painful defecation before age 3. Partin, Hamill, Fischel, and Partin (1992) reviewed records of 227 children presenting to a pediatric gastroenterology clinic between 1981 and 1990 with difficult defecation. More than 50 percent of the children of school age who came in with fecal soiling or chronic fecal impaction had experienced painful defecation before age 3 and had a history of withholding stool. In another study of children treated in a tertiary Encopresis clinic over the course of twenty years, Fishman, Nurko, Rappaport, and Schonwald (2003) reported that over half of the children referred to the clinic were constipated and soiled every day, with most of them soiling in school and up to 58 percent soiling at night in their sleep.

Psychological stressors may be a risk factor for constipation and Encopresis (e.g., parental discord, getting a new sibling, or a family move). A child cannot control these events so may try to control something he can control, such as passing of stool (Mason et al., 2004). Younger children may have a higher incidence of soiling or Encopresis than older children. Mason et al. (2004) state soiling or Encopresis occurs in about 3 percent of 4-year-olds and 1.5 percent of 10-year-olds.

Hackett, Hackett, Bhakta, and Gowers (2001) studied South Indian children with Enuresis and/or Encopresis, interviewing parents of 1,403 randomly selected children ages 8 to 12. They found 4 percent of the children having "had an episode of Encopresis in the past year." These researchers found that Encopresis in this population was associated with male sex, physical and psychiatric symptoms, poor academic achievement, early separation from parents before the age of 4, not having a toilet (which is common in some areas in underdeveloped countries), and the use of physical punishment for discipline.

One older theory proposes that Encopresis is due to the mother having trouble separating from the child and becoming overinvolved to the point the child is undifferentiated from the mother. Blaming the mother created guilt in mothers who began to feel powerless, helpless, and defeated. Riccelli (2005) describes work with parents to recognize, then decrease these feelings. Riccelli points out that contributing factors to Encopresis could include the too-busy world of parents today allowing for little time and patience with toilet training.

The disorder is more common in males compared to females.

5. **What kinds of treatments are currently commonly being utilized to treat children with constipation, and what treatments are used for Encopresis?** Fishman, Nurko, Rappaport, and Schonwald (2003) found that treatment of Encopresis before the child is referred to their clinic had not changed a lot in recent years, although fewer children are given enemas and about a fifth receive no treatment. The favorites remain mineral oil, laxatives, suppositories, and toilet sitting.

There are guidelines for treating constipation, which are described in an article by Mason et al. (2004). Treatment begins with education of the family that treatment will take as long as six to twelve months. The rectum is cleaned out in the first week of treatment through a series of enemas or high doses of oral medication. These authors suggest that children usually do better with the oral doses than the enemas. If the child refuses the oral therapy, a nasogastric solution of polyethylene glycol may be given often on a hospitalized basis. During the six to twelve months, the child receives oral laxatives and a high-fiber diet, fluids, and behavior modification.

Behavior modification consists of a toilet schedule, which is usually twenty minutes two to three times a day after meals to utilize the gastrocolic reflex. A timer can be used to deter the child from asking when they can get up. The child's feet are placed on the floor. A calendar and recording of stool passed gives the child some evidence of any success. Parents are taught to increase the fiber in the child's diet by adding high-fiber cereals, breads, and crackers and fresh fruits and vegetables. In a weaning phase the child is weaned off of laxatives but is encouraged to continue the high-fiber diet and to get adequate fluid intake. Increased fiber in the diet causes increased water in stool contents, making the stool bulkier and softer.

Mason et al. point out that there are treatment failures in about 20 percent of the children treated for constipation, and these failures are often those with a long history of constipation or those who have found secondary gain. Perhaps attention that is normally hard to come by or the sense of control that is difficult to achieve in some families or situations comes with the failure to pass stool in the toilet. A question arises about whether children with only constipation are more successful in treatment with fiber versus those with constipation and Encopresis combined. Loening-Baucke, Miele, and Staiano (2004) conducted a study of the dietary fiber glucomannan: a fiber gel polysaccharide made of tubers of the Japanese Konjac plant versus placebo. These authors found that 69 percent of children with constipation only were treated successfully with fiber and only 28 percent of those with constipation and Encopresis. These findings and others that some children do not respond to physical treatment suggest that some subset of children may need a nontraditional approach or an innovative individualized psychological approach.

6. **Define and discuss reflexology as a treatment for Encopresis.** Reflexology is a "specialized pressure massage of reflex zones of specific areas of the body, particularly the feet." The feet have various zones each corresponding to some area of the body. It is believed that massaging a zone correctly will put the corresponding

body part, or organ, into balance (i.e., create, facilitate, maintain homeostasis) (Bishop, McKinnon, Weir, and Brown, 2003). Reflexology has been utilized in Asian countries more than the United States, but is gaining popularity in the United States.

Bishop, McKinnon, Weir, and Brown (2003) describe a study combining traditional treatment with reflexology. It was conducted in a pediatric department in Cheshire, England, and is described as consisting of removal of impacted feces with a phosphate enema followed with laxatives to keep the stool soft. In addition the usual treatment would consist of advisement by the dietitian. Sixteen children who would have received this traditional treatment were selected for a nontraditional pilot study using reflexology as a treatment alternative to the administration of an enema to a child.

Each child in the study received one half-hour a week of reflexology. Before the study 78 percent of the group was soiling at least once a day and 16 percent were soiling one to three times a week and 6 percent had no soiling in the prior seven days. After reflexology the 78 percent soiling daily was reduced to 20 percent and those soiling one to three times a week increased from 16 percent to 30 percent and 48 percent now had no soiling over a week. Overall, soiling after reflexology had declined.

7. **Theera's Aunt comes to visit him. She asks you to tell her what the doctor has said about Theera's problem. She also tells you that she wants to give you some information about Theera and the family. What is your response to her request for information and her offer to give you information?** You need to advise the aunt that you cannot share information with her about her nephew unless his parents sign an official release of information for her to receive information or she is with the parents and they orally request information be shared in their presence. You are bound by your nurse practice act, standards of practice, hospital rules and regulations, and the law to maintain confidentiality. You may want to discuss the importance of confidentiality with nursing peers to avoid the problems that could occur if the sister approaches any of them and someone breaches the confidentiality.

You can receive information from the aunt or anyone else who wants to freely give it.

8. **What do you think about the social worker's idea of talking to the child about being boss over the poop?** Thinking about who is the boss is something that a young child could understand. Children are concrete thinkers and relate to things they know. Children this age understand the concept of a bully, and given enough confidence in themselves and their strengths, they can be boss over the bully.

Riccelli (2005) at Stanford University Psychiatry Department described using this "boss over poop" technique with a large number of children diagnosed with functional Encopresis. The children know Riccelli as "the poop lady." She describes the anguish that parents present with, having many times been blamed, or feeling they have been blamed, for their children's failure to defecate in the toilet. The child is acting as if there is no problem, the same way they have been taught by their parents to ignore a bully on the playground. She points out that this is what the child is doing with the poop bully in the gut. The child is ignoring it. If he poops and hides it, the parents ask: "Did you poop?" And he says: "No." If the poop smells, he acts like he doesn't smell it. She points out that the poop bully loves ignoring. He loves the warm cozy tummy or squishy warm of the underpants. She paints poop as wanting to be boss over the child. She asks the child: "Do you want to be the boss over the poop?" Riccelli empowers children to believe in themselves as capable of being the boss over their poop and empowers parents to help them. One technique she uses is a chart with two columns: one column is entitled: "I'm the Boss over Sneaky Poop" and the other is "Sneaky Poop is the Boss over Me." This chart helps the child work toward being boss. While the child is in the hospital, Riccelli does things to help the child develop strengths by such methods as asking the child if they can run and timing them in running and getting them to better their time. This makes them feel their strength and also strengthens the idea they can make it to the toilet in time to defecate in the toilet.

9. **The mother mentions that she has gone to the Buddhist temple to take food and robes for the monks, light incense, and get a wish about Theera offered up to Buddha. She says she thinks this problem with his not going to the toilet may have something to do with Theera's past lives. What would be an acceptable response given that you are not of the Buddhist religion?** A good response would be to simply listen and accept that

there are people in the world whose religious beliefs are not the same as yours. Other people's beliefs are often as strong and as important to them as yours are to you. An attitude of respect for their right to practice their own religion is helpful to them. Some nurses may be strong in an atheist belief, others may be agnostic, and some may hold a strong belief in one of the various religions of the world. If clients or their families ask you to pray with them and you feel comfortable doing this, it can be therapeutic. You must always ask yourself if your actions are professional, therapeutic, and in the client's best interest. As you must know by now, health care is not about making the nurse feel better; it is about serving the client.

10. **What assessments would you do? What nursing diagnoses and treatment goals would you likely write for Theera? What interventions do you think would be helpful for this child and his family?** It would be helpful to have some baseline data on Theera's bowel movements. You do not know at this point if Theera has constipation associated with his Encopresis or not. It is important for the nurse to always know the status of any client in terms of elimination. Sometimes nurses fail to check on this important aspect of a client's health status. You need to know what his usual diet is, and you need to document what he eats in the hospital and how this affects stools. You will want to know what his intake and output are. It is important to gather information about his strengths and limitations and his interests as well. You will want to gather information about family dynamics as well as where he is in terms of developmental tasks.

Nursing diagnoses may include but are not limited to:

- Situationally low self-esteem
- Impaired elimination
- Knowledge deficit in regard to prevention of constipation
- Ineffective coping
- Powerlessness

Treatment goals may include such goals as:

- No instances of constipated stool
- Number of soft, well-formed stools to be one per day or every other day, and no instances of defecating in inappropriate places
- Will state feels power over "poop"
- Will be able to state pride in one or more abilities

The nursing interventions can include such actions as:

- Build a trusting relationship with parents and child.
- Educate the parents about ways to help their child build confidence in himself and to identify and build on his strengths.
- Educate the parents about diet, the use of bulk and fluids, and regular exercise to prevent constipation.
- Orient the parents and child to the hospital rules and schedule and give them choices in selected aspects of the schedule whenever possible to give them a sense of ownership in the schedule and some sense of control.
- Present the rules in positive manner whenever possible (e.g., "If you comply, the reward is ___" instead of "If you don't comply, this punishment will happen"). This sets an expectation that the child will comply.
- Use positive reinforcement to shape behavior rather than negative reinforcement and model this for the parents.
- Play age-appropriate games with child and model for parents how to help children learn through games and the importance of play to children.
- Help the parents to develop a schedule for home that provides adequate time for toileting and a sense of consistency from day to day.
- Encourage attendance at parenting classes for the parents. Provide information about such classes in the local area.
- Encourage parents to continue family therapy after hospitalization.

The treatment team will decide which approaches to use with this child. As one of the nurses you will have input. You may want to provide information about reflexology as an alternative treatment for Encopresis. Being Thai, the parents will be familiar with reflexology, and this might be something they would want to try in addition to other approaches.

References

American Psychiatric Association. (2000). *Diagnostic and Statistical Manual of Mental Disorders, 4th ed.* Text Revision. Washington, DC: American Psychiatric Association.

Bishop, E., E. McKinnon, E. Weir, and D.W. Brown. (2003). "Reflexology in the Management of Encopresis and Chronic Constipation." *Paediatric Nursing* 15(3): 20–22.

Fishman, L., S. Nurko, L. Rappaport, and A. Schonwald. (2003). "Trends in Referral to a Single Encopresis Clinic Over 20 Years." *Pediatrics* 111(5): 604–608.

Hackett, R., L. Hackett, P. Bhakta, and S. Gowers. (2001). "Enuresis and Encopresis in a South Indian Population of Children." *Child Care Health and Development* 21(1): 35–46.

Loening-Baucke, V., E. Miele, and A. Staiano. (2004). "Fiber (Glucomannan) Is Beneficial in the Treatment of Childhood Constipation." *Pediatrics* 113(3): 259–261.

Mason, D., N. Tobias, M. Lutkenhoff, M. Stoops, and D. Ferguson. (2004). "The APN's Guide to Pediatric Constipation Management." *The Nurse Practitioner* 29(7): 13–19.

Partin, J.C., S.K. Hamill, J.E. Fischel, and J.S. Partin. (1992). "Painful Defecation and Fecal Soiling in Children." *Pediatrics* 89(6): 1007–1009.

Riccelli, A. (2005). "Memoirs of a 'Poop Lady.'" *The Journal of Collaborative Family Health Care* 21(1): 109–118.

Penny

GENDER	**SPIRITUAL/RELIGIOUS**
Female	
AGE	**PHARMACOLOGIC**
7	■ Desmopressin (DDAVP) tablets or spray
SETTING	**PSYCHOSOCIAL**
■ School nurse's office	■ Does not accept invitations for overnight stays from peers due to bedwetting
ETHNICITY	**LEGAL**
■ White American	
CULTURAL CONSIDERATIONS	**ETHICAL**
PREEXISTING CONDITION	**ALTERNATIVE THERAPY**
	■ Alarm to alert of wetness at night and behavior modification
COEXISTING CONDITION	■ Relaxation therapy
	PRIORITIZATION
COMMUNICATION	
	DELEGATION
DISABILITY	
SOCIOECONOMIC	

MODERATE

ENURESIS

Level of difficulty: Moderate

Overview: Requires an understanding of Enuresis and its possible causes. Requires patience, empathy, and ability to use creative thinking to develop interventions utilizing a knowledge of the way children think and behave according to their developmental level.

Client Profile

Penny is a 7-year-old girl who wets the bed at night, nearly every night, and has done so since she was a baby. Her father is upset with her because he says he is tired of the smell of urine-soaked sheets and her mother having to get up at night to help her change her bed. The father often drinks several beers after work at night. He tends to be angry with her when he is drinking. When he is drinking too much, he makes Penny get out of bed at night and wash her own wet bedsheets. Penny's father calls her lazy and stupid and says she will never learn to get out of bed and go to the bathroom at night and she won't ever have a boyfriend or a husband because no one wants a bed wetter.

Penny is upset with herself not only because of what her father says to her but also because she cannot stay overnight with anyone from school or have anyone stay overnight with her until she stops wetting the bed. Her self-esteem and confidence in herself is so low that she never tries to make friends. Penny stays dry during the day, but at night she awakes with her pajamas and bedsheets wet. Penny's mother wet the bed when she was Penny's age, but she has not talked with Penny about it as she is embarrassed and is afraid of her husband being angry. She feels guilty and ashamed about this secret.

Case Study

In school one day, Penny asks the teacher if she can go to the bathroom and the teacher asks her to wait until she finishes a spelling test. Penny wets her underpants and is sent to the school nurse's office to get cleaned up. The school nurse encourages Penny to talk about how she feels about wetting her underpants and then asks her if she realizes that this happens to lots of other children. The school nurse reveals that when she was a child, she wet her own bed at night for several years. Penny replies that this is the first time that she has wet her underpants in the daytime but that she does wet her bed at night too. She wishes that she could stop doing this, but she says she will probably wet her bed all her life because her father said she would. The school nurse offers to talk to Penny's parents and to try to get them to help her stop wetting the bed at night: "Please let me talk to them about helping you stop bedwetting. I believe you can stop the bedwetting. It may take some time and some work, but it can be done."

Questions and Suggested Answers

1. **What is Enuresis? Are there subtypes of Enuresis?** Robson (2005) explains that the word Enuresis is derived from a Greek word meaning to make water. In North America, Enuresis is used to refer to wetting either in the day or at night. Nocturnal Enuresis is the term used for night time wetting. For a client to be diagnosed with Enuresis, the client must exhibit the essential feature of the disorder, which is repeated urinating into the bed or clothing during either the day or at night. This voiding into bedclothes or clothing can be either voluntary or involuntary. The client must have demonstrated this behavior at least twice a week for at least three months in a row or have "clinically significant distress or impairment in social, academic (occupational) or other important areas of functioning" (APA, 2000). The client must be at least 5 years old or equal to this in developmental age. The voiding into bedclothes or clothing must not be due only to the direct effects of a substance such as a diuretic or a general medical condition such as a seizure disorder or diabetes.

    There are three subtypes of enuresis. The subtypes are: 1. Nocturnal only, 2. Diurnal only, and 3. Nocturnal and Diurnal. The nocturnal type of Enuresis is the most common subtype. The child with this type has voiding in bedclothes and clothing only at night and typically only during the first third of the night, although sometimes voiding takes place during REM sleep and the child remembers a dream in which they were urinating (APA, 2000).

2. **If you were the school nurse and you had wet the bed as a child, would you share with a child that you had also wet the bed?** Disclosing personal information is to be done only after careful consideration. The nurse must have a good reason or reasons for disclosing information and should do so only when it is therapeutic for the client. In this case, if you decided that you would disclose your experience, this decision to disclose the personal information seems sound based on the knowledge that most children who wet the bed feel totally alone with this problem. Robson (2005) writes that family members with a history of nocturnal Enuresis should be encouraged to share their experiences and offer moral support. In this case, the threat of the father's anger may keep the mother from sharing her experiences. The disclosure by the nurse has promise for reassuring the child that others have had the same problem and have resolved it and suggests that the nurse may have some help to offer. The mother may be more apt to share with her daughter after hearing of the nurse's example, particularly if the father can be educated about Enuresis.

If you decided you would not disclose the personal information, that is acceptable too. As the nurse in this case, you could decide to disclose later if you believe it serves a purpose in the work with this child and her family. Many times nurses decide not to disclose at all after evaluating the need as they conclude it will distract from the work to be done.

3. **If you were the school nurse, how would you approach getting the parents to discuss what to do for Penny?** One problem is how to get the parents to meet with you, and another is how to get the parents to form an alliance to help Penny. What are your options for solving the first problem? You could ask the parents to come to the school and meet with you. A second option would be to ask them to come to the school and have an official meeting with not only you, but with the teacher, school psychologist, and principal. A third option would be to ask for a short time to have coffee and visit at their home. There are probably many other options you could think of, but keep in mind that coming to the school can be very intimidating to some parents. A visit to the home (i.e., the parent's own "turf") may work better than a meeting at school.

To get the parents to open up, you might want to spend a few minutes thanking them for visiting with you and in small talk about something of interest to them, as well as finding something to commend them for as being good parents. You could print out the information for parents on the American Academy of Child and Adolescent Psychiatry website entitled "AACAP Facts for Families #18" (www.aacap.org/publications/factsfam/bedwet.htm). This information is brief and in language parents can understand. This website offers five things parents can do initially to see if they can help resolve the problem before seeking professional help.

4. **If Penny's parents refuse to meet with you and refuse to get her treatment, will her bedwetting at night resolve itself? What can Penny's parents and others like them try in order to resolve their child's bedwetting? Will this take a commitment on the part of the parents and mean a change in their behavior?** Whether Penny's bedwetting at night will resolve itself or not depends on the cause of the bedwetting. In almost all cases of functional enuresis, the problem will resolve itself by puberty (www.aacap.org/publications/factsfam/bedwet.htm). Since Penny is age seven, puberty is several years away, and this could mean five or six more years of being embarrassed, not being able to have sleepovers, enduring the father's anger, and feeling low self-esteem. The main reason to treat is to "minimize the embarrassment and anxiety of children and the frustration of parents" (Robson, 2005).

Parents can do the following: 1. Limit fluids in the evening before bedtime (e.g., one glass of liquid at the evening meal and one glass in the next two hours and nothing liquid within two hours of bedtime); 2. Take the child to the bathroom before bedtime; 3. Praise the child if they are dry in the morning; 4. Avoid any punishment; and 5. Wake the child during the night to urinate (www.aacap.org/publications/factsfam/bedwet.htm). This behavior will take a commitment on the part of the parents. You as the nurse can provide encouragement and assurance that you believe the parents can and will do it. This encouragement is usually important in motivating the parents and modeling the setting of positive expectations. You can also model the use of positive reinforcement by praising the parents anytime they come close to meeting an expectation. The father has to learn to use positive reinforcement rather than punishment or negative reinforcement.

Is making a child change their bedsheets in the middle of the night punitive? This activity can be punitive but with a change in tone and a matter of fact manner, the changing of the bed becomes a sharing of responsibility rather than punishment.

The American Academy of Family Physicians Website (http://pediatrics.about.com/od/bedwetting), suggests an alarm, reward system, having child help change sheets, and having the child hold urine for longer and longer times in the daytime to stretch the bladder.

Suggestions similar to those of AACAP are offered on Madera's Suggestions website (http://Seaknet. ne.alasla.edu/~/eigh). Madera was a camp nurse in Oregon and a school nurse for the Washington County ESD. She had two to twelve campers each week with night-time bedwetting. She had campers meet in support groups and had them drink freely until 6 P.M., except they could have no caffeine drinks and no milk after lunch. They would go to the bathroom before bedtime and in the middle of the night and practiced relaxation exercises before bedtime. She would send campers home free of nocturnal Enuresis.

5. **What is the usual course of Enuresis?** According to the American Psychiatric Association, there are two different courses that Enuresis can take (APA, 2000). The first type of course is called a "primary" type and involves a client that has never had urinary continence. The second type of course is called a secondary course, in which the problem involves a disturbance that began after a time of established urinary continence. The first type begins at age 5 and the second type between the ages of 5 and 8 but may occur at any time. The rate of spontaneous remission ranges between 5–10 percent per year after the child is 5 years old. Almost all children will be continent by age 15, but some clients will be incontinent into adulthood.

6. **Does Enuresis typically run in families, and does it occur equally in both genders or in one more than the other? What is the incidence of Enuresis?** Robson (2005) points out that a family history is found in 50 percent of the families of children with secondary nocturnal enuresis.

According to the American Academy of Child and Adolescent Psychiatry website (www.aacap.org/publications/factsfam/bedwet.htm), "many more boys than girls" have bedwetting after age three.

Robson (2005) presents the reported prevalence rate in males as being 9 percent in boys age 7 and 10 percent in boys age 10, whereas the percentage is 6 percent in girls age 7 and 3 percent in girls age 10.

Not all cases are reported or treated, as there is a perception by many parents that their child will grow out of their bedwetting, so figures on the incidence of Enuresis could be low in relation to the true number of cases. El-Radhi and Board (2003) have described nocturnal Enuresis as affecting sixty million people in the world, about 1 percent of the population, and over half a million children in the United Kingdom.

The American Academy of Child and Adolescent Psychiatry website (www.aacap.org/publications/factsfam/bedwet.htm) states on their website that approximately 15 percent of children wet the bed after age 3.

Robson (2005) reports that 23 percent of 5-year-olds have nocturnal Enuresis.

7. **The parents do meet with you, and the father asks you "What causes bedwetting? Is it laziness?" What would you tell the father?** You would stress with the father that bedwetting is not caused by laziness and that bedwetting has many causes. Some medical causes would include: urge syndrome/dysfunction voiding, urethral obstruction, neurogenic bladder, ectopic ureter, diabetes mellitus, diabetes insipidus, and others.

If Penny had daytime Enuresis, you would share that, according to Neveus (2003), the most common cause of daytime urinary incontinence is instability of bladder muscles; however, this father's child has nocturnal Enuresis.

Psychological problems are an important cause of secondary nocturnal Enuresis, according to Robson (2005), who also points out that psychological problems are almost always a result of primary nocturnal Enuresis and only rarely the cause. Penny would appear to have primary nocturnal Enuresis, so you would not mention psychological problems as a cause or effect at this time. You could look at this as you further assess this client and the client's family.

You could share with the parents that nocturnal Enuresis, as bedwetting not due to medical causes, has some prominent causal theories at present. One theory described in an article by Neveus (2003) is children who have Enuresis have low arousability, and this could be due to the "autonomous nervous system and to a disturbance in the upper pons" of the brain. This article calls Enuresis a disorder of sleep with "high arousal threshold being one of three major pathogenic factors." The other two factors are nocturnal polyuria and detrusor hyperactivity.

Why nocturnal polyuria, or production of more urine at night? A possible cause is a deficiency in production of antganine vasopressin (AVP), an antidiuretic hormone, the hormone that decreases urine production at nighttime. In some children the deficiency of AVP results in an increase in nocturnal urine output that exceeds the functional bladder.

Another causal theory is described by Robson (2005), who points out that in a Danish family with nocturnal Enuresis, chromosome 22 was identified as the site of nocturnal Enuresis loci in 1995. He also points out the later reports have linked differences in chromosomes 8, 12, and 16 to nocturnal Enuresis in other families. He further states that autosomal dominant transmission is usually involved in nocturnal Enuresis.

8. **The mother asks if it is possible that Penny's bedwetting is due to a medical cause. How would you respond if you were the school nurse?** The mother having had nocturnal Enuresis as a child would suggest that this client's nocturnal Enuresis is not due to a medical cause, but the nurse has not been let in on the mother's secret yet. The nurse's answer to mother is that of course the possibility exists that a medical condition could be present, but that in most children, it is not a medical condition causing the problem. If you can get the parents to take Penny for a checkup by the pediatrician to rule out medical causes, it would put to rest any fears of a medical condition by the family and/or the child, and if there is something wrong, early intervention will be helpful. Robson (2005) points out that a urinalysis is the most important screening test in a child with nocturnal Enuresis and usually if that is normal no invasive tests need be done. A voiding log may be given to the parents for recording the client's voiding for several days. In some rare cases additional testing needs to be done. If the parents refuse to take the child to a pediatrician, you need to at least assess for any symptoms of a urinary infection, and if present, suggest this as a possibility and get the parents to take her to the pediatrician. You can educate the parents about the signs and symptoms of urinary infection.

9. **The parents would like to know if there is some treatment for bedwetting. The mother has heard that one of the neighbor children took some pills to stop it. What are the current treatments for Enuresis?** Skoog and Andriole (2004) suggest behavior modification provides the best long-term success. This would include decreasing the amount of fluids in the evening before bed as described above, emptying the bladder before bed, awakening child in the night to go to the bathroom, and using positive reinforcement for a dry bed.

A second type of treatment would be use of an alarm positioned on the child's pajamas at night with a sensor in the underwear. The alarm is triggered by contact with urine. When the alarm sounds, a parent is to take the child to the bathroom to finish emptying their bladder. The bed linens are changed and the alarm reset, and ultimately this procedure will lead to the client awakening due to a full bladder. It may take up to four months for this to happen. Skoog and Andriole require twenty-five nights dry before removing the alarm device.

A third type of treatment would be medication. Skoog and Andriole state that the children with the most severe bedwetting of six or more nights per week of wetting the bed will do well on the alarm, oral desmopressin (DDAVP), no fluids at least two hours before bedtime, along with voiding prior to bedtime. Robson (2005) says that desmopressin acetate (DDAVP) is the preferred medication to treat children with nocturnal Enuresis. It decreases nocturnal production of urine and may have effects on arousal. It comes in tablet and nasal spray form with both having similar efficacy, but the tablets have several advantages. The nasal spray does not work well when children have nasal congestion, and the tablet is more discrete in sleepovers. The tablet has less serious adverse side effects. Desmopressin is not recommended for children under 6 years of age. Two other types of medications are used for the treatment of enuresis. One type is the anticholinergic agents such as oxybutynin (Ditropan), hyoscyamine (Levsin), tolterodine (Detrol), and flavoxate (Uripas). None of the anticholinergic drugs except for hyoscyamine is recommended for children under 12. Hyoscyamine does come in a pediatric dose and can be given to young children. The third type of medication is the tricyclic antidepressant imipramine (Tofranil), which decreases bladder contractility and increases outlet resistance as well as inhibiting the reuptake of norepinephrine and serotonin at the presynapic neuron.

Madera, the camp/school nurse who worked with kids with Enuresis, also taught the children to use meditation before bedtime.

10. **What assessment information would you like to have in order to write a nursing care plan on this client?** Getting information from the family may be a sensitive issue and is best approached in a sensitive manner. You want to try to find out about the labor and delivery, early developmental milestones for the child, history of when toilet training began and how it was approached, as well as the history of Enuresis, including any family members who had Enuresis and their history. An assessment of any stressors in the child's life would be helpful. A medical history should be taken, including the history of any health problems and medication the child is taking, Assess the child's strengths and limitations and developmental level. The nurse needs to assess the family dynamics and coping skills used by family members. If possible, the nurse needs to assess the father's use/abuse of alcohol and the effect this has on the family psychologically, physically, and financially.

11. **What nursing diagnoses and goals would you likely write for this client and her family? What nursing interventions would you likely initiate?** Nursing diagnoses could include:

- Situational low self-esteem
- Ineffective family coping skills

Goals could include the parents reporting an increase in the number of nights per week that the client's bed remains dry. When this is accomplished, the goal will be revised to a dry bed 100 percent of the time. Short-term goals need to be achievable.

Nursing interventions would include:

- Build a trusting therapeutic relationship with client and client's parents.
- Provide client and parents with information about Enuresis and ways to help a child resolve this problem.
- Educate the family about the alarm system if it is used or about any medication prescribed for her.
- Encourage parenting classes and providing information on where to get parenting classes at no or low cost.
- Encourage the family to get no or low-cost therapy and providing information on where to get it.
- Help the parents and child find support groups so they can meet with others who have similar problems.
- Provide information on support groups for family members of alcoholics if the father's drinking is such that this is warranted.
- Work with the teacher to educate him or her about Enuresis and the child's needs in terms of permission or reminders to go to the bathroom. Requests to go to the bathroom and reminders could be a secret signal between teacher and child to eliminate the embarrassment of asking or being told verbally in front of others.
- Find opportunities for the client to engage in fun activities with other children and encourage participation.
- Enlist teacher's help in getting the client to have a friend in class through work pairs assignments or other means.

There are many innovative things that you might think of. Some of these might include: suggesting a program on Enuresis to the president of the school PTA and helping him or her find a speaker or volunteering to be that speaker, starting support groups for children after school, and/or working with the parents to get Penny mentored through the Big Brother, Big Sister Program or a similar program available in the community.

References

American Psychiatric Association. (2000). *Diagnostic and Statistical Manual of Mental Disorders, 4th ed.* Text Revision. Washington, DC: American Psychiatric Association.

El-Radhi, A.S. and C. Board. (2003). "Providing Adequate Treatment for Children with Nocturnal Enuresis." *British Journal of Community Nursing* 8(10): 440–447.

http://familydoctor.org/handouts/168.html. Accessed June 17, 2006.

http://pediatrics.about.com/od/bedwetting. Accessed June 18, 2006.

http://Seaknet.ne.alasla.edu/~/eigh. Accessed March 20, 2005.

Neveus, T. (2003). "The Role of Sleep Arousal in Nocturnal Enuresis." *Acta Paedeatrica* 92(10): 1118–1124.

Robson, W.L. (2005). "Enuresis." Available at www.emedicine.com/ped/topic689.htm. Accessed March 20, 2005.

Skoog, S.J. and G.L. Andriole. (2004). "How to Evaluate and Treat Pediatric Enuresis." *Urology Times* 32(5): 46–49.

www.aacap.org/publications/factsfam/bedwet.htm. Accessed March 20, 2005.

Hannah

GENDER

F

AGE

89

SETTING

- Home of client's daughter

ETHNICITY

- Black American

CULTURAL CONSIDERATIONS

PREEXISTING CONDITION

- Pernicious anemia

COEXISTING CONDITION

COMMUNICATION

- Requires hearing aides to hear

DISABILITY

- Difficulty hearing

SOCIOECONOMIC

- Upper middle class

SPIRITUAL/RELIGIOUS

- Methodist

PHARMACOLOGIC

- Anticholinergic medication
- Donepezil (Aricept)

PSYCHOSOCIAL

- Sits with old friends in Sunday school and with daughter in church: cannot recall events of the past or read bible verses but sings old familiar songs of her childhood

LEGAL

- Claiming power of attorney for a parent or declaring parent incompetent and getting guardianship

ETHICAL

- Ethical issue around making decisions for grown parents

ALTERNATIVE THERAPY

- Music therapy

PRIORITIZATION

DELEGATION

MODERATE

DEMENTIA OF THE ALZHEIMER'S TYPE

Level of difficulty: Moderate

Overview: Requires the nurse to be knowledgeable about Alzheimer's Disease and its stages. Nurse must do more explanations and teaching with the client's caregiver since the client has difficulty understanding or recalling what the nurse has explained to her. The nurse needs to determine when and if it is appropriate to see that the caregiver gets information about declaring the client incompetent or getting the power of attorney and about respite care.

Client Profile

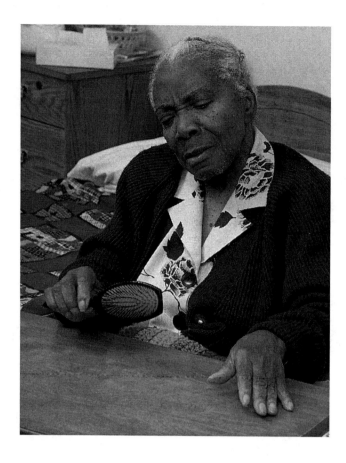

Hannah is an 89-year-old woman who had been living in her own home for years and fiercely protecting her independence from her five grown children. Hannah drove her car until she was 87 and did her own cooking, but had a cleaning woman come once a week. Women friends came on Sunday to take her to Sunday school and church. Hannah had been married three times, and one day in Sunday school she was asked to tell about her last husband who was now dead. She could not recall anything about him, including his name, so she said to a friend: "You tell about him." She did enjoy singing old familiar hymns and being with her women friends of many years. Hannah began to get even more forgetful, frequently forgetting the names of the grandchildren and her own children and covering this by calling them all "sugar." She began to pay some of her bills more than once, and when the daughter, Jean, found this out, she hired someone to live in with her mother and took over the bill paying. Jean decided to let her mother keep her car keys, but secretly took the battery out of the car. Hannah tried to start the car every day and would call Jean to tell her the car wasn't working, and Jean would say she had called someone to come repair it. The next day Hannah would forget that the car wasn't working and would try to start it again.

Within a week of Jean hiring someone to live with her, Hannah fired the woman. Jean decided to take her mother to live with her, about a ninety-minute drive from Hannah's home. Jean works out of her home and believed she could work and look after her mother without any problem; however, problems started as soon as Hannah arrived at Jean's home. Hannah begged people who called or came to visit her daughter to take her home. She would offer them money and say she was kidnapped. She fell and decided to stay in her bed and refused to get up. The daughter was unsure if her mother had broken her hip or not. Jean was concerned that her mother might be anemic because she had been diagnosed with pernicious anemia and was receiving B12 injections monthly before coming to live with Jean. Hannah lost five pounds after moving in with her daughter

Jean. The weight loss was puzzling since her mother had a voracious appetite and seemed to eat enough for two people, demanding food several times a day in between meals and telling people "that woman is starving me." Jean decided to call a home health service that would send a home health nurse and a health care providers to the home and would draw blood for lab tests and send a mobile x-ray unit.

Case Study

A home heath agency nurse has come to visit Hannah at her daughter's home. Hannah offers the nurse a hundred dollars to take her home. Hannah whispers to the nurse that if she had car keys, she would drive herself home. The nurse fluffs up Hannah's pillows and chats with her awhile about her little dog. The nurse talks Hannah into letting him look at her hearing aids and check the batteries and into agreeing to wear the hearing aides. Hannah tells her daughter that she will wear the hearing aides "because that nice nurse wants me to wear them." After awhile the nurse gets Hannah to agree to have blood drawn for CBC, HIV, and thyroid tests. A portable x-ray technician is called to come and get an x-ray of Hannah's hip.

The nurse asks Jean if she has any old pictures of Hannah's parents or siblings and discovers a wedding picture of the parents. Hannah immediately identifies her parents. The nurse tests Hannah's orientation and finds she does not know the year, month, or day. Hannah thinks it is 1941. She refers to her daughter as "that woman who kidnapped me." The nurse does a Mini Multi-State Examination (MMSE).

The nurses talks to the client before leaving and tells her that a "nice doctor" will read the x-ray and review the results of the lab tests and make a home visit to see her. The nurse adds: "You will like the doctor."

In private, Jean shares with the nurse that her mother has been demanding and is wearing her down. Jean says her mother sleeps until noon, but stays up until dawn watching television, which she misinterprets because she can't hear it (e.g., Hannah thought the television said that local onions were poisoned and then she accused Jean of poisoning her). Jean describes efforts to be nice to her mother. She took her out to eat, but the next morning the mother did not recall going out to eat and accused Jean of starving her and holding her "prisoner in a dark place."

Hannah's son comes to visit, and in a moment of clarity she calls him by name and says, "Oh my, that woman in there must be your sister and she is trying to help me." Later Hannah refers again to Jean as "that woman" and does not seem to know her.

After reviewing the x-ray and lab tests, as well as the MMSE and the past health history, and examining Hannah, the health care provider decides Hannah's hip is not broken and notes that she has a history of pernicious anemia and probably has Alzheimer's Disease. He writes orders for a B12 injection every week for three weeks, then every month; a home health aide for assistance with hygiene tasks; and prescribes 5 mg of donepezil (Aricept) daily.

Questions and Suggested Answers

1. **Why did the nurse take time to chat with Hannah about her dog and fluff up her pillows? Why did the nurse check the batteries of the hearing aides and want her to wear the hearing aides? What else does the nurse need to do at this point?** The nurse was building rapport with the client. Hannah loves her pet, and the nurse showing interest in the pet provides a good chance to communicate on a nonthreatening topic. Fluffing the pillow shows care and concern for Hannah as a person. You would not have to do the same things, but it would be helpful to build rapport in some way before assessing the client. Building rapport helps to allay fear and suspicion. Clients with dementia can be suspicious and fearful and/or can become agitated. A gentle, slow approach helps the client feel safer with the nurse.

   The reason the nurse checked the hearing aides was to be sure the batteries were working properly before having Hannah put them on. It is important that Hannah be able to hear what the nurse says. The nurse needs to assess whether Hannah's daughter knows how to care for the hearing aides and batteries and how to check and insert the batteries. If she does not know any or all of this, the nurse needs to teach, demonstrate, and have a return demonstration. In addition the nurse needs to enunciate clearly, use simple words, face the client, and use short sentences when talking to a client who is suspected of having dementia or has been diagnosed with dementia. A person with a short-term memory problem does not understand the communication when the nurse gives a lengthy set of instructions or a lot of information at once.

2. **Why could the client identify her parents from an old picture and not recall the names of her children or grandchildren or the day, month, or year? Why can she recall words of songs, and what implications does this have for interventions?** Individuals with dementia tend to have better recall of names and events from the distant past as compared to recent days. This is true in clients with dementia of the Alzheimer's type. It is comforting to a client to have pictures from the distant past around them. Some more recent pictures labeled well may also help recall. A large calendar and clock is also helpful for reorientation. Hearing and singing familiar songs can be comforting. The client can recall songs because a different part of the brain is involved in recalling music than the part of the brain involved in recalling names or events.

3. **Why did the nurse make a point of telling Hannah that the health care provider who would come would be very nice? What would you do or say differently if you were the nurse in this case? What in particular are the provider and nurse hoping to learn from the CBC, thyroid and HIV laboratory tests?** The nurse was planting the idea with Hannah that she would like the health care provider. The nurse does not want to be the only one that Hannah has rapport with, as it will take more of the team to care for her than just the nurse. The nurse has established a beginning trusting relationship and is in essence saying, not only can you trust me, but there is someone else you can trust too.

   The provider and the nurse need good rapport with the client in order to do tests looking for various causes of dementia and not assume that it is a result of Alzheimer's Disease. Many things can cause dementia, and some of these are reversible, such as vitamin B12 deficiencies, head trauma, thyroid problems, and neurosyphillis. Brain tumors and HIV and many other medical conditions can cause or mimic dementia. Alzheimer's Disease is the most common form of irreversible dementia. The health care provider and nurse know that other causes of dementia need to be ruled out before a probable diagnosis of Alzheimer's can be made. If the problem is other than Alzheimer's, then that problem needs to be treated.

4. **The health care provider has diagnosed pernicious anemia for this client. Do you have any reason to believe that pernicious anemia is the cause of this dementia? What is pernicious anemia?** This client has had a diagnosis of pernicious anemia in the past and was receiving B12 injections. She began to gradually have difficulty with memory while she was getting B12. If the dementia clears when the client receives B12 injections again, it may be that the dementia is due to the anemia. If it does not clear, then it is more likely that this is Alzheimer's Disease.

   Pernicious anemia is a medical problem where the parietal cells lining the stomach are atrophied, and this leads to a lack of intrinsic factor in the stomach. Normally people get B12 from foods including liver, meats, milk, milk products, and legumes. When a person eats these foods, B12 gets attached to intrinsic factor in the stomach and the B12 and intrinsic factor complex goes to the intestine where the vitamin B12 is absorbed into the blood. When there is no intrinsic factor, the B12 passes out of the body and is not absorbed.

5. **What do you think of Jean's idea of taking the battery out of the car and letting Hannah try to start it every day?** It may seem like an unkind act or unethical to you for Jean to trick Hannah into believing something is wrong with the car; however, the important issue here is safety—Hannah's safety and that of other people she might encounter should she be allowed to drive.

6. **If you were the nurse, would you mention to Hannah's daughter the possibility of having her mother declared incompetent in court at some point and becoming her mother's legal guardian?** This is a situation where you would not make a recommendation and providing information has to be done carefully, if at all. You are not in the role of deciding if Hannah is competent or not, although at some point it may seem perfectly clear that she is not. The laws about declaring someone incompetent vary from state to state and change from time to

time. You could talk with the health are provider to see if he thinks Hannah is competent or not. If he thinks that Hannah is not mentally competent, he may want to discuss this with the daughter, Jean. The process for declaring a relative incompetent will likely require someone to file a notice of application with the court and to get a sworn statement in writing from at least one medical practitioner and someone who knows the client citing behaviors that are evidence of incompetence (www.legal-info-legale.nb.ca/pub-manage-afairs.asp).

If the client is currently competent, the daughter may want to try to get her mother to give her power of attorney for business and health matters. The mother's dementia may get worse, and the daughter may need this power of attorney to carry on business on behalf of her mother. The attitudes and wishes of Jean's siblings may influence what Jean does in terms of getting a power of attorney or guardianship. The daughter may want to consult with an attorney about the laws in her state in regard to attaining guardianship or power of attorney and the benefits and problems associated with each of these actions.

7. **The client's daughter asks you to explain what Alzheimer's Disease is. She also wants to know about the stages and incidence of Alzheimer's Disease. How would you respond to these questions?** Alois Alzheimer first described this disorder in 1907. It is a slow, progressive type of dementia involving impairment in memory as an essential feature for the diagnosis and involving other impairments in areas such as language, decision making, judgment, cognitive function, and personality. The human brain involves a communication network that has billions of nerve cells called neurons. These tiny neurons communicate with each other and are like a trail over which information is gathered and sent to various places in the brain. In people with Alzheimer's Disease, these pathways breakdown and eventually cells die. When these cells die, then various aspects of brain function controlling such areas as personality, memory, behavior, and other functions are impaired or lost. Alzheimer's involves protein deposits in the cerebral cortex. (http://health.allrefer.com/health/alzheimers-disease-info.html). On autopsy the "neuropathological findings include amyloid plaques and neurofibrillary tangles" (Tavee and Sweeney, 2002).

The first stage of Alzheimer's Disease lasts two to four years and the symptoms are mild. The person tends to have recent memory loss, which can affect the way they do their work. Some people forget what they have been told to do or what they are supposed to do. Confusion about places can be present and the person can get lost. The individual's spontaneity may be diminished or gone. There can be mood and personality changes. The person may be anxious about their symptoms and avoid people. They may have poor judgment and take longer with routine chores and have trouble handling money and paying bills.

The second stage lasts about two to ten years after diagnosis and the symptoms have increased in severity to a moderate level. There is increased memory loss and confusion. The attention span is shorter. The person begins to have trouble recognizing close family members and friends. The individual may be restless, especially late in the afternoon and at night. The person may confabulate (make up answers) when unable to recall things. There may be loss of impulse control. The individual may be suspicious as well as irritable. They may fidget or be teary or silly. There may be problems with reading and writing. There may be weight loss. The person may be afraid to take a bath or just not bathe and may hear or see things that are not present.

The third stage is the terminal stage. In this stage the person may not recognize himself or herself in the mirror. They may not recognize family members. The person may lose weight while eating a good diet. They may sleep a lot. There may be difficulty swallowing. Choking is a risk. The person can become dehydrated. There may be very little self-care taking place. The person may have trouble communicating with words. They may put everything in their mouths or touch everything. There can be a loss of bowel and bladder control (www.alz-nca.org/aboutalz/phases.asp).

About 100,000 victims of Alzheimer's Disease die each year, and 360,000 new cases are diagnosed each year. It is estimated that by 2050 the number of cases in the United States will reach 14 million and by 2020 there will be 30 million people worldwide with this disorder (www.ahaf.org/alzdis/about/adabout.htm).

Marwan Sabbagh of the Sun Health Research Institute in Sun City, a facility for the study of dementia, points out that in Arizona in the last four years, the number of people with Alzheimer's Disease increased by 9 percent and was up from 78,000 in 2000 to 85,000 in 2004 with predictions of 130,000 in 2025. These increases are thought to be due partly to baby boomers aging, partly to people retiring to the western states, and partly to better techniques for diagnosis (Vaccine Weekly, 2005a, b).

8. What are the diagnostic criteria for dementia of the Alzheimer's type, and do you think this client matches those criteria? To meet the criteria for dementia of the Alzheimer's type:

1. The client must have developed more than one cognitive deficit shown by both memory impairment in learning new information or recalling information learned in the past and at least one of the following cognitive disturbances: aphasia (language disturbance), apraxia (impairment in motor activities even though motor function is intact), agnosia (not recognizing or identifying objects even though sensory function is intact), and disturbance in executive functioning, which includes such things as ability to plan, organize, sequence things, and abstract.

2. The cognitive deficits have to cause significant impairment in social or work functioning and clearly be a significant decline from previous functioning level.

3. The course of the disorder is a gradual onset and ongoing cognitive decline.

4. Any cognitive deficits are not due to another disorder of the central nervous system or a systemic condition that causes dementia or a substance-induced condition.

5. The cognitive deficits do not occur only during a delirium.

6. The problem is not accounted for by a mental disorder such as Major Depressive Disorder, Schizophrenia, or other mental disorder.

The Dementia of Alzheimer's type is subcategorized as being with or without behavioral disturbance and of early onset or late onset subtypes (APA, 2000).

Hannah has had difficulty recalling information about her family and about her finances and difficulty organizing bill payments. She has had significant impairment in her social functioning as well as in doing housework. Hannah has had a gradual onset of, and ongoing, cognitive decline. The medical team is in the process of ruling out other causes for her deficits. Her ability to sequence will be assessed on the MMSE. Further assessment will help in determining if Hannah meets the criteria for the diagnosis of Dementia of the Alzheimer's type or not. The nurse can test to see if Hannah can abstract by asking her to interpret a short proverb such as "A rolling stone gathers no moss." People who are unable to abstract interpret this proverb quite literally (e.g., when you push a stone off a hill, when it gets to the bottom, it has no green on it). Inability to abstract is just one clue to Dementia of the Alzheimer's type. It is also found in so called "normal" people who have just not developed the ability to abstract and in people with various mental disorders.

9. Is there a definitive test for Alzheimer's Disease? What is the Mini Multi-State Exam that the health care provider ordered for Hannah? At the present time there isn't a definitive laboratory test or scan or other means of definitely determining a person has Alzheimer's disease. The probable diagnosis is most often made by the history, ruling out of other causes, and by scores on the MMSE. A PET scan will demonstrate differences in the brain of a person with probable Alzheimer's compared to so-called normal persons. On autopsy histological examination of tissue can provide a conclusive diagnosis.

The MMSE is a short standardized means to grade cognitive mental status. A total score is attained to place the person on a scale of cognitive functioning. The total score does vary by age and education. A chart depicting variations by age and education (comparing fourth grade education with eighth grade, high school, and college) is available at www.nemc.org/psych/mmse.asp. The MMSE assesses orientation, immediate and short-term recall, language, and the ability to follow simple verbal and written commands. It begins by asking the client some questions to determine whether they are oriented or not and in what way. The questions include: "What is today's date? What is the month? What is the year? What is the day of the week? What is the season? What is the name of this place? What floor are we on? What country are we in? What state are we in?" Each question gets a point. The next section tests immediate recall by asking the subject to recall three specific words. The following section asks the client to do serial sevens. This task involves counting backward by sevens from one hundred. Next the client is asked to spell "world" backward. Asking the client to recall the three words you gave him or her earlier tests delayed recall. The client is tested on naming by showing him or her a pencil and a watch and asking him to name these objects. The client is given a three-stage command. He or she is given a piece of paper and told: "Take the paper in your hand, fold it in half, and put it on the floor." Each part of this instruction when completed earns one point. The client is given a card with the written instructions: "Close your eyes." One point is earned if the client closes his or her eyes. The client is then asked to write a sentence. It need not be grammatically correct but needs a subject, verb, and to make sense to earn points. The MMSE needs to be given by someone trained in its administration. You can see and download the MMSE standard version form by Folstein, Folstein, and McHugh (1975) from www.medafile.com/mmses.htm. The normal MMSE is around 24–30 depending on age and education. A score of 20–23 is said to be mild dementia, 10–19 is moderate, 1–9 is severe, and 0 is profound. This examination requires that the person be able to read, see, and hear.

10. **What are the current theories of causation of Alzheimer's Disease?** According to Beckman (2005) researchers have discovered seventy-two genes that possibly relate to risk of late onset Alzheimer's Disease and mutations in three others that cause Alzheimer's Disease in younger middle-aged adults; however, only one gene has been consistently found to increase the risk in older adults. The e4 variant of a gene called apoE, a gene involved in fat metabolism, has been found to increase the risk of getting Alzheimer's Disease by three to fifteen times. Beckman also points out that some researchers have found a gene in this same region as apoE called UBQLN1 that could interact with presenilinoa, a protein implicated in Alzheimer's Disease. A variation of UBQLN1 called 8i is about 1.5 to 2 times more common in clients with Alzheimer's Disease. David Secko (2005) says the "risk for (late onset) Alzheimer's disease may come down to expression of various forms of human apolipoprotein E gene (apoE)" and describes Jean-Cosme Dodart and colleagues having injected a variant of apoE into mice brains and finding this had an effect on the formation of the amyloid plaques found in Alzheimer's Disease. This work provided more evidence that apoE will prove to be a major risk factor for Alzheimer's Disease.

11. **What treatments are currently being used with Alzheimer's clients?** Bates, Boote, and Beverly (2004) state that dementia treatment is "divided into two main categories": "psychopharmacological treatment underpinned by medical model of care and nonpharmacological psychosocial and other alternative approaches reflecting a more holistic vision of person-centered dementia care."

The pharmacological approaches include acetyl cholinesterase drugs like donepezil and rivastigmine.

According to Hashimoto et al. (2005), the only approved pharmacological approach for symptomatic treatment of Alzheimer's Disease in Japan is the use of donepezil hydrochloride. These authors further state that recent in vivo and in vitro studies have suggested the possibility that cholinesterase inhibitors could slow the rate of hippocampal atrophy in Alzheimer's Disease. Hashimoto et al. did a study with fifty-four patients with Alzheimer's Disease who received donepezil and ninety-three control subjects who did not receive anti-Alzheimer's Disease medications. MRI was done twice a year at a one-year interval, and the rate of hippocampal atrophy measured for the year. They found that the treated subjects had significantly smaller hippocampal volume loss than controls.

The nonpharmacological treatments include validation therapy, which is a method of communicating with elderly people with Alzheimer's Disease and related dementias, developed by Naomi Feil between 1963 and 1980. Feil classified people with cognitive impairment as being in one of four stages that are on a continuum of dementia (Briggs, 2003). Validation therapy involves the theory that the elderly struggle to resolve unfinished life issues before death. Validation is a way of classifying behaviors into four progressive stages, which are: 1. Malorientation: "expressing past conflicts in disguised forms"; 2. Time confusion: "longer holding onto reality but retreating inward"; 3. Repetitive motion: "movements replace words and are used to work through unresolved conflict"; and 4. Vegetation: "shutting out world completely and giving up on trying to resolve living." Validation therapy includes forming groups of five to ten individuals designed to stimulate energy and interaction socially as well as social roles.

A trained health care professional uses techniques including careful listening, pacing body rhythms, and good eye contact to enter the client's world and listen for underlying life themes. A major idea of validation therapy is that a trained person can and will build a relationship of mutual trust and respect with the older person because empathy builds trust, trust increases strength, and strength reduces stress and assists in restoring a feeling of well-being and joy.

In addition, there are ten principles of validation that are similar to some of the ten principles of mental health that have been taught in many nursing programs and some are similar to what is included in the philosophy of some nursing programs. Could it be that nurses need not only to learn these principles but to apply them as well? These principles are:

1. All people are unique and should be treated as an individual.
2. All persons are valuable, no matter how disoriented.
3. There is a reason behind the behavior of disoriented old people.
4. Behavior in old age is not only a function of changes in brain anatomy but reflects physical, social, and psychological changes that take place during the life span.
5. Behaviors of old people can be changed only if the person wants to change them.
6. Old people should be accepted nonjudgmentally.
7. Each stage of life has particular life tasks to be completed and failure to complete them may lead to psychological problems.
8. When recent memory fails, older adults restore balance to their lives by retrieving memories of the past.
9. Painful feelings that are expressed, acknowledged, and validated by a trusted listening will diminish. Painful feelings ignored will gain strength.
10. Empathy builds trust, decreases anxiety, and restores dignity" (www.vfvalidation.org/whatis.html).

The benefits of validation therapy are said to be restoration of self worth and lessening of the degree of withdrawal as well as promotion of communication and interaction, decrease in stress and anxiety, facilitation of independent living, and stimulation of potential that has been dormant.

Music therapy has been used with clients with dementia. Some clients who know how to play a musical instrument retain the ability to play the instrument. Some clients recall words to songs they knew in the past and can sing along when the song is played and sung by others.

Reminiscence therapy is also utilized with people who have dementia. Sometimes videos of family events in the past are shown to the person or photo albums are shown. Old pictures can be displayed in the person's room. In group therapy, pictures are sometimes shown of the town or city several decades in the past and people are encouraged to discuss memories of the past.

A method used in some facilities treating Alzheimer's clients is referred to as Snozelin. This therapy is described as a multisensory stimulation therapy providing sensory stimulation for the senses of sight, hearing, touch, taste, and smell through such means as music for meditation, the feel and smell of relaxing oils, lighting effects, and tactile surfaces. Verkaik, VanWeert, and Francke (2005) reviewed a number of psychosocial methods used to treat clients with dementia and stated that there is some evidence Snozelin in a multisensory room decreases apathy in people who are in latter phases of dementia.

12. **If you were the nurse in this case, what teaching would you do with Hannah and Jean about donepezil (Aricept)? What do you need to know about the drug? If this client refuses to take her Aricept when offered by her daughter, what would you recommend?** You can talk to Hannah about the medicine improving her memory. She cannot deal with large amounts of data so the teaching with Hannah has to be in short sentences and small amounts at a time. The majority of the teaching is with her daughter, Jean. You would tell Jean that donepezil is an anti-Alzheimer's agent, a cholinesterase inhibitor, and you could tell her why inhibiting cholinesterase is helpful. In addition you would tell Jean that this medicine has been found to temporarily decrease symptoms of dementia, but it will not cure Alzheimer's. Jean needs to know that the medication should be given daily at the same time and may be given with or without food. If a dose is missed, it should be skipped, and her mother should have no more than ordered (i.e., giving more medicine will not increase the benefits but may increase the side effects). Also advise Jean that the medication may cause dizziness and to notify you or the health care provider if Hannah experiences any nausea, vomiting, diarrhea, changes in stool color, or any new symptoms or if previous symptoms worsen.

As the nurse, you need to realize that this medication may cause bradycardia and you need to periodically monitor heart rate. Adverse reactions reported for this medication can be reviewed and are so varied that if Hannah has any new signs or symptoms, they need to be reviewed again to see if the medication could be causing them.

You will need to get a baseline measurement on cognitive function (memory, attention, ability to perform simple tasks, use of words, reasoning) and periodically reassess to see if there have been changes.

If the client refuses to take medication that she needs, you could recommend that the daughter distract her by suggesting tea and cookies and reoffering the pill in a few minutes. It is better to say: "It is time to take your medicine" instead of "Would you like to take your medicine?" If Hannah continues to refuse, the daughter may choose to put the medication in pudding or ice cream. While this creates an ethical problem in giving someone something they have refused, the daughter is acting in her mother's best interests and often this is the only way relatives can get confused persons to take medication.

13. **The client's daughter says she has a fear and a reoccurring nightmare that she will eventually need to place her mother in a facility that cares for people with Alzheimer's, but she wants to keep her at home. Keeping in mind black American culture, what questions, comments, or suggestions would you have for Jean at this time? Do you think Jean needs support, and if so, what kinds of support would you suggest?** In black American culture, it is a cultural practice to keep relatives who are sick or old in the home. Family and spirituality are important in the culture and need to be assessed and kept in mind in working with this client and her daughter. Jean wants to keep her mother at home rather than in a treatment facility, and you need to be careful to support this as long as it is safe and feasible. You must keep to yourself personal views you might have in regard to what you would do if you were in Jean's place. You could tactfully encourage Jean to visit some treatment facilities, designed to care for clients with Alzheimer's Disease, while the mother is in a day program or getting respite care. Visiting facilities may help alleviate fears of such facilities and help Jean be prepared should she reach the point she feels she has to put her mother in such a facility.

You can ask Jean what she will do if her mother says and does things that are frustrating and she feels like retaliating. Help Jean make a plan and a back-up plan, such as calling a trusted neighbor to watch her mother while she takes a break, asking Hannah's church friends for help get her to Sunday school and church, calling the home health agency and talking with you, or distracting her mother with a different activity such as singing. Help Jean make a list of sources of respite care and encourage her to call them.

Some of Hannah's confusion may be due to relocation stress syndrome. It often takes at least a month for a person to adjust to new surroundings. A second move at this time could bring increased confusion, depression, agitation, and other undesired behavioral changes. Any change in routine needs to be made gradually and carefully. This is similar to taking a small child to the school several times to acquaint them with the surroundings and the teacher before the start of school.

Christenson (2002) states that providing support for the caregiver is essential because 50 percent of all caregivers will suffer depression. Another reason for support is to keep the caregiver from getting burned out and/or being verbally and physically abusive to the person with Alzheimer's Disease due to being physically and emotionally exhausted.

You can be supportive to Jean by listening to her and letting her know that you realize it is not easy caring for her mother and by offering encouragement and positive reinforcement as well as information that is helpful to her. Being empathetic and listening to Jean will be helpful in building trust and strength.

In addition to being empathetic and listening, if your assessment determines that the client could benefit from a day program, you can suggest that Jean begin to look at day programs for people with Alzheimer's Disease, as this would provide some respite for her and would help her mother socialize and have reorientation activities by trained people. You may need to provide her with a list of programs for her to call and visit, or she may be able to do this on her own. You will need to follow up and see if she has contacted these programs and whether she needs more assistance from you. There may also be an Alzheimer's Disease support group locally that Jean could join. She could possibly start a small group if there is none.

14. What assessment data would you like to have if you were the nurse writing a nursing care plan for this client? What nursing diagnoses, goals, and interventions would you likely write for this client? You need some baseline vital signs, and you need to find out what physical health problems the client currently has and what health problems she has had in the past. You would want to know what her strengths and limitations are as well as what her interests are. You would want to assess mood, orientation, and ability to abstract. You would want to assess for any psychosis (hallucinations or delusional thinking). You would want to know the condition of her skin and whether it is intact and free of redness or bruising and whether she has any edema or not. All body systems would be assessed.

Nursing diagnoses would likely include:

- Risk for injury to self
- Thought processes altered
- Risk for relocation distress syndrome
- Fear
- Anxiety
- Powerlessness
- Depression
- Knowledge deficit

Goals will likely include the following:

- Will be safe from injury
- Skin will be intact
- Will bathe daily, brush teeth daily, and accept assistance with activities of daily living (ADLS) as needed
- Will remain out of bed during the day except for any scheduled rest/nap time
- Will participate in a day program that accepts people with dementia and offers socialization and reorientation as well as other appropriate activities

Interventions would likely include, but not be limited to, the following:

- Make efforts to orient client by providing a large clock and calendar in an area where client can easily and often see them.
- Put a picture on client's door that she will recognize. It could be a copy of the wedding picture of her parents. Display old comforting pictures in the house.
- Show family videos or movies of family outings or events if these are available.
- Put the day, month, and year on a bulletin board or the refrigerator or somewhere that client will see it.
- Remove all hazards such as rugs that slide.
- Encourage fluids. Measure intake and output to assure that both are adequate to prevent dehydration and reduce chances of decubitus ulcers.
- Provide exercise appropriate to age and condition.
- Provide opportunities to socialize within client's abilities and needs (e.g., day program or continued attendance at Sunday school and church).
- Use positive reinforcement.
- Schedule time and events for beauty efforts such as hair care, skin care, manicures, and pedicures as this improves self-esteem, may improve mood, and instills a sense of being cared for.
- Assess causes and level of fear and use creative means of reducing fear. Remain with client during bathing/showering and assist as necessary as may be afraid of showering. Also increase lighting in the house and decrease shadowy areas as this can cause fear at night
- Assist client with oral hygiene and other hygiene chores and dressing, limiting choices in clothing to two at most.
- Speak clearly, slowly, and in concrete terms while facing client and keep hearing aides in working order and assist client in putting them on.

- Provide teaching about medication to client and caregiver.
- Assess caregiver periodically for adequate support and offer ideas for respite care.

References

"A-Beta Immunization Protects Against Cognitive Impairment." (2005a). *Vaccine Weekly*, March 23, 10–12.

American Psychiatric Association. (2000). *Diagnostic and Statistical Manual of Mental Disorders, 4th ed.* Text Revision. Washington, DC: American Psychiatric Association.

Bates, J., J. Boote, and C. Beverly. (2004). "Psychosocial Interventions for People with a Milder Dementing Illness: A Systematic Review." *Journal of Advanced Nursing* 45(6): 644–659.

Beckman, M. (2005). "New Link to Alzheimer's Identified." *Science Now*, March 3, 4–6.

Briggs, N.M. (2003). "Validation Therapy for Dementia Review Update." *Cochrane Database Systematic Review* (3) CD 001394.

Christenson, D.D. (2002). "Practical Principles for the Management of Alzheimer's Disease." *Primary Care Companion to Journal of Clinical Psychiatry* 4(2): 63–69.

"Diagnosis of Alzheimer's Disease Expected to Increase." (2005b). *Vaccine Weekly*, March 23.

Hashimoto, M., H. Kazui, K. Matsumoto, Y. Nakano, M. Yasuda, and E. Mori. (2005). "Does Donezepil Slow the Progression of Hippocampal Atrophy in Patients with Alzheimer's Disease?" *American Journal of Psychiatry* 162(4): 676–682.

http://health.allrefer.com/health/alzheimers-disease-info.html. Accessed February 1, 2006.

Secko, D. (2005). "Alzheimer's Disease: Genetic Variables and Risk." *Canadian Medical Association Journal* 172(5): 627.

Tavee, J. and P.J. Sweeney. (2002). "Alzheimer's Disease." http://www.clevelandclinicmeded.com/diseasemanagement/neurology/alzheimers/alzheimers1.htm. Accessed July 17, 2006.

Verkaik, P., J.C. VanWeert, and A.L. Francke. (2005). "The Effects of Psychosocial Methods on Depressed, Aggressive, and Apathetic Behaviors of People with Dementia: A Systematic Review." *Institute Journal of Geriatric Psychiatry* 20(4): 301–314.

www.ahaf.org/alzdis/about/adabout.htm. Accessed April 3, 2005.

www.alz-nca.org/aboutalz/phases.asp. Accessed April 3, 2005.

www.legal-info-legale.nb.ca/pub-manage-afairs.asp. Accessed April 4, 2005.

www.medafile.com/mmses.htm. Accessed February 1, 2006.

www.vfvalidation.org/whatis.html. Accessed February 1, 2006.

GENDER		SPIRITUAL/RELIGIOUS

Male

AGE

15

SETTING

- Alternative high school health classes with school nurse

ETHNICITY

- White American and Black American

CULTURAL CONSIDERATIONS

PREEXISTING CONDITIONS

- Learning disabilities

COEXISTING CONDITIONS

- Alcohol abuse

COMMUNICATION

DISABILITY

SOCIOECONOMIC

- Ward of state; qualifies for free school lunch

SPIRITUAL/RELIGIOUS

PHARMACOLOGIC

PSYCHOSOCIAL

- Current: sexually aggressive with girlfriend
- Early childhood: Father in prison
- Mother charged with neglect
- Multiple foster care situations

LEGAL

- On probation after serving sentence in juvenile justice system

ETHICAL

- Nurse contemplating adoption of client

ALTERNATIVE THERAPY

PRIORITIZATION

DELEGATION

DIFFICULT

CONDUCT DISORDER

Level of difficulty: High

Overview: Requires adhering to mental health principles that all people have worth and that all people can and do change. Requires maintaining a professional and helping therapeutic manner without losing sight of the need for setting consistent limits.

Client Profile

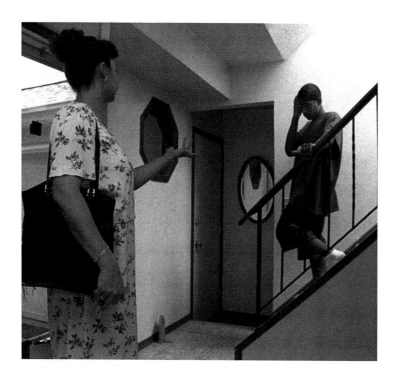

Elias is a 15-year-old male. His father is white American and his mother is black American. His father suddenly left the family when Elias was 7 years old. He later learned his father is in prison. Elias's mother tried to raise him and work two jobs. Elias started hanging out with a group of boys with a reputation for skipping school and drinking when he was 12 years old. A neighbor accused him of trying to drown her cat. He denied this, saying he was only trying to see if the cat could swim. The neighbor reported Elias's mother for neglect based on this and other instances of Elias getting into trouble while his mother was working. Elias became a ward of the state and was placed with a series of foster families. He has a reputation for starting fights and cutting a boy's face with his ring. The school expelled him because an ex-girlfriend accused him of threatening to hurt her if she didn't come back to him and have sex with him. The previous year a male student had killed his ex-girlfriend under similar circumstances, and the school was not about to risk a reoccurrence. In the past Elias has done some minor shoplifting without getting caught. About a year ago, he and some of his friends stole a car and decided to put on masks and costumes and rob people at knifepoint on Halloween. However, he chose an off-duty policeman to rob, and this ended in his being overpowered and arrested. He went to a state prison facility boot camp and a halfway house, then was placed with another foster family and returned to the public school system. He was not in the juvenile prison system long enough to get a GED and job training, but he did learn to live in a very structured system. Although he has learning disabilities, he made some progress in the prison education system in his reading skills.

Case Study

Elias is taking classes at an alternative high school with more flexible hours and programs for high school students who need to work, who have children, or who have been discipline problems and respond better in a structured, goal-oriented environment. Elias is taking a health course from a school nurse. The schools nurse gives Elias extra duties in the classroom and extra homework projects. He willingly completes the tasks. The school nurse tells Elias she is interested in his reading progress and offers to help him in reading or to assign a student with good reading skills to help him. The school nurse experienced trouble reading when she was a child, but received a lot of help and managed to compensate for some learning difficulties.

The school nurse receives a notice that she needs to come to a meeting of Elias's teachers and support staff. Elias has been having some discipline problems in one of his classes. The school nurse is surprised to hear this as Elias behaves well in health class.

In the faculty lounge waiting for the meeting about Elias to begin, the school nurse supervisor overhears two teachers talking about Elias. The general theme of their conversation is that they read his school records from the state juvenile corrections system and discovered that he has a diagnosis of Conduct Disorder (CD). One of the teachers says Elias is never going to amount to anything because he has Conduct Disorder. The other teacher says Elias is draining resources from other students as he will eventually go to prison. When the school nurse tries to talk with the teachers about Elias's good qualities, one of them suggests the school nurse adopt Elias if she likes him so well. The school nurse is not sure if the teacher is serious or not and begins to think the idea over.

Questions and Suggested Answers

1. **If you were the school nurse in this case, would you have difficulty relating to Elias if he had been in prison for robbing someone at knifepoint? Would you treat him any differently if he had been imprisoned for doing or selling drugs? Describe an attitude and approach you and other nurses need to take with an adolescent like Elias.** Nurses can feel apprehensive working with a client who has threatened or hurt someone else with or without a dangerous weapon. There are some nurses who would feel challenged while others will want to "mother" the client or rescue him. It is reasonable and healthy for nurses to be anxious and even fearful. Nurses need to be cautious and professional with all students before, during, and after building a therapeutic nurse-patient (nurse-student) relationship. As far as you know, this client is not on drugs and is not psychotic, but he could be. Sometimes the client we are aware of as having threatened someone or being on drugs is not as dangerous as the one we don't know anything about. Nurses can be biased against someone who is on or has been on drugs or has sold drugs and/or biased against someone who has threatened or hurt someone else regardless of their present state of rehabilitation. These biases and negative feelings as well as empathetic feelings can arise because of past personal experiences or the experiences of family and/or friends. It is important to keep in mind a basic mental health principle that people can and do change and deserve a chance to change. Another mental health principle to keep in mind is that all people have worth. If you were working with this client, you would need to put aside personal biases and stereotypes and treat this client as an individual worthy of your nursing help. You would need to stay focused on being therapeutic as well as safe and resist any thoughts or feelings of anger and any desire to give up on this client.

2. **Was the nurse's approach consisting of asking for assistance and offering to help with learning to read an acceptable approach or not? Provide a rationale for your answer. If you were the nurse in this case, how could you begin to work on developing empathy for Elias?** The approach by the school nurse was acceptable. In this case, the school nurse is tapping into Elias's need to be helpful. Being helpful is something that most, if not all, humans feel good about. It helps build self-esteem. It can help a person feel as if they belong. The nurse is also demonstrating caring by offering help and by taking an interest in this client. All humans need someone to care about them, and this client may especially need it. He will probably do much better in class if he has a sense that he belongs in the class.

Being empathetic means using your imagination to put yourself in another person's place (in this case Elias's place): to imagine yourself in their life and what that would be like, what it would feel like, and what it would take to help you reach your maximum potential (in this case as Elias). It is good to imagine yourself in the client's place and then step back as yourself and think about what is needed from you as a professional and therapeutic person.

3. What criteria did Elias have to match to be diagnosed with Conduct Disorder? What behaviors does he have that match this diagnosis? Is it possible to have a mild case of Conduct Disorder, and what are the subtypes of Conduct Disorder? The person with Conduct Disorder has a persistent behavioral pattern of violating basic rights of other people and violating rules as well as major societal norms. There are four main groupings under which behaviors fall, and there are fifteen behaviors scattered throughout these four main groupings. A person has to have at least three of the fifteen characteristic behaviors.

The fifteen characteristic behaviors are grouped under four main categories: 1. aggression toward people and animals; 2. property destruction; 3. theft or deceitfulness; and 4. serious violations of rules. Elias has demonstrated behaviors that seem to fall under the first category: aggression toward people and animals. A neighbor accused him of trying to drown a cat. He may have picked a physical fight or two, and he is known to have pulled a knife on victims at Halloween. He did seriously threaten his former girlfriend.

In the second group of symptoms (property destruction), Elias seems lacking. As far as we know, he did not engage in fire setting or deliberately destroy property. He does have some symptoms under the category of theft or deceitfulness. He has engaged in shoplifting and tried to rob people at knifepoint. Under the category of serious violation of rules, Elias has had times when he ran away from home or was truant from school; however, running away from home does not count if the child was running away from physical or sexual abuse. This is an area for further data gathering. Was Elias abused in addition to being abandoned?

Behaviors of Clients With Conduct Disorder	Does Client Have These Behaviors?
Aggressive acts toward people and animals	
1. Frequently is found to be bullying, threatening, or intimidating to others	Yes, he has threatened his girlfriend and been intimidating to her
2. Has often started physical fights	Has started some fights or at least engaged in fighting
3. Has used a weapon with potential to bring serious physical damage to others (e.g., gun, knife, broken glass, brick, bat, etc.)	He tried to rob someone at knifepoint
4. Has engaged in physical cruelty to people	
5. Has engaged in physical cruelty to animals	Possibly tried to drown a cat
6. Has confronted someone and stolen from them (e.g., stealing a purse, armed robbery, mugging)	Confronted someone with a knife and attempted to steal but was overpowered and arrested
7. Had forced sexual activity with someone against their will	Tried to force sexual activity with ex-girlfriend
Destruction of Property	
8. Deliberate fire setting with purpose of causing serious damage	No, as far as is known
9. Deliberate destruction of someone else's property (by means beside fire setting)	No, as far as is known
Deceitfulness or theft	
10. Breaking into another person's home, building, or vehicle	No, as far as is known
11. Frequently engages in lying to get goods or favors or get out of obligations (cons others)	Need to evaluate
12. Stealing things of nontrivial value but not confronting victim (e.g., shoplifting or forgery)	Has done some shoplifting

(Continued)

Behaviors of Clients With Conduct Disorder	Does Client Have These Behaviors?
Serious violations of rules	
13. Frequently remains out at night even though parents prohibit this, starting before age 13	Needs evaluation. Was running with a group who skipped school and drank alcohol. Assess whether out at night before age 13.
14. History of running away from home and staying away overnight two or more times or one time without returning for a long time	Need to evaluate. If he has a history of running away due to abuse, it would not count in meeting this criteria.
15. Frequently truant from school starting before age 13	Yes

(Adapted from APA, 2000)

It is interesting that the diagnosis of CD has severity specifiers of mild, moderate, and severe depending on the number of characteristics a person has and the severity of effect on others. It is possible to have a mild case of Conduct Disorder, but it is also possible to have a moderate case or a severe case. There are also two subtypes: childhood onset with at least one characteristic before age 10 and adolescent onset type.

4. **Describe what keeps Elias from being diagnosed with Oppositional Defiant Disorder or Antisocial Personality Disorder instead of Conduct Disorder.** People with Oppositional Defiant Disorder do not have the persistent patterns of abusing the basic rights of others and/or breaking age-appropriate social rules or norms. People with Antisocial Personality Disorder must have exhibited behaviors consistent with those of Conduct Disorder beginning before age 15 and must be at least 18 years of age. Elias is too young to receive a diagnosis of Antisocial Personality Disorder. It may be that these three disorders—Oppositional Defiant Disorder, Conduct Disorder, and Antisocial Disorder—are on a continuum, with the behavior getting more entrenched and the abuse of others' rights increasing with time. On the other hand, they may be completely unrelated with unrelated causes.

5. **What are some theories about the cause of Conduct Disorder? What is the prevalence of Conduct Disorder?** Kelly (2002) describes adolescents with Conduct Disorder as having social information processing deficits as well as other cognitive deficits. She suggests that normally developing peers shun the adolescent with CD, and because of this shunning and the weak attachment to their parents, these adolescents with CD then attach to deviant peers. This idea is consistent with the fact that many with Conduct Disorder also have learning disabilities, and as many as 60–90 percent of clinic-referred children also are diagnosed with ADHD (Frick, 2001). Some theorists have suggested CD may be a variant of ADHD in some cases.

There appear to be both genetic and environmental factors influencing the development of Conduct Disorder. After a review of the research, Frick (2001) found that the research "suggests that CD is multi-determined and for most children and adolescents who develop CD, it is the end result of a complex inter-action among many types of causal mechanisms." Frick identified some of these causal mechanisms as: a person's individual vulnerabilities, problems in the environment the child is being reared in, and stressors in larger social ecology, such as poor educational opportunities or crime. Frick further suggested that children and adolescents with CD are heterogeneous in regard to causes of their behavioral problems with different causal pathways. It has also been suggested that those who develop CD as children have causes that differ from those that develop it as adolescents, suggesting that perhaps those who develop it younger have more biological causes and those developing it later have more environmental causes. Having multifactorial causes has implication for individualized treatment that addresses the client's individual biological and environmental problems.

Looking at risk factors for Conduct Disorder, the American Psychiatric Association (2000) pointed out that children with a biological or adoptive parent who has Antisocial Personality Disorder or a history of Conduct Disorder or who have a brother or sister with Conduct Disorder are at greater risk of developing

Conduct Disorder. Other risk factors for Conduct Disorder include having biological parents who have a dependence on alcohol, a mood disorder or Schizophrenia, or a history of Attention-Deficit/Hyperactivity Disorder. Risk factors also likely include a history of abuse or neglect and having learning disorders and/or developmental disorders.

The literature suggests the following: Conduct Disorder has increased in the past few decades, is probably higher in urban settings, is more common in males but is on the rise in females, and is one of the top diagnoses in mental health facilities (inpatient and outpatient). The prevalence has been reported in the range of less than 1 percent to more than 10 percent. In mental health facilities for inpatients and in facilities for outpatients, Conduct Disorder is one of the most often diagnosed conditions (APA, 2000).

6. **What are learning disorders? Are learning disorders more common in adolescents with Conduct Disorder?** The learning disorders, which used to be called Academic Skills Disorders in the diagnostic and statistical manual (APA, 2000), include:

1. Reading Disorder (includes accuracy, speed, and/or comprehension). People with Reading Disorder (referred to as Dyslexia) have distortions, substitutions, and/or omissions when reading orally. They experience mistakes in comprehension and are slow in reading silently or out loud.
2. Mathematics Disorder includes a number of different skills, one or more of which is impaired, such as understand and/or naming terms, clustering objects into groups, copying numbers right, remembering to add in carried numbers, counting objects, sequencing mathematical steps, and learning multiplication tables.
3. Disorder of Written Expression (the term Dysgraphia seems to be used in the literature and in popular use). "The disorder of written expression is rare when not associated with other Learning Disorders" (APA, 2000).
4. Learning Disorder Not Otherwise Specified.

It is likely that learning disorders are more common in adolescents with Conduct Disorder. Not being able to read and write and not being successful in learning in school may bring out the worst in a student's behavior and may cause a student to drop out of school and to get into legal trouble. The Texas Youth Commission serves 4,200 youth offenders in its juvenile corrections centers. Those serving sentences are ages 10 to 21 with the average age being 16. Dr. Forrest Novy (2004), director of special education for TYC, stated at the Texas Learning Disabilities Conference that 25 percent of incarcerated youth have learning disabilities. Forty-three percent are in special education. Many cannot read, and most are school dropouts. Not all those incarcerated have a diagnosis of Conduct Disorder, but it is a common diagnosis in the Texas youth served by the state juvenile corrections system. Other states may have similar statistics.

7. **What data do you think would be most helpful to gather on this client? What nursing diagnoses and goals would you write for this client? What interventions would be helpful? Who do you need to work with in carrying out interventions?** One of the most helpful pieces of information to have is a list of the client's strengths. John Willson, director of a Wilderness Camp in North Carolina, speaking at the Texas Learning Disabilities Conference in 2004, said, "Carrying around a list of your strengths helps in dealing with challenges." This is true for all kinds of diagnoses and for people without diagnoses as well as for kids with Conduct Disorder and learning disorders. Robert Brooks, psychologist and faculty member at Harvard, told a story at the 2004 Learning Disabilities Conference of Texas. His story was about a boy who was refusing to come to school. The principal asked what he liked to do and was good at. The boy said: "Take care of my dog." Once the principal enlisted the boy's help to be a pet monitor for the school, he was always there and never late.

Along with strengths, you want to gather data about things that Elias needs help with, for example, interpersonal skills such as communication and building friendships. This student may need help in self-esteem building.

Elias has had some abuse of alcohol in the past. The nurse needs to get a history of alcohol and other drug use from this client, as well as any education and treatment received for problems with alcohol abuse.

It would be helpful to get information about any pattern of abusing rules in the past or currently. The client may or may not have a need for help dealing with addictive behaviors. The nurse could assess the foster family to see what support they are giving or are willing to give this client and could work with the family to maximize support and enhance client's strengths.

Likely nursing diagnoses include:

- Chronically low self-esteem
- Ineffective coping
- Risk for loneliness
- Impaired social interaction
- Risk for other-directed and self-directed violence

Self-esteem may improve through success in meeting goals. Self-esteem may improve through the pride that comes with coping more effectively with problems. A goal might be to demonstrate use of problem-solving skills each day. The nurse can present theoretical or real situations in which a person normally gets angry and have the client think through how to respond to these situations more appropriately.

In regard to loneliness and impaired social interaction, the goal might be to participate in a school activity or a school group. The nurse who is teaching the health class can carefully select someone to work with this client to complete in-class assignments or can assign small group work, which she can supervise. The nurse can share what she is doing with the other teachers so what is working can be duplicated in other classes.

The goal for dealing with high risk for violence would be something like "no instances of violence toward self or others." Another goal might be for the client to journal a page a day about feelings or to use a special signal to the nurse or teacher when feeling out of control. Interventions might include talking about feelings and what to do with them on an individual and on a class basis. It might be possible to have the client participate in peer conflict management training or assign the client to research peer conflict management and to help set up some training in conflict management. There are many imaginative/creative ways to help this client resolve nursing diagnoses.

The nurse also needs to work with the parents (natural, stepparents, or adoptive) or guardians of the child to teach them ways to help the child. The nurse needs to support and provide education and encouragement to parents, who often feel blamed for their child having behavioral problems and frustrated when they can't find a way to get their child to get to school on time or even attend school at times. These frustrated parents are further frustrated when they are fined for their children's nonattendance at school (Wood, 2002).

Parents/caregivers of adolescents with traits of conduct disorder are often frustrated because their pleas for the adolescent to stop unacceptable behaviors are futile. The nurse can explain that interacting with this adolescent may be like being in a car with a driver who has faulty brakes. You ask the driver to stop and he can't, but if you ask him to turn, he can. The nurse can help the foster parents to provide Elias with more guidance in how to deal with situations, rather than ongoing threats if he does not stop (e.g., problem solving on how to get to school rather than threats if he doesn't get there).

When developing a plan of care and implementing it, the nurse needs to work with the school administration, faculty, and support staff who are educationally responsible for Elias. The nurse needs to work with the Child and Family Services caseworker or whoever is working with Elias as a ward of the state. The nurse needs to work with the parents. All these parties may attend planning conferences for Elias, and this is an opportunity for the nurse to share ideas and concerns, to educate, and to suggest interventions. Everyone working with Elias needs to be consistent in applying rules as well as rewards for good behavior and consistent in providing the structure and support he needs.

8. **What therapies are currently being used to treat Conduct Disorder? What is the likelihood that treatment of Conduct Disorder will have success?** Individual behavior modification programs initiated in a variety of settings, with training for teachers and parents to maintain the program after discharge, have been used in the past and continue to be used, as they are successful in many cases. Failure often occurs at the point the

parents or teachers don't continue the program. Small classes with caring, well-trained teachers are recommended and being used today in some schools. Parents with children who have Conduct Disorder traits early on often seek out special schools or private schools, which provide small classrooms and special teaching methods. Wood (2002) has said that Conduct Disorder is especially hard to treat and cites the National Assembly for Wales in 2001 in stating that educational models of intervention appear to have more success than therapeutic models. Key supporting points for this idea is that school can: 1. Motivate adolescents to learn and meet education goals, which boost their self-esteem; 2. Offset negative effects of family risk factors; and 3. Be a force for giving a message of societal norms at a time when the adolescent has stopped looking to family for role models. Some juvenile justice programs are stressing small classes with caring teachers, attainment of high school equivalency diplomas, and work training. The Texas Youth Commission boot camp also stresses self-esteem and self-worth and respect for others, personal accountability, physical fitness, self-improvement, constructive use of time, and appropriate discipline (www.tyc.state.tx.us/programs/boot_camp.html).

Many programs utilize family therapy in treating Conduct Disorder. Parents are often taught how to provide structure and how to include the child in developing rules and consequences for breaking rules. Children and adolescents often develop tougher rules and consequences for breaking them than do parents. Helping develop rules helps the client be more committed to the rules. Parents are taught how to get input from their children and how to discourage manipulation. These clients need to be held to completing homework by a given deadline and to going to bed at a certain bedtime.

Frick (2001) describes interventions for children and adolescents with Conduct Disorder. He points out that limited effectiveness of programs in the past have been due to the "failure to address causal mechanisms implicated in the development of Conduct Disorder." Treatment approaches described by Frick include: 1. Contingency management programs based on the premise that children with CD have not been exposed to a consistent and contingent environment, with treatment being a structured behavioral management system; 2. Parent management training; 3. Cognitive behavioral skills training including teaching methods to inhibit impulsive or angry responding; 4. Stimulant medication (Ritalin and others) as between 60–90 percent of "clinic referred" children and adolescents with Conduct Disorder also have ADHD; and 5. Specially designed, multicomponent programs such as the Fast Track Program designed by Conduct Problems Prevention Research Group. This program targets intensive intervention during the kindergarten year. Another special program described by Frick is Multi-Systemic Therapy (MST), which has been used to treat severe antisocial behavior in juveniles with multiple arrests. MST begins with comprehensive assessment looking at the child's level and severity of problems and the family and larger societal context of these problems. Treatment is individualized depending on assessment findings and could involve treatments such as marital therapy for parents, family therapy, peer intervention, social peer groups such as scouts or athletics, academic remediation, facilitation of parent-teacher communication, and other treatments as deemed appropriate.

Shamsie (2001) claims that "even with the best-known treatment, the success rate on follow-up does not exceed 74%" and that "failure in treatment often results in the adolescent becoming an adult with Antisocial Personality Disorder." While Antisocial Personality Disorder is an even more difficult condition to treat than Conduct Disorder and not a good outcome, it is encouraging that three-fourths of treated clients will have a successful outcome and well worth the investment of resources. With more resources devoted to treatment of CD and research on CD, the success rate could improve.

9. **Where would nurses encounter children and adolescents with diagnoses of Conduct Disorder other than the public school system?** Nurses working in any area where children and adolescents are cared for will encounter some clients who meet the criteria for a diagnosis of Conduct Disorder. Of course nurses working in residential psychiatric treatment centers and psychiatric inpatient units, as well as the juvenile justice system, will encounter clients with this diagnosis more often. Nurses will encounter people in their personal lives who could meet this diagnosis or who want advice or help in dealing with their children who have this diagnosis. Sometimes a student in nursing school will admit in class that they had this diagnosis or firmly believe they could have met this diagnosis, but that they somehow changed their attitude and behavior, usually because of an adult or adults who cared about them and made a difference in their life.

10. **Why is it important to care about and for children and adolescents who have a diagnosis of Conduct Disorder or who have traits of the diagnosis?** There are many reasons why nurses and others need to care about and for these children, so almost any answer you gave will be right. One of the most important reasons is that we need to care for all clients who need our help, not just the ones who have an acute medical problem that will respond quickly to treatment.

Another reason is that without help, children and adolescents with Conduct Disorder are at risk of committing violent acts toward others, damaging property, developing depression, hurting themselves or committing suicide, as well as having problems with employment, family relationships, and the law (Frisch and Frisch, 2006). While not all adolescents who take weapons to school and who threaten, hurt, or kill others at school have Conduct Disorder and while not all kids with Conduct Disorder are violent, national publicity about school shootings and other acts of violence at school have demonstrated the urgent need to care for the kids who don't fit in and who are aggressive.

11. **What do you think about the nurse's thought of adopting this client? What would you do in her place?** It is not unusual to want to rescue a client from their less-than-perfect situation. It is not unusual to want to provide resources for a client. What actions a nurse takes on these thoughts need to be well thought out. It is important to remind yourself that you are the professional nurse, and it is generally unacceptable in a workplace for a nurse to adopt a client. It is almost always better to work on helping the client learn to resolve problems, on finding resources, and on advocating for the client, rather than rescuing the client and taking over their care. It is essential to therapeutic nursing care to keep the relationship with the client at a professional and therapeutic level rather than on a friendship level.

In addition, as the nurse in this case, you might begin to want to provide the client better clothing or make the client lunch or provide other recourses. Almost always, it is better to encourage the client to get ongoing resources through social service programs than to personally give the client money, food, or other resources. The relationship changes when the client begins to depend on you for money or goods or anything outside the usual professional relationship.

Keep in mind that this child still has parents who may want to work toward getting him back into their care at some point in time. He is a ward of the state. His caseworker would know if adoption is possible whether it is prudent or not.

References

American Psychiatric Association (APA). (2000). *Diagnostic and Statistical Manual of Mental Disorders, 4th ed.* Text Revision. Washington, DC: American Psychiatric Association.

Brooks, R. "Video Theater: Look What You Have Done—Learning Disabilities and Self-Esteem." Presentation at the Learning Disabilities Association of Texas Annual Conference, Austin, Texas, November 2004.

Frick, P.J. (2001). "Effective Interventions For Children and Adolescents with Conduct Disorder." *Canadian Journal of Psychiatry* 46(7): 597–609.

Frisch, N.C. and L.E. Frisch. (2006). *Psychiatric Mental Health Nursing, 3rd ed.* Albany, NY: Thomson Delmar Learning.

Kelly, M.K. (2002). "Attachment and Affect Regulation: A Framework for Family Treatment of Conduct Disorder." *Family Process* 41(3).

Novy, F. (2004). "Incarcerated Youth with Learning Disabilities: There Is Life after Second Grade." Presentation at the Learning Disabilities Association of Texas Annual Conference, Austin, Texas, November 2004.

Shamsie, J. (2001). "Conduct Disorder: A Challenge to Child Psychiatry." *Canadian Journal of Psychiatry* 46(7): 593–594.

Willson, J. "Positive Behavior Development Techniques and Strategies for Youth Diagnosed with ADHD." Presentation at the Learning Disabilities Association of Texas Annual Conference, Austin, Texas, November 2004.

Wood, C. (2002). "Supporting the Parents of Adolescents with Conduct Disorder." *Paediatic Nursing* 14(8): 24–27.

www.tyc.state.tx.us/programs/boot_camp.html. Accessed December 17, 2005.

GENDER

Male

AGE

7

SETTING

- Community mental health center

ETHNICITY

- White American

CULTURAL CONSIDERATIONS

PREEXISTING CONDITION

COEXISTING CONDITION

COMMUNICATION

DISABILITY

SOCIOECONOMIC

SPIRITUAL/RELIGIOUS

PHARMACOLOGIC

- Methylphenidate hydrochloride (Concerta)

PSYCHOSOCIAL

LEGAL

ETHICAL

ALTERNATIVE THERAPY

PRIORITIZATION

DELEGATION

DIFFICULT

ATTENTION-DEFICIT/HYPERACTIVITY DISORDER

Level of difficulty: High

Overview: Requires the nurse to keep an open mind about whether a child with Attention-Deficit/Hyperactivity Disorder (ADHD) might benefit from stimulant medication. Requires the nurse to discipline herself to neither advise for or against the medication, but to use the nursing process to assess an individual child's behavior, determine the child's problems (nursing diagnoses), and intervene in appropriate ways. Critical thinking is required to come up with creative ways to keep the child and others around him safe and to help him succeed in school when he has impulsivity, hyperactivity, and a short attention span.

Client Profile

Martin (Marty) is a 7-year-old boy who has a history of being so active that his family and others describe him like he is battery or motor-driven. He lives with his divorced father, two uncles, an aunt, and grandparents. His mother was given custody in divorce proceedings, but she changed her mind about caring for him as a single parent and left him with the father. Since that time Marty has only seen his mother once. The father intends to go to court for custody when he has money to pay the lawyer and court costs.

Marty has gone nonstop from the time he gets up until he goes to bed at night since he was a toddler. Marty seems to have no concern for safety. At age four he bit into a live lamp cord, resulting in a serious burn and scarring of his lip. This condition was corrected by plastic surgery. On a walk with a cousin, he suddenly climbed over the fence around an electrical transformer station and refused to get out. His attention span is short, and he goes from activity to activity quickly. One minute he is pointing a bow and arrow at a family member and the next jumping on the furniture. When he was four years old, he discovered the fun of doing somersaults in the tub, and those supervising him fear he is going to hit his head on the faucets. The family takes turns watching him as he quickly tires a person out. Family members have noticed when they send him to get something he forgets to bring it back.

His teacher at school has sent notes home and had conferences to communicate his behavior at school, including interrupting others, not wanting to wait his turn, and not following directions like other children. His hand is frequently up, and he has something to say whether it is relevant or not. When other children are finishing work, he is doing something else. He gets out of his seat frequently. When the teacher gets him to sit in his seat and do his work, she notices his hands and feet are very "fidgety" and he makes careless mistakes. He seldom turns in assigned homework. His grandparents try to get him to read for them, but he says: "I don't want to." They find it nearly impossible to get him to sit and play quietly. The family and the teacher have all noticed that he is easily distracted by anything happening in his environment. He is an attractive child with a handsome smile. People tend to like him even though they don't like some of his behavior.

Case Study

Marty and his father have come to the community mental health center. Several people have suggested to the father that Marty might have ADHD. If he has this disorder, the father wants to see if the child psychiatrist will prescribe some medication and/or offer other help to increase Marty's attention span and slow him down a bit. Marty is into everything in the waiting room. He takes things out of the trash receptacle, throws some toys at the desk, climbs over and under chairs, turns the lights off and on, and then he runs behinds the desk and grabs one of the donuts the nursing staff have for coffee break. The father says to the nurse: "I'm sorry. Do you think he has ADHD?"

The nurse weighs Marty, measures his height, and gets vital signs and a preliminary history. The psychologist does some testing and asks a lot of questions and verifies the diagnosis of ADHD. The child psychiatrist also sees Marty and his father and prescribes methylphenidate hydrochloride (Concerta). The nurse does some teaching with the father and answers his questions. Next, the nurse asks the father about Marty's mother. The father reveals that the mother has custody of the child, but that the child lives with him. The nurse gets a release of information from the father so the treatment team can share information and obtain information from the mother. The nurse contracts the mother in regard to the medication. The mother says, "I don't want Marty to have Ritalin or any other drug that messes with his mind. I won't sign giving permission for him to be on drugs." She says: "I have read that Ritalin is prescribed for kids that don't need it. Marty just has more energy than most kids his age. He will grow out of it."

Questions and Suggested Answers

1. **If you were the nurse in this case, what would you say to the father when he asks: "Do you think he (Marty) has ADHD?"** In some states master's prepared clinical nurse specialists in mental health psychiatric nursing may be trained and permitted by law and facility policy to make psychiatric diagnoses. A staff nurse does not diagnose but can give acceptable and helpful answers. One possible answer would be: "You are in the right

place to get this answer, although it will take some special assessments to decide whether Marty has ADHD or not." Another possibility is: "It sounds like you have thought about ADHD as a possibility." This statement invites the father to talk about behavior he has observed that suggests ADHD or to address whatever questions and concerns he might have. This simple statement suggests the nurse has time and interest in his concerns. The nurse can also assess what the father knows about ADHD, verify his correct knowledge, gently correct any misconceptions, and can provide additional education as needed.

2. **If you were the nurse in this case, what could you and other staff members do to make the time in the waiting room easier for the father and this very active child?** You could direct the father and child to a location with age-appropriate toys, if there is one. You could suggest an activity such as throwing paper wads into a wastebasket with the idea of starting close to the basket and then increasing the distance as more of a challenge. Dad could be enlisted to help with this activity. You could model self-esteem building statements by using positive verbal reinforcement for things like good enthusiasm or great style or good attempt when the child misses. Applauding can occur when the child makes a basket. Student nurses and staff nurses are capable of being quite creative in suggesting activities to keep children busy as they wait in health care facility waiting rooms. By watching nurses modeling ways to keep children engaged in activities that are therapeutic, and then mirroring the nurses' behavior, the father will learn techniques that can be utilized at home and in other settings.

3. **What behaviors does Marty have that match the criteria for Attention-Deficit/Hyperactivity Disorder (ADHD)? Looking at the criteria, what type of ADHD do you think he would most likely have?** The criteria for ADHD is directed to not only determining if the client has Attention-Deficit/Hyperactivity Disorder but to determining if it is Predominantly Inattentive Type or Predominantly Hyperactive-Impulsive Type or a Combined Type (meeting criteria for inattention and hyperactivity and impulsivity).

Criteria for ADHD	Does Client Meet This Criteria?
1. Meet either six or more listed symptoms of inattention or six or more listed symptoms of hyperactivity-impulsivity	Yes.
Inattention:	
Making careless mistakes or failing to pay close attention to details	Yes, the teacher has noticed he makes careless mistakes in his schoolwork.
Frequently has trouble remaining attentive to tasks and play activities	Yes. The teacher describes his inability to sit in his seat and stay attentive.
Frequently does not appear to listen when someone speaking directly to him or her	
Frequently does not finish instructions and fails to finish work (not due to oppositional behavior or not understanding instructions)	Yes, he seldom turns in homework or finishes work in class.
Frequently has trouble organizing tasks and activities	
Frequently voices dislike or demonstrates reluctance or avoids doing tasks requiring sustained mental effort (e.g., homework)	Yes, avoids homework and says: "I don't want to" when grandparents ask him to read at home.
Often loses items needed for tasks or activities	Yes
Distracted by extraneous stimuli	Yes, teacher and his family have noticed that any extraneous stimuli distracts him from his activity.
Frequently forgetful in daily activities	Yes. When family members send him for something, he forgets to bring it back.

(Continued)

Criteria for ADHD	Does Client Meet This Criteria?
Hyperactivity-impulsivity symptoms:	
Hyperactivity:	
Frequently restless in seat or fidgets with hands and/or feet	Yes, a teacher has noticed he is "fidgety" in his seat when she can get him to stay seated.
Gets out of seat in class or other places where children are expected to remain seated	Yes, the teacher describes him doing this.
Frequently runs about or climbs more in situations in which it is inappropriate	Yes. He climbed over a fence and into an electric transformer area. He tries to run about in the classroom.
Frequently has trouble playing or engaging quietly in leisure activities.	Yes. His grandparents describe difficulty getting him to play quietly.
Frequently talks to excess	
Impulsivity:	
Frequently shouts out answers before someone is finished asking the questions	
Frequently has trouble waiting his/her turn	Yes, teacher has described Marty having trouble waiting his turn.
Frequently interrupts or intrudes, for example, interrupting or butting into games	Yes, teacher has sent notes home from school saying that he frequently interrupts others in class.
2. Some symptoms of hyperactive impulsivity or inattention causing the impairment were identified before child was age seven.	Yes, he bit the light cord and had plastic surgery at age four. According to his father, Marty has gone non-stop all day long since he was a toddler.
3. Impairment from symptoms is seen in at least two settings (e.g., school and home).	Yes, his family and the teacher have noticed impairment from symptoms.
4. Significant impairment in some area of functioning (social, school, work).	Yes, he is having significant impairment in school.
5. The symptoms are not exclusively during or better accounted for by a course of pervasive developmental disorder, Schizophrenia, or other mental disorder.	To be assessed but yes as far as is known

(Adapted from APA, 2000)

This client has demonstrated behavior addressed in the criteria for both Hyperactivity and Impulsivity-Inattention type and will likely be determined to have a Combined Type of ADHD.

4. **What would you tell the father about Concerta the medication prescribed for his son?** The effects of Concerta (methylphenidate hydrochloride) last twelve hours, so it is given once daily in the morning and can be taken with or without food. Concerta is a capsule that must be swallowed whole and not chewed, crushed, or divided. The starting dose is usually low and gradually increased. The FDA first approved this drug in 2000. It was the first true long-acting medication, which enabled the child to take the medication before going to school and not have to go to the nurse's office during the school day to get medication.

The father does need to know that the active ingredient of Concerta is Ritalin (methylphenidate hydrochloride). Haber (2003) describes how Concerta works. A nondissolvable capsule is coated with regular methylphenidate hydrochloride (Ritalin), and this coating begins to dissolve shortly after the capsule is swallowed. The inside of the capsule is a paste-like methylphenidate. The capsule has a tiny hole drilled in the top and the bottom has an "expander" material. As the capsule goes through, the intestine fluid comes through the walls of the capsule and the expander swells and pushes small doses of the medication out the top of the capsule.

Side effects reported for Concerta include headache, stomachache, and sleeplessness. If the headache and/or stomachache do not disappear with rest or distraction and persist, the medication can be changed. For the sleeplessness, over the counter Benadryl is often used and discontinued after a short time when the sleeplessness resolves.

5. **If you had the opportunity, what would you say to the mother who is refusing to allow Ritalin for Marty and stating he just has more energy than other boys and will grow out of his hyperactivity?** You need to talk with the mother in a way that conveys respect and facilitates building a trusting relationship. You want to get the mother to talk with the health care provider about the diagnosis and possible treatments, including a discussion of medication for ADHD. You can share that you understand her concern about the diagnosis and about the medication and that it is important for her to talk with you and with the provider about her concerns. It is not the nurse's role to decide if Marty should have medication or not. This is the role of the health care provider. It is then the custodial parent who decides whether to let the child have medication or not. As the nurse in this case, you can listen to the mother, assess her knowledge base of ADHD, and provide any needed information about the disorder and treatment. You could point out that Concerta helps reduce impulsivity, inattention, and hyperactivity. It could help to remind her of Marty's behavior, especially his impulsivity and how this has placed him and others in danger (e.g., biting a plugged-in light cord and burning his mouth and shooting arrows at others). This is a difficult situation since the mother is the custodial parent and at present has the right to decide what treatment Marty receives, but has not lived with him since the divorce from Marty's father. She may not be fully aware of Marty's impulsive, inattentive, and hyperactive behaviors. You could mention to the mother that researchers did a study involving four hundred children with ADHD. The children were divided into two groups: those on Concerta and those on placebo. The researchers concluded that the children on Concerta did better on attention span, hyperactivity, impulsivity, and schoolwork over a twelve-hour period (Haber, 2003).

6. **Discuss the debate as to whether ADHD is overdiagnosed and Ritalin and similar stimulants are overprescribed for ADHD. Is Ritalin or other psychostimulants sometimes necessary for children? Why or why not?** Many people think that ADHD is overdiagnosed, and stimulant drugs overprescribed, based on studies and media reports. An article in the journal of the American Academy of Pediatrics (2001) points out that the use of Ritalin and similar drugs by children and adolescents has increased sevenfold between 1990 and 2000. Haber (2003) points out that in some areas "the greatest increase (in the use of stimulant medication) is in the lower socioeconomic populations, where medication has become a replacement for adequate educational remediation and psychological and family services." On the other hand, Haber suggests that overprescription of stimulants may also occur in schools in affluent areas or private schools because it increases the ability to focus, which is viewed as a tool to better grades. ADHD has become the most prevalent neurobehavioral disorder in children between the ages of 6 and 12, with 30–50 percent of children presenting to the offices of mental health professionals for the diagnosis and treatment of Attention-Deficit/Hyperactivity Disorder (Haber, 2003). A number of neurobiologists and child neuropsychiatrists including Haber suggest that factors involved in increased numbers of children diagnosed with ADHD may include: underdiagnosis in the past; an increase in children with neurological deficits resulting from such causes as drug abuse by parents before and during the fetal growth period and increasing numbers of premature babies surviving at earlier ages and lower birth weights than in the past; as well as advertisement from drug manufacturers pushing new drugs for ADHD.

Some authors advocate for not giving any child medication for ADHD. John Breeding's (2003) book, *The Wildest Colts Make the Best Horses*, is dedicated to convincing parents that no child needs to be medicated for ADHD. Breeding is a psychologist who advocates behavioral interventions and acceptance of a wider spectrum of children's behavior, as his book title would suggest. Support groups exist in larger cities for parents who don't believe in giving medication to children for ADHD. Parents can obtain parental training for working with children with ADHD. The parents work on finding ways to increase attention, decrease impulsivity, and decrease hyperactivity without medication.

Some people fear side effects of medication used to treat ADHD. Kluger (2003) discusses medications used in treating ADHD and presents a look at the side effects of these medications as well as the benefits. Although Kluger urges caution especially when symptoms are mild, he presents some true stories of actual kids who have ADHD: kids who realize the medication flattens their personalities but make it possible for them to succeed in school and be in enough control to play sports. One boy who was so fidgety that he could not play baseball or do schoolwork took stimulant medication that made it possible for him to become a straight "A" student and play ball. Another self-report from a high school honor student, diagnosed in kindergarten with ADHD, describes how in kindergarten she was sent to time-out about three times a day for not being able to control what she said or when she said it. She was started on Ritalin in first grade. This seriously decreased her appetite causing her to lose weight, but gave her a lot more focus. She became a straight "A" student, which she says she never would have been without medication. She is now on Adderall, and describes behaving very different when she is on it than when she is off of it. On it she does not talk to others at school and keeps to herself, but when off of it at home, she is spontaneous and outgoing and funny. This student says that she chooses to be on this medicine because she enjoys how she can focus and apply herself. She says she does not take the medicine when she goes to parties so she can be more spontaneous and outgoing and make friends.

Coghill (2004) makes a case for not withholding effective treatments from individuals diagnosed with ADHD saying it is "unjustifiable" given that there is a "wide range of negative outcomes. These include low self-esteem, poor academic achievement, impaired occupational status, poor peer relationships, and impaired family functioning, and increased injury rates, disruptive and antisocial behavior, substance abuse, and mood and anxiety disorders." Coghill points to scientific studies showing that stimulants produce a positive effect on both biological and cognitive processes. He calls attention to the fifty-year use of methylphenidate and dexamfetamine to treat symptoms of ADHD in millions of kids, without serious adverse events.

7. **What other medications besides Ritalin could the health care provider prescribe for ADHD?** Methylphenidate, amphetamines-related drugs, and some antidepressants are used in treating ADHD.

Methylphenidate has a number of brand names including Ritalin, which is available as a generic drug. The short-acting regular Ritalin starts working in thirty minutes, peaks in about two hours, and loses its effectiveness in four hours, which means that to cover a school day the child usually has to take medication at school.

Dexmethyphenidate (Focalin) is a new formulation of, and short-acting form of, methylphenidate, which also begins to act in thirty minutes, but lasts about five hours. A long-acting form may be available soon.

There are also other formulations of methylphenidate, including intermediate-acting and long-acting formulations. The intermediate medications include: Metadate ER, Methylin ER, and Ritalin SR.

Long-acting formulations of methylphenidate include Metadate CD, Concerta, and Ritalin LA. Concerta was discussed earlier. Ritalin LA is a capsule containing two sets of beads containing medication. The capsule releases one set of beads in about half an hour and the second set is released after about four hours. The effect of the medication is around nine hours. This capsule can be used with children who cannot swallow a capsule as it can be opened and mixed with food and followed up with a glass of water (Haber, 2003). Metadate CD is similar to Ritalin LA in that it also has two sets of beads in a capsule; however, 30 percent of the medication is released immediately and 70 percent over the next eight hours. It can also be sprinkled on food.

The amphetamine-related drugs include Adderall (a mixture of amphetamines), also available as Adderall XR, and dextroamphetamine (Dexedrine and Dexedrine Spansules).

Antidepressants may be used when: 1. Children have coexisting anxiety, depression, or other mood problems; 2. Stimulant medications don't seem to work; or 3. Side effects from stimulant medications are intolerable. Antidepressants used include imipramine (Tofranil), bupropion (Wellbutrin), and more recently atomoxetine (Strattera).

Strattera is the first nonstimulant medication to be produced primarily to treat ADHD. Atomoxetine HCl (Strattera) is thought to be involved in the "selective inhibition of presynaptic norepinephine transport" (Spratto and Woods, 2006). It is classified as a selective serotonin reuptake inhibitor (SSRI). Unlike the stimulants that require a written prescription for each month's medication since they are controlled substances, Strattera can be written as a regular prescription as it is not a controlled substance. This drug takes two or three weeks to produce an effect and is designed to be given on a regular basis and not to be stopped on holidays, weekends, or at vacation time. Strattera has not been found to cause insomnia, although it can cause sleepiness and diminished appetite with a temporary decrease in weight that generally resolves in about twelve weeks (Haber, 2003). Editors of *Pain and Central Nervous System Week* (American Academy of Pediatrics, 2004) reported that patients on Strattera fell asleep about ten times faster than those on methylphenidate. Patients on Strattera also slept longer.

8. **The father asks: "What causes ADHD?" How would you answer this question?** There are a number of causes for the cluster of symptoms that the American Psychiatric Association has decided to call ADHD, which in the past has had other names, including Minimal Brain Injury, Minimal Cerebral Dysfunction, and Hyperkinetic Syndrome. There appears to be two major sets of causation, one of which is genetic. Haber (2003) suggests that in perhaps as much as 40 percent of those children with true ADHD, you can find a clear and strong family history of ADHD. The child will have a close relative or relatives with the disorder. Parents who bring their child with ADHD for diagnosis and/or treatment will often say things like: "I had this same behavior (or I had these same problems) when I was a child." Children with ADHD of a genetic type have somewhat "different wiring" in the brain. As Haber explains it, there are "misconnections causing problems in how the brain carries messages and interprets information, particularly in the areas of paying attention, modulating activity, being organized, doing things in sequence, linking one piece of information to another, connecting facts to meaning, interpreting social signals in all environments, and responding to the feelings of others." The National Genome Project has found some differences on the eleventh chromosome in some individuals with ADHD. This finding offers some promise for development of a test to identify understand genetically transmitted ADHD.

   In contrast to children who appear to have inherited their ADHD, there are others diagnosed with ADHD who appear to have developed it as a result of central nervous system and brain injury. Prematurity or low birth weight for any reason puts a child at risk for ADHD. Parental prenatal use of drugs and alcohol can put a child at risk for brain injury and ADHD. Technology and advances in medical and nursing care have made it possible for smaller and smaller babies to survive, and the use and abuse of alcohol and other drugs in the United States has increased over past decades. These factors could account for some increase in the numbers of kids diagnosed with ADHD.

9. **Marty's father shares an observation that all the children he knows that have ADHD seem to be boys. He asks: "Do girls also have ADHD? What is the ratio of girls to boys who have ADHD?" How would you answer this father?** You could share with the father that his observation that ADHD is more common in boys is correct. Depending on the type of ADHD (hyperactivity-impulsive vs. inattention vs. both) the ratio of boys to girls is from two to one to nine to one. Girls who have ADHD are more likely to have inattention type than the hyperactivity-impulsivity type. Children seen in the clinic are more likely to be male (APA, 2000). This would make sense as a parent would probably be very concerned about the hyperactivity and impulsivity that puts children at risk for accidents and wears parents and caretakers down. A parent would be more apt to work much longer at home with the child who has inattention type of ADHD before seeking professional help, if help is sought at all.

10. **If you were to help write a care plan for this client, what information would you like to gather?** It is good to assess Marty's strengths or what experts working with children who have learning disabilities call "islands of competence" and to build on these. You will want to know what Marty's interests are. You will want to know about behavioral patterns that cause Marty difficulty at home or at school. Your assessment will include finding out more about the family dynamics and how much and what kind of structure Marty has at home. You will want to know what a typical day is like at home for Marty as well as what a typical school day is like for him. You will want some baseline information on height and weight so you could determine if it is within the normal range for his age. You would want some idea of what Marty's diet consists of on a day-to-day basis.

11. **What nursing diagnoses and goals would you likely write for this client? What interventions, other than medication, do you think would be helpful for this client?** Nursing diagnoses for this client could include

   - Chronic low self-esteem
   - Risk for loneliness

- Risk for injury due to impulsivity
- Risk for caregiver role strain

Likely goals for this client include:

- No instances of injury as a result of impulsivity
- No instances of placing others in danger or injury to others as a result of client's impulsivity
- Maintain friendship with at least one peer of same age

Interventions include providing structure, as children with ADHD need structure. Parents may need to be taught the importance of a scheduled time to go to bed and to arise each day and a consistent schedule from day to day insofar as possible. Having written family rules is another good intervention. Written schedules for the child to use as a checklist are often helpful. Parents can help children learn social skills by providing socialization opportunities with another child outside of class, as well as role playing with their child. The parent can play the role of a peer and encourage his or her child to ask questions to indicate an interest in someone outside themselves.

Helpful strategies for teachers and parents include using positive reinforcement for behavior that is moving toward or has reached what is expected. In addition to these strategies, the teacher and parent can work out secret codes to let the child with ADHD know when the child needs to focus on the task at hand or go to a quiet time-out place. The teacher or parent could pull on their ear or put their hand on their chin or use any number of actions as a secret code message.

Some teachers have decided that students who are inattentive and/or easily distracted can do better in the classroom if they have a headset and listen to music. One of these teachers, Edna Nation, said: "My students with ADHD seem to realize when I am giving instructions and they take the headsets off for that time" (Edna Nation, 2006).

You could look at Marty's dietary intake to see if dietary changes would be helpful to this client. In the mid 1970s the Feingold or Kaiser Permanente diet was popular in treating hyperactivity associated with Attention-Deficit/Hyperactivity Disorder. This diet involved eliminating foods with natural salicylate ash and food coloring. An FDA study found that about ten out of one thousand children would respond to this diet (Haber, 2003). Diet has not been the final answer to treating hyperactivity, but you can encourage parents and teachers to be observant for any connection between certain foods and hyperactivity and to encourage them to reduce or eliminate these foods if possible. Sometimes teachers and parents find that some children are more hyperactive after eating sweets. It would make sense to eliminate sweets, at least during school time.

References

American Academy of Pediatrics. (2001). "Clinical Practice Guidelines: Treatment of the School-Aged Child with Attention Deficit/Hyperactivity Disorder." *Pediatrics* 108(4): 1033–1044.

_____. (2004). "ADHD Study Patients Fall Asleep Faster on Strattera Versus Methylphenidate." *Pain and Central Nervous System Week,* May 31, 21–23.

American Psychiatric Association. (2000). *Diagnostic and Statistical Manual of Mental Disorders, 4th ed.* Text Revision Washington, DC: American Psychiatric Association.

Breeding, J. (2003). *The Wildest Colts Make the Best Horses, 3rd ed.* Austin, TX: Eakin Press.

Coghill, D. (2004). "Use of Stimulants for Attention Deficit Hyperactivity Disorder." *British Medical Journal* 329(7471): 907–908.

Haber, J.S. (2003). *ADHD: The Great Misdiagnosis.* Lanham, MD: Taylor Trade Publishing.

Kluger, J. (2003). "Medicating Young Minds." *Time,* November 3, 46–56.

_____. (2004). "Long Term Data Suggest Changes in Effectiveness of Stimulant Medication Over Time." *Brown University Child and Adolescent Behavior Letter* 20(6): 1–3.

Nation, E. (2006). Personal communication. Austin, Texas.

Spratto, G.R. and A.L. Woods. (2006). *PDR Nurse's Drug Handbook.* Clifton Park, NY: Thomson Delmar Learning, 113.

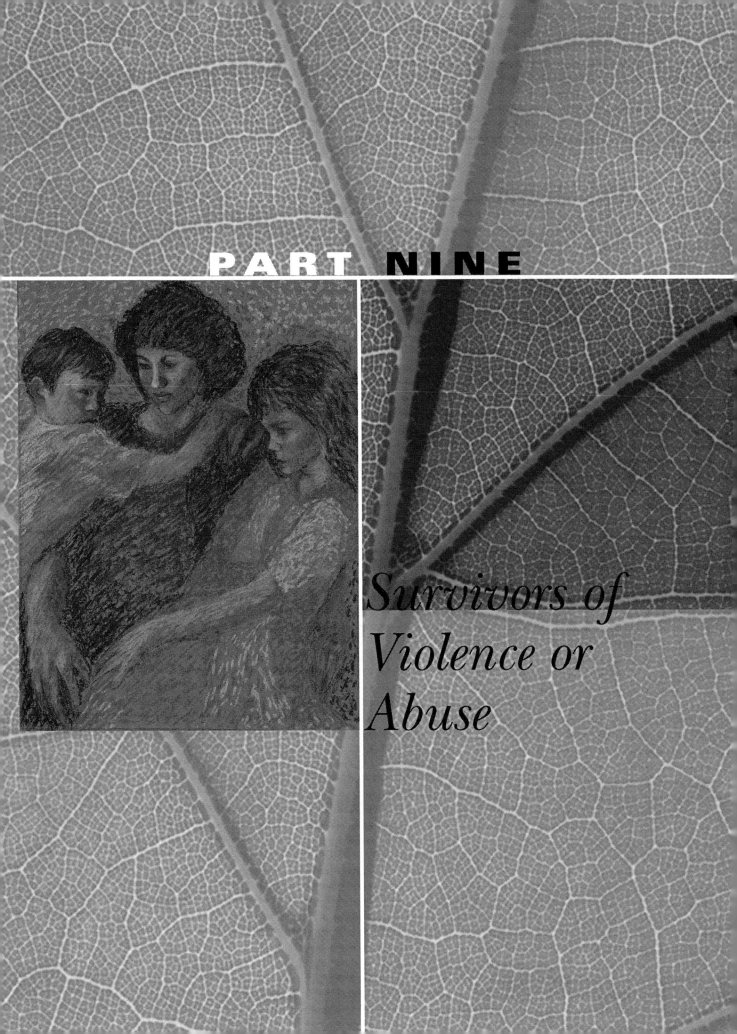

PART NINE

Survivors of Violence or Abuse

GENDER

Female

AGE

10

SETTING

- Home setting with visit by home health nurse

ETHNICITY

- White American

CULTURAL CONSIDERATIONS

- Southern
- Rural
- Military

PREEXISTING CONDITIONS

COEXISTING CONDITIONS

COMMUNICATION

DISABILITY

SOCIOECONOMIC

- Lower middle class

SPIRITUAL/RELIGIOUS

- Belongs to Seventh-Day Adventist church but not attending

PHARMACOLOGIC

PSYCHOSOCIAL

LEGAL

- Legal requirement to report "suspected" abuse
- Confidentiality

ETHICAL

- Child and mother's need to report suspected child abuse to ensure safety.

ALTERNATIVE THERAPY

PRIORITIZATION

DELEGATION

MODERATE

PHYSICAL ABUSE OF A CHILD

Level of difficulty: Moderate

Overview: Requires understanding of what constitutes child abuse and critical thinking to determine if there is sufficient evidence to warrant a suspicion of abuse. Requires knowledge of the legal requirements and process for reporting child abuse.

Client Profile

Reata is a 10-year-old girl living with her parents in their rural home. Her mother suffers from Manic Depression and Panic Disorder with Agoraphobia and smokes two packages of cigarettes a day. When agitated or angry, the mother hits Reata or burns her with cigarettes and tells her that she was/is an unwanted child. Reata's mother was raised in the Seventh-Day Adventist Church by the grandparents who live in a nearby city and still attend church. Reata's mother does not attend due to her Agoraphobia and her mental illness, which, combined with living in a rural area, greatly isolates the family.

Reata's father is a member of a military guard unit and is gone from home for long periods of time. When the father is home, he punishes Reata for such things as not doing chores perfectly, not having better grades, imperfect table manners, and for many small infractions of his strict rules. She is beaten with his belt and sent to her room hungry. One time she tried to run away, but her father killed her dog and put his head on the fence for her to see when he found her and brought her back home. She is afraid of her father and more so of his belt.

During the time that the father is gone, Reata tries to stay away from home as much as possible and to hide from her mother when she is at home. She feels safer when the visiting nurse is in the home and comes out of hiding due to curiosity and in hopes of getting some food or candy without being beaten or burned.

Case Study

The visiting nurse knocks on the door, which is opened by Reata, who is wearing a cast on her arm. The nurse is a visiting nurse from the county health department who has come to care for Reata's mother. The nurse asks Reata: "How are you today?" The child whispers in a low voice: "Hungry." The mother yells: "I heard that. It is not mealtime yet. Go get the nurse and me a glass of ice water, you stupid girl." The mother tells the nurse: "She just wants to eat all the time. I can't fill her up no matter how hard I try."

The nurse says: "Reata seems very thin." The mother does not respond, and the nurse asks how much Reata weighs. The mother responds: "Oh, I don't know how much she weighs, but the worthless child eats all the time and just runs it all off. She is always running. Don't worry about her. Take my blood pressure." The nurse starts getting out her stethoscope and sphygmomanometer. She quietly slips Reata a sandwich from her bag while the mother is walking toward her chair and not looking. The nurse can see Reata in the next room, sitting under the table and eating the sandwich in a few quick bites, without her mother being aware of it.

Midway through the visit, the nurse says: "I notice that Reata has a cast on." The mother does not reply, and the nurse says: "Tell me about the cast." The mother explains: "She is a clumsy girl. Always climbing trees and falling out. She also climbs out her window and jumps off the roof [one-story roof]." The nurse notices a burn on the dorsal side of Reata's left hand, but says nothing about it at this time, focusing instead on the client, Reata's mother. Just before leaving, the nurse says: "Reata has a burn on her hand." "Just a cooking accident because she is stupid," replies the mother.

Questions and Suggested Answers

1. **If you were the nurse in this case, making a first visit and not knowing what was going on in the family, what would you think when you see Reata's cast and her thinness and hear her say she is hungry? What would you think as you hear the mother's explanations for these observations and for the burn on the child's hand?** You might be thinking that it is not unusual for active children to have a cast or for children to fall from trees or off the roof. Perhaps you were an active child yourself or know a "tomboy" type of girl and find this mother's explanation plausible. Maybe you know some 10-year-olds who are thin and always hungry so you would not find it strange for this young girl to complain of hunger to a stranger.

On the other hand, you probably recognize that it is somewhat unusual for a child to hide to eat and to have a burn on the dorsal side of the hand. If children burn themselves, it is usually on the palm surface of the hand as they try to touch something hot. It is not inconceivable that the child touched the dorsal side of the hand to something hot; however, what probably troubles you is not any one of these findings by itself, but the pattern of findings, which are suggestive, but not proof, of physical abuse and neglect.

2. **If you were the nurse, would your visit focus only on the mother's care or would you be concerned with her child? Did the nurse do the right thing in giving the child a sandwich, and what did the nurse learn by doing this?** The agency you work for is undoubtedly paying you for a limited amount of time with the mother and expects you to focus on this client. You could have some ethical decisions as you consider whether to focus on the immediate physical needs of the client and stay within your allotted time for the visit or work with what may be critical (even life-threatening) family issues. You are probably aware that it is in your client's best interests if you protect her from harming a child. It is also in the child's best interests and yours professionally and personally to protect any children of the client.

Giving the child a sandwich was a judgment call. The nurse had a sandwich, and it worked out all right to secretly give it to Reata. The nurse learned that Reata was indeed hungry and seemed to be hiding the sandwich from her mother. The nurse could have asked the mother's permission to give the daughter a sandwich. The mother could have said "no," which would be cruel to the child: wanting an offered sandwich and being denied it. Another option would be to ignore the daughter's comment about being hungry as, after all, the home visit is about the mother, isn't it?

3. **Briefly describe the therapeutic communication tools used by the nurse in this home visit and a rationale for using them. What strategy does the nurse use to get information about the daughter from the client? Do you agree with this strategy, and if so, why? If not, what strategy would you like to use?** One therapeutic communication tool used was *observation* (e.g., "Reata seems very thin" and "I notice that Reata has a cast on"). The nurse also uses *encouraging* (e.g., "Tell me about the cast"). These techniques are nonthreatening, open-ended, encourage the mother to talk, and do not suggest answers. These techniques have been tested over time and are often successful in getting information.

The nurse in this case is trying to get information from the mother about the daughter without letting the mother know that the goal is to find out if the daughter is being maltreated and particularly physically and/or emotionally abused. The nurse does not ask a series of questions, but instead uses therapeutic communication techniques keeps moving the focus back and forth from a brief focus on the daughter's situation to a longer focus on the client's physical needs and concerns. This keeps the client from becoming defensive or angry, or even possibly asking the nurse to leave. This appears to be a good strategy on the part of the nurse. You may have another strategy you would like to use in this case. An alternative strategy would be to say something like: "Many parents have questions about problems they are having with their children or on discipline." You would stop and use the therapeutic technique of silence, giving the mother an opportunity to say something in response. Silence is a good tool for nurses to use, though it is one of the more difficult tools for most nurses who tend to be uncomfortable with silence and want to fill any silence by saying something.

4. **If you were the nurse in this case, what would you do to build a trusting relationship with Reata and help her other than reporting your suspicion of abuse? Provide a rationale for your actions.** You could give the child small bits of attention that are not obvious to the mother (e.g., a small quick smile when the mother is not looking, eye contact, and calling the child by name). The mother appears to want the focus to stay on her and may abuse the child if you divert too much obvious attention to Reata.

You could help the child by getting her to a safe place. You could suggest to the mother that she get a rest from child care so she can focus on her own needs more. You could work with her to get a grandparent or perhaps someone from the church to take Reata into their home for a while. The Seventh-Day Adventist Church is family focused, and one of its customs/practices is for members to take relatives and others into their homes when there is a need.

You could work with the mother to get her to permit the child to have a mentor or to increase her contact with the community in whatever ways are available. The less isolated the child is, the more likely she will reveal the abuse and/or neglect, if it is occurring, and the healthier it will be for the child. The mother may realize that contact with those outside the family brings increased risk of the child revealing family secrets, and she may resist your attempts. You need to overprovide attention to the mother to be able to provide some attention to the child. If the mother perceives you are focusing more on the child, she may "fire you."

5. **Discuss the federal act that names and defines four major classifications of maltreatment of children. As the nurse in this case, your observations and assessment in the home would best support a suspicion of which one or more of the four types of abuse described in the federal act?** The Federal Child Abuse Prevention and Treatment Act (CAPTA, PL. 93-247), passed in 1974, provides a basis for each state in the United States to describe offenses against children within their civil and criminal codes. This act outlines minimum requirements in child protection that each state must meet if they are to be eligible for federal funding. CAPTA recognizes and defines four major classifications of maltreatment of children: 1. Physical abuse; 2. Child neglect; 3. Sexual abuse; and 4. Emotional abuse. *Physical abuse* is "inflicting of physical injury from punching, beating, kicking, biting, burning, shaking, or otherwise harming a child." *Child neglect* is "failing to provide for the child's basic needs including physical, educational, or emotional." *Emotional abuse* is defined as "acts and omissions of parents or care-givers that caused or could lead to behavioral, cognitive, emotional, or mental disorders. Emotional abuse underlies other forms of abuse." *Sexual abuse* is "performing sexual acts ranging from fondling genitals, and exhibitionism to intercourse, rape, sodomy, and exploitation through prostitution or production of pornographic materials" (Massey-Stokes and Lanning, 2004, 193).

Your observations and assessment in the home provides a cluster of data or a pattern that best support a suspicion of physical abuse (broken arm and burn on hand). You have some observations that suggest possible neglect (e.g., child complaining of hunger and hiding to eat). You have observations that support emotional abuse (e.g., instances of mother referring to child as stupid and clumsy). It is possible that Reata is being sexually abused, but so far you have nothing to support a reportable suspicion of sexual abuse.

6. **What are some of the common characteristics of parents who abuse or neglect children? Do Reata's parents or family have any of these characteristics?** Parents who abuse or neglect children tend to be socially isolated, lack a support network, be suspicious of others, have many personal and marital problems, be under economic stress, show little interest in the child's well-being, have been abused or harshly punishment when a child themselves, blame the child for any injuries they incur, be critical of their child or children, use excessive punishment in dealing with their own children, use a different health care provider and/or facility for each new injury requiring treatment, exhibit moralistic thinking, and abuse alcohol or other drugs currently or have abused them in the past (www.safechild.org/childabuse2.htm; Mulryan, Cathers, and Fagin, 2004; Rinehart et al., 2005).

The family seems to be isolated, living in a rural area with the father in the military guard and gone a lot and the mother having mental illness and Agoraphobia. The mother and child are definitely isolated unless many people are visiting the home, which is unlikely.

The mother criticizes the child and blames the child's "stupidity," high activity level, and type of activities for the injuries she has sustained. The mother has mental illness. A study by the Substance Abuse and Mental Health Services Administrations (SAMHSA) looked at the correlation between mother's child abuse potential and current mental health symptoms using the Child Abuse Potential (CAP) Inventory and found that "current mental health symptoms were the strongest predictor of mothers' scores" on the CAP. This study also found that substance abuse stands out as one of the strongest predictors of child maltreatment (Rinehart et al., 2005). One in four children in this country is believed to be subjected to alcohol abuse or dependence in their family. You would want to assess for alcohol and other drug abuse in the family.

The nurse in this case has yet to learn about the father's harsh discipline, strict standards for the child, or putting the head of her dog on the fence when she attempted to run away. These behaviors are abusive behaviors.

7. **What are some behaviors frequently found in children who are abused? What conditions could a child have that might mislead a nurse into thinking the child was being abused when they are not experiencing abuse?** Newton (2001) described abused children as easily startled, having difficulty in attention and concentration, and having academic difficulties. Some abused children exhibit aggressive behaviors and engage in lying or stealing and may use alcohol and other drugs. Some abused children seem anxious, exhibit shyness, and display fear of certain adults. Some children begin bedwetting while others chronically complain of pain. Some children display regressed behavior such as thumb sucking.

Conditions that might mislead a nurse into thinking a child is being abused when they are not include Osteogenesis Imperfecta, Attention Deficit Disorder with Hyperactivity, and Autism. Carol Brown (2004), an LVN, asks nurses to be aware of a genetic defect known as Osteogenesis Imperfecta, a condition in which bones break easily and sometimes for no apparent reason. The author's grandson had six fractures by age 5. It is always good to keep an open mind and be aware of any conditions that can mislead the nurse into falsely suspecting child abuse. There is more information about Osteogenesis Imperfecta at www.oif.org.

A small number of children with Attention Deficit Disorder with Hyperactivity are so impulsive that they engage in high-risk behavior without thinking of the consequences, unintentionally bringing injuries to themselves—injuries that might be falsely attributed to the parents. Autistic children can also suffer injuries because of lack of thought toward consequences of their actions and problems with coordination (Brown, 2004). There have been instances in which neighbors' observations of a child's injury or injuries were the only thing that saved a parent or caregiver from being reported for abuse and/or neglect.

8. **What short-term and long-term effects could occur if this child is being abused and neglected and this continues because you don't report your suspicions to the proper authorities?** The result of not reporting could be that the child would die or be seriously injured because of the parent's abusive or neglectful actions. You have not caused the death or injury, but you will wonder if you contributed or could have prevented it. One instance of slamming a child hard against a wall or hitting a child in a vulnerable location, and the child can be a death statistic. This child could also inflict self-injury, attempt suicide, or complete suicide. It is not uncommon for abused children to begin to cut or burn themselves or to think about killing themselves.

Growing up in an abusive family tends to cause a person to have difficulty completing the life task of trust versus mistrust, leading to difficulty in trusting others and in forming and maintaining healthy relationships.

Growing up in abusive families puts a person not only at immediate risk, but also lifelong risk for a wide variety of physical and mental problems, including but not limited to depression, anxiety disorders, cancer, diabetes, and early death, according to a team of scientist from UCLA who analyzed more than ten years of research on how the family's environment influences physical and mental health (www.eurekalert.org/pub_releases/2002-03/uoc-cf032102.php). Repetti, the lead researcher for this study, says: "While many people separate physical and mental health, research shows that physical and mental health may not be as separate as is often assumed, and that our brains and bodies may be more closely connected." She also states that "the research studies reveal that a child's genetic predispositions interact with the environment, and in risky families, a child's genetic risk may be exacerbated. This combination can lead to the faster development of health problems, which may be more debilitating than they would be in a more nurturing family."

9. **Are all nurses legally obligated to report suspected child abuse? Does the nurse have to gather sufficient data to prove child abuse? Are you as a nurse protected from civil and criminal liability if, acting in the interest of a child, you report suspected child abuse or neglect? How can you find out the procedure to follow to report child abuse and neglect?** All fifty states, Washington, D.C., Puerto Rico, and the U.S. Virgin Islands have laws mandating nurses who are aware of, or suspect, child abuse to report it. Each state and territory designates an agency to receive these reports. The agency designated by the state is often the state or county child protective services unit.

All nurses need to be aware of the particular statutes in their state dealing with requirements for reporting child abuse and/or neglect or suspicion of it. There are laws in place in all the states and territories that protect you from civil and criminal liability if you act on what you believe to be true in regard to suspicion of child abuse or neglect.

An example of a state statute, described by Dean and Montagno (2005), advises Florida nurses of the particular section of the Florida statues that "requires any person who knows, or has reasonable cause to suspect that a child who has been abused, abandoned, or neglected by a person, legal custodian, care giver, or other person responsible for the child's welfare, to report their knowledge or suspicion." The nurse need not have proof of abuse, a suspicion warrants reporting. If you knowingly make a false report (i.e., a report you know at the time is not true), you are not legally protected by the law and may be prosecuted for this malicious and unprofessional behavior; if proven in a court of law, the penalty for the offense varies from state to state. Martinez (2005a) reported in the *Austin American Statesman* that Texas, in the 2004 legislative session, increased the punishment for intentionally making a false report of abuse or neglect to Child Protective Services. The penalty was raised from a class A misdemeanor to a felony jail time, meaning that a person can be fined up to $10,000 and jailed from 180 days to 2 years. The sponsor of the bill for this legislation admitted that very few cases of false reporting go to court in Texas. It is very difficult for prosecutors to prove a person did not act in good faith and intentionally made a false report. Proponents of the stronger penalty say it discourages false reporting by spouses and ex-spouses in child custody battles and others as well, and helps reduce the caseload of child and family services caseworkers.

There are various means for finding out where to report suspected child abuse: you can ask your supervisor, read your agency policy and procedure on reporting abuse and neglect, or call the county child protective services agency and ask about the reporting procedure. You can call USA's National Child Abuse Hotline at 1-800-4-A-CHILD and talk with counselors who can give you the phone numbers for reporting abuse by state. The website of the U.S. Health and Human Services has links to information about child abuse and neglect and reporting at www.acf.dhhs.gov/programs/cb/.

The National Clearinghouse on Child Abuse and Neglect phone numbers are 1-800-394-3366 or 703-385-7565 and their website is www.prcvent.childabuse.org. From this source you can get information on your state's child abuse and neglect definitions and the state's reporting procedures.

10. **What do you think bothers nurses the most about reporting suspicion of abuse and neglect? If you report that you suspect Reata is being abused and neglected and she is taken from the family and placed in foster care, how would you feel? On the other hand, if you report suspected abuse and neglect and the authorities decide your suspicions are unwarranted or that the child is in no danger and better off staying with her parents, how would you feel and what would you do?** You may worry about the parents becoming angry and harming you. Frisch and Frisch (2006) state, "Ideally, nurses should tell abusing parents that they are legally required to report the suspected child abuse in an attempt to keep lines of communication open." However, nurses "should not put themselves at risk for injuries if they think that informing the families [about reporting abuse] would lead to personal harm."

You may be worried about reporting suspected abuse and being wrong about the abuse. Sometimes suspicions seem well founded, but a full investigation finds that the child or children are not being abused or can't determine if abuse is occurring or not. Sometimes families move away before the investigation is complete. The statistics for the Texas Child and Family Services Agency for 2004 showed 76 percent of the 138,587 investigations of child abuse complaints were unconfirmed (Martinez, 2005b).

You may be worried about causing the child or children to be taken away from the family and being emotionally harmed by this. The child protective services caseworkers have options, during an investigation of a complaint of suspected child abuse, depending on their findings. A child or children can be removed from the home immediately and permanently, removed temporarily until the parents meet certain conditions, or retained by the parents with certain conditions placed upon the parents.

Hopefully you will feel all right with the child protective services decision. Safety of children is important. The parents will likely be able to get their children back if they indicate a willingness to provide good parenting and back this up by doing positive things such as attending parenting classes and going to family therapy. If the parents are not willing to change or work with the child protective services, that is their decision. While you may feel badly initially about the children being taken away, think about whether you need feel guilty if the parents are unwilling to do some therapy or educational work to prove that the home will be safe.

If you feel strongly about the child being in danger and Child and Family Services disagrees or takes no action, you may worry about the child's welfare or you may be angry with the authorities investigating the case. You may be angry with the parents. In spite of your feelings and how strong they may be, you must abide by the law and accept the findings of the investigating agency and perhaps the court, for now. If you are still working with the family, you can keep assessing for any signs of abuse or neglect and can work with the mother to build tools and strengths to avoid abusing and neglecting behaviors. If the family is not working with you any longer due to not trusting or anger or any reason, having another nurse make visits can also be helpful in that they can assess the family and add another set of observations, which may match with yours or not.

11. **What other means of getting information can you think of to confirm your suspicion of physical abuse and neglect, or to rule it out?** You need to collaborate with the school nurse and the child's primary health care provider. These professionals may have had some clues to child abuse in the past and may or may not have reported their suspicions, although health care providers, school nurses, and teachers are required to report suspected child abuse. You will have to get a release of information from a parent or parents to share information and get information from teachers, the school nurse, and the health care provider. It will challenge your skills to get a release of information form signed. It will be helpful to you to have other professionals to collaborate with and to help take some responsibility for the child and mother's welfare.

12. **Making the child as well as the mother, who is the official client of the nurse, the focus of nursing process, what additional assessments would you do? What nursing diagnoses and goals would you likely write for this child if you continue working with the family and child? What interventions would be helpful?** Additional assessments could include assessing the degree of isolation of the child and mother; the child's strengths and limitations as well as those of the mother; whether the family has adequate food or not and if not, what can be done to resolve this; the mother and child's support system to see if the child has a teacher, relative, or other adult that she trusts and the mother has a means of obtaining groceries and receiving emotional support. An examination of the child's skin for bruising or other injuries would be helpful. You will want to assess the child and the family for alcohol abuse or other drug use or abuse.

Possible nursing diagnoses include:

- Risk for other-directed violence
- Risk for self-mutilation
- Anxiety
- Fear
- Powerlessness
- Risk for loneliness
- Imbalanced nutrition: less than body requirements
- Chronic low self-esteem

Some appropriate goals you could set include but are not limited to the following goals:

- Will not experience harm from others
- Will not engage in self-harm behavior (e.g., self-mutilation, risky sexual behavior, or use alcohol and other drugs)
- Will develop an appropriate relationship with at least one adult
- Will develop a friend relationship with at least one peer
- Will evidence weight gain

Interventions could include the following interventions:

- Encourage mother to temporarily have the child stay with a family member (who is not likely to abuse) or with someone in the church.
- Report the suspected abuse and neglect.

- Build a trusting relationship with the child, but do not become the child's only resource.
- Get a release of information to work with the grandparents, the school nurse, the pastor, the family health care provider, and anyone likely to be a resource to the child and to the mother also.
- Get a community mentor for the child. The mother might accept Reata having a community mentor, such as a mentor from an organization like the Big Brother-Big Sister organization, provided you approach her when she is receptive and in a manner that encourages her approval of this plan.

References

Brown, C. (2004). "Fractures and Child Abuse." *Nursing* 34(12): 8.

Dean, K., and J. Montagno. (2005). "Mandatory Reporting of Child Abuse and Liability for Inadequate Staffing." *Florida Nurse* 53 (1): 12.

Frisch, N.C. and L.E. Frisch. (2006). *Psychiatric Mental Health Nursing, 3rd ed.* Albany, NY: Thomson Delmar Learning.

Martinez, M.M. (2005a). "Change in Abuse Law May Do Little." *Austin American Statesman*, June 16, B1, B6.

Martinez, M.M. (2005b). "CPS: Judge and Jury. Austin American Statesman February 19." Available at http://www.infowars.com/articles/ps/cps_judge_jury.htm. Accessed June 18, 2006.

Massey-Stokes, M. and B. Lanning. (2004). "The Role of CSHPs in Preventing Child Abuse and Neglect." *Journal of School Health* 74 (6): 193–194.

Mulryan, K., P. Cathers, and A. Fagin. (2004). "How to Recognize and Respond to Child Abuse." *Nursing* 34(10): 52.

Newton, C.J. (2001). "Child Abuse: An Overview." *Therapist Finder.net Mental Health Journal*. Available at www.therapistfinder.net/childabuse. Accessed June 2005.

Rinehart, D.J. et al. (2005). "The Relationship Between Mothers' Child Abuse Potential and Current Mental Health Symptoms." *Journal of Behavioral Health Service and Research* 32(2): 155–166.

www.acf.dhhs.gov/programs/cb. Accessed June 15, 2005.

www.eurekalert.org/pub_releases/2002-03/uoc--cf032102.php. (2002). "Children from 'Risky Families' Suffer Serious Long-Term Health Consequences, UCLA Scientists Report." Accessed June 18, 2006.

www.oif.org. Accessed June 14, 2005.

www.safechild.org/childabuse2.htm. Accessed June 14, 2005.

GENDER	SPIRITUAL/RELIGIOUS

GENDER

Male

AGE

77

SETTING

- Gerontologist's office

ETHNICITY

- White American

CULTURAL CONSIDERATIONS

PREEXISTING CONDITION

COEXISTING CONDITION

COMMUNICATION

- Hard of hearing; has hearing aides

DISABILITY

SOCIOECONOMIC

MIDDLE INCOME

SPIRITUAL/RELIGIOUS

PHARMACOLOGIC

- haloperidol (Haldol)

PSYCHOSOCIAL

- Daughter controls access of client to others

LEGAL

- Legal requirement in most, if not all, states for nurses to report abuse/neglect of elderly
- Confidentiality
- Right to make decisions unless declared incompetent

ETHICAL

- Professional manner with a person suspected of abusing the elderly
- Daughter giving client medication without his consent

PRIORITIZATION

DELEGATION

PHYSICAL ABUSE OF ELDERLY CLIENT

Level of difficulty: High

Overview: Requires knowledge of signs and symptoms of elder abuse. Requires keeping an open mind while using therapeutic communication skills to determine if there is enough evidence to warrant reporting suspected elder abuse.

Client Profile

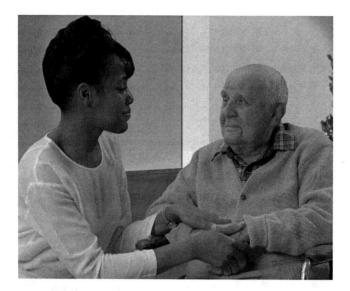

Francis, described as a cantankerous old man by family and neighbors, lived alone until recently, when he reluctantly moved to another city to live with his daughter Alline. He has five living children, none of whom particularly like him, remembering him as being humorless and even mean to them when they were growing up. Francis feared going to a nursing home and got his daughter Alline to promise to keep him out of nursing homes by saying he would leave her some money when he dies.

Alline thought it was a good idea to have her father move in with her, but it soon became evident that he required a lot of care, could not be left alone safely, and was never quite satisfied with anything she did for him. Alline also had to care for his dog that he brought with him, and she did not like the dog. Alline began to resent her siblings not helping her with their father's care. One day she became so angry with her father, the dog, her siblings, and the situation that she shoved her father. He fell, broke his glasses, broke a bone in his foot, and acquired a few bruises. There was some question about whether the foot was broken or not, but Alline decided it probably was not broken. She thought it would be a lot of trouble to get the foot x-rayed, so she did not. A few days later Alline lost control again and hit her father several times, giving him even more bruises. Francis has hearing aids, but his daughter has not put batteries in them. He is usually restrained in a wheelchair when his daughter goes to the store to get groceries. Francis often feels like he is drugged and wonders if his daughter is slipping something into his pudding to calm him down. He usually slips the dog at least half his pudding. Francis is correct in his suspicions. Alline's neighbor gave her a bottle of Haldol after her husband died and no longer needed it. Alline has been putting half a crushed Haldol pill into the pudding.

Case Study

Francis's daughter and a younger brother, who came from another state on an unannounced visit, bring Francis to a gerontologist's office. The brother tells the nurse that he is concerned about Francis's swollen foot, his complaint of pain, the bruising, and Francis thinking it had been at least three years since he had last seen a doctor. The brother mentions that Francis cannot see well because his glasses were broken and he does not hear well because his hearing aids don't work. After weighing Francis, the nurse tells the family she is taking him to an examination room for his physical examination. Alline jumps up to go with them. Francis yells, "No, don't come!" Alline insists on accompanying her father and says: "The nurse will have trouble understanding you and you will have trouble understanding and remembering, so I had better come too."

Questions and Suggested Answers

1. **What are some possible reasons this elderly client might not want his daughter with him during his physical examination?** Possible reasons for not wanting his daughter to be with him during the physical examination include modesty, wanting to retain some control, and/or elder abuse. Francis has lost a lot of control due to age, health problems, and moving in with his daughter, so it could be a control issue. The elderly are vulnerable to abuse. A high percentage of elder abuse is perpetrated by a relative, usually an adult child or a spouse. The abuser often does not want the abused person to talk to people when he or she (the abuser) is not present.

   Unless you have good reason to believe the client is not legally competent (e.g., the daughter says she is his legal guardian), you will honor the client's decision. You will take him alone to the exam room area, measure his weight and height, and get his vital signs and get a health history from him along with his chief complaints. If he does not know what medications he is on, you will have to go ask the daughter to list the medications for you. If the client is legally incompetent, the health care provider and nurse will still try to talk with an elderly client alone when elder abuse is a possibility. The mentally ill and mentally retarded are especially vulnerable to abuse, as people may assume they will not be believable if they claim abuse. If this or any other client describes abuse, it usually is a good idea to have another health care team member hear what the client says.

2. **The client is hard of hearing. What actions will you take to enhance his ability to hear you?** You need to ask the client if he hears out of one ear better than the other, and if he does, you would speak to him on that side. Talking louder is not helpful. Face the client when talking to him so he can see your lips and so the sound goes directly to him. You would ask him about whether or not he has a hearing aid or hearing aids. You would learn that he has them, but they are not working. This is something to discuss with the daughter, his caregiver. You can work with her to get his hearing aids functional by asking her to do whatever is needed: repairing, replacing, or getting new batteries installed. You would instruct her to bring the hearing aids to the next visit.

   You need to try different tones of voice and loudness until you find one the client seems to hear and understand best. Talk slowly and pronounce your words clearly. Since 90 percent of communication is unspoken, watch your body language. Keep your arms unfolded and choose gestures that you think will clarify what you are saying but will not be viewed as threatening.

3. **What approach will you take with this client whom you suspect might be the victim of elder abuse? Are there questions that need to be asked of the caregiver and the client separately? If so, what are these questions and what is your rationale for interviewing the client and others separately?** In cases of possible abuse, you need to talk with the people involved, separately. You are working in a health care provider's office so you need to talk with the provider about who is going to ask questions. Will the provider ask them or will you? Will you both ask questions separately or will you ask them together?

   You need to try to build a little rapport with the daughter and find out how stressful caring for her father is and how she might make that less stressful. You could say something like: "It seems to me that it could be difficult and maybe even stressful caring for your father." Hopefully she will admit to the difficulty of caring for her father, and you can then ask: "Have you thought about some ways to get a respite from caring for your father or to get help with his care?" If she has not thought about this, you could brainstorm with her to come up with some ideas. The client's daughter could refuse all suggestions for getting help, and it may take some outside pressure (e.g., Adult Protective Services) to make her realize she has to make some changes.

   In talking with this client you must avoid leading him (i.e., you must not put false ideas into the client's mind). You can use therapeutic communication techniques (e.g., "Tell me about your bruises" or "I notice you have a number of unusual bruises"). If this is not productive, you may need to go to direct questions. Gray-Vickery (2004), a nurse, suggests the following direct questions to ask the caregiver and the client separately: "When did it happen?" "How did it happen?" "How often has this happened?" Differing answers may mean that one or the other is attempting to cover up the true story, or it could mean poor memory or confusion. It is often hard for an adult client to admit that one of their children is abusing them.

Sellas and Krouse (2006), emergency medicine health care providers, point out that the American Medical Association recommends that doctors routinely screen for elder abuse and interview client and caregiver separately. Sellas and Krause provides a list of direct questions to use for the various types of elder abuse. To screen for physical abuse she suggests: "Are you afraid of anyone at home?" "Have you been struck, slapped, or kicked?" "Have you been tied down or locked in a room?" "Have you been force-fed?" To screen for neglect, she suggests these questions: "Do you lack items such as eyeglasses, hearing aids, or false teeth?" "Have you been left alone for long periods?" "Is your home safe?" "Has anyone failed to help you care for yourself when you needed assistance?" To view the complete list of questions suggested by Sellas and Krouse, go to www.emedicine.com/emerg/topic160.htm.

4. **Define elder abuse, elder physical abuse, and elder neglect. Give examples of caretaker behavior that constitutes elder physical abuse and elder neglect. What is the incidence of elder abuse? Are more men than women victims of elder abuse?** Elder abuse is an urgent problem and is underrecognized, underreported, and undertreated (Lang, 2004). The National Center on Elder Abuse points out that for every one case of elder abuse, neglect, exploitation, or self-neglect reported, about five more go unreported and that current estimates of the frequency of elder abuse range from 2–10 percent of the elderly population. This implies that for every one hundred clients seen in a gerontologist's office, somewhere between two and ten have experienced some form of abuse from a caretaker (www.elderabusecenter.org/default.cfm?p=statistics.cfm). Machuca (2005) cites Rozell, chairman of the Kern County, California Elder Abuse Prevention Counsel, as saying: "Nationwide an estimated 15 to 20 millions cases of elder abuse are believed to take place each year"; "only one out of every 20 abuse cases is reported" and "85% involve a family member."

A variety of sources point out that female victims constitute the majority of elder abuse cases. The National Center for Elder Abuse reported finding 62 percent of the elderly abuse cases involved female victims (Moody, 2005).

Types of elderly abuse include physical abuse and neglect, but also emotional and sexual abuse, exploitation, and abandonment. Legal definitions of elder abuse may vary from state to state. You need to look at the definition your state uses. The definition from the National Center on Elder Abuse defines elder abuse as any knowing, intentional, or negligent act by anyone that results in "harm or a serious risk of harm to a vulnerable adult" (http://www.elderabusecenter.org/default.cfm?p=faqs.cfm, 2005).

Another definition proposed by a panel convened by the U.S. National Academy of Sciences defines elder abuse as "(a.) Intentional actions that cause harm or create a serious risk of harm (*whether or not harm is intended*) to a vulnerable elder by a caregiver or other person who stands in a trust relationship to the elder or (b.) failure by a caregiver to satisfy the elder's basic needs or to protect the elder from harm" (Lachs and Pillemer, 2004).

Elder physical abuse is using physical force that may result in bodily injury, physical pain, or impairment of an elderly person. Examples of elder physical abuse include: striking the elderly person with or without an object, pushing or shoving, hitting, pinching or slapping, kicking, burning, inappropriately using drug and physical restraints, force feeding, and giving out physical punishment (http://www.elderabusecenter.org/default.cfm?p=faqs.cfm, 2005).

Elder neglect takes place when the caretaker fails to provide for the elderly person's basic needs. Examples of neglectful caregiver behavior include failing to provide eyeglasses, dentures, hearing aids, and adequate nutrition and hydration as well as failure to insure the elderly person is clean, dressed warm or cool enough, has adequate shelter, and is safe from harm.

5. **What are the risk factors for elder abuse? Which of these risk factors are present in this case? What are the signs and symptoms of elder physical abuse that you would look for? What are the signs and symptoms of neglect you would be observing for?** Some of the risk factors you may have thought of and that are listed by Wynne-Jones (2005), and that are present in this case, include: social isolation and a poor relationship between the elderly person and the person caring for them. Other risk factors that need to be assessed for include a history of previous abuse in the family; dependence of the caregiver on the elderly person for

financial, emotional, or accommodation assistance; mental health problems; alcohol and other substance problems; or personality disorder in the caregiver.

You would look for the following signs of possible elder physical abuse:

- Bruising, especially bruises in various stages of healing
- Lacerations, burns, fractures, and other injuries
- Black eyes, rope burns, welts
- Statements by the client that suggest abuse
- Broken eyeglasses and frames as well as broken hearing aids
- Caregiver not wanting the person to be alone with others
- Sudden change of behavior when caregiver comes into room

Signs and symptoms you would look for in terms of possible neglect include:

- Dehydration
- Decubitus ulcers
- Deterioration of health
- Malnutrition
- Glasses or hearing aids in poor repair, broken, or missing
- Poor hygiene
- Burns from urine
- Lice or scabies
- Clothing inappropriate to weather or situation or in bad repair

6. **If this client says nothing to you or to the health care provider about abuse and he is being abused, why isn't he telling you about the abuse and getting it stopped? Are you as a nurse required to report suspected elder abuse, and how do you report it?** One possible reason for not complaining about the abuse is that they love the person who is abusing them in spite of the person's actions and they don't want to get their caregiver in trouble. A client like the one in this case may fear going to the nursing home and think it is better to remain with someone who periodically abuses them than to be in a nursing home. Another possibility is that abuse has been going on a long time in the family and it feels familiar. Other reasons include faulty memory or threats from the caregiver.

In most states, nurses and other health care professionals are required to report elder abuse. You need to be familiar with the laws pertaining to elder abuse in your state, as well as the policies and procedures of your workplace that address elder abuse.

The Administration on Aging (www.aoa.gov/eldfam/Elder_Rights/Elder_Abuse/Elder_Abuse.asp) states that legislatures in all states have set up reporting systems. Generally Adult Protective Services (APS) is the agency that you report elder abuse to, and it is the agency that investigates the reports of suspected abuse of an elderly person. There will be a twenty-four-hour hotline number to call to report suspected elder abuse.

7. **If you report suspected elder abuse and it is substantiated, can the abuser be punished by the legal system? What percentage of reported suspected elder abuse cases are substantiated, and what is the type of elder abuse most often substantiated?** The law applying to, and the civil and criminal penalties for, different types of elder abuse vary from state to state. Law enforcement officers and prosecutors are trained on elder abuse and aware of civil and criminal laws and can use these laws to prosecute those who abuse the elderly. It is possible, but not certain, that if elder abuse is reported in this case, the charges will be substantiated and the client's daughter will be charged with abuse and/or neglect.

In some cases that are reported to Adult Protective Services, the elderly person is allowed to remain in the home if the abusers meets certain conditions, which could include such things as getting respite care, getting help with care, attending anger management classes, and/or going to a support group for caregivers of the elderly. In other cases, for reasons of safety, the elderly person will be removed from the home temporarily or permanently.

Your responsibility as a nurse is to follow the state law and your agency policies and procedures in regard to reporting suspected abuse of the elderly to the proper authorities. You may feel badly that you are reporting someone who might get into legal trouble, but realize you only know a part of the story. It could be worse than you realize, or there may no abuse or neglect at all. A trained investigator for Adult Protective Services will investigate to determine the actual situation. Keep in mind that by reporting suspected abuse, you could prevent the abuser from actions that will result in the client's death, which would put the abuser into greater legal trouble.

Most of the reported suspected elder abuse cases are substantiated. About 70 percent of the elder abuse cases substantiated by Adult Protective Services are cases of neglect, while 25 percent of the cases substantiated are physical abuse, 35 percent of substantiated cases involve emotional abuse, and 30 percent of cases involve financial abuse (i.e., exploitation) (Gray-Vickery, 2004). The elderly are often subjected to more than one type of abuse by their caregiver.

8. **If the client and his daughter hold firm in that nothing abusive is occurring in the household, what is your course of action?** One course of action would be for you and/or the health care provider to report suspected abuse on the basis of the bruises and the broken bone in the foot, the lack of health care, and the hearing aids in disrepair. The daughter and brother can be educated about what constitutes abuse of the elderly, and you can ask them for their plan on ensuring that the client is not subjected to abuse.

9. **The client says he thinks his daughter is putting pills in his pudding. Alline admits to getting the deceased neighbor's Haldol and putting it into her father's food. What actions do you need to take? Given what you know and suspect about how Alline is treating her father, how would you now feel about working with Alline and her father?** You need to impress upon the client's daughter the dangers of giving a major tranquilizer to an elderly person. You will impress upon her the importance of working with the health care provider to get whatever prescriptions her father needs. The provider needs to know every medication the client is taking to avoid drug interactions and drug overdosing. The daughter also cannot medically restrain her father against his will legally. You can assure her that if her father needs something to calm him and the provider prescribes it, that you will work with her to educate her father about the need for the medication and approaches to get him to accept it.

You may feel angry and not want to work with Alline. You may just want to turn this situation over to Adult Protective Services by reporting suspected elder abuse and neglect. On the other hand, you may realize that Alline and her father both need your help. He needs your help to prevent his being harmed. Alline needs to be protected from hurting her father. You do need to report this case, but you can still work to educate Alline, her father, and the father's brother about what constitutes elder abuse and how to prevent it. You can serve a role in helping both the client and caregiver to find ways to get their needs met appropriately. If the client has a return visit to the gerontologist, you need to treat the client and his caregiver in a professional and therapeutic manner.

10. **Nurses in some health care providers' offices may not write care plans; however, some likely nursing diagnoses will come to your mind. What are those nursing diagnoses? What goals and interventions would be helpful to this client?** Some likely nursing diagnoses include the following:

- Powerlessness
- Relocation stress syndrome or at risk for relocation stress syndrome if moved again
- Impaired skin integrity
- Pain

Some likely goals include:

- Will be free of bruises and any other skin impairment
- Will state he feels safe in his environment
- Will state he feels he has some control in his life
- Will report he is free of pain

Interventions that would be helpful include:

- Educate family and client about what elder abuse is and the prevention of elder abuse.
- Provide information about opportunities for respite care and encourage family to look into other opportunities for respite care.
- Find a support group for caregiver.
- Find a day program for the elderly client.
- Teach caregiver to give some options to elderly to give a sense of control.
- Report suspected elder abuse to APS.

11. **What do you especially need to document in this and other cases of suspected abuse?** It is important to document objectively what you observed, such as the size of bruises and the pattern of bruises and other injuries as well. It is important not to document your subjective opinions but instead to document findings and any quotes of what the client said that pertain to abusive actions. Many facilities have a form with a drawing of two outlines of the body: one representing the front and the other the back of the client. The location of the injuries can be marked on these drawings with the type of injury and size and description labeled.

References

Gray-Vickery, P. (2004). "Combating Elder Abuse." *Nursing* 34(10): 47–53.

Lachs, M.S. and K. Pillemer. (2004). "Elder Abuse." *Lancet* 364:1263–1268.

Lang, S.S. (2005). "Elder Abuse Cited as an Urgent Problem." *Human Ecology* 32(3): 23.

Machuca, M. (2005). "Agencies Team Up to Battle Abuse of Elderly." Available at www.ebcoalition.org/Articals/01-02-01%20Agencies%20team%20up%20to%20battle%20abuse%20of%20elderly. Accessed January 18, 2006.

Moody, E.F. "Elderly Abuse." (2005). Available at www.efmoody.com/miscellaneous/elderlyabuse.html. Accessed June 20, 2006.

Sellas, M.I., and L.H. Krouse, L.H. (2006). "Elder Abuse." Available at www.emedicine.com/emerg/topic160.htm. Accessed June 20, 2006.

www.aoa.gov/eldfam/Elder_Rights/Elder_Abuse/Elder_Abuse.asp. Accessed July 2, 2005.

_____. National Center for Elder Abuse Frequently Asked Questions. http://www.elderabusecenter.org/default.cfm?p=faqs.cfm.

www.elderabusecenter.org/default.cfm?p=statistics.cfm. Accessed July 1, 2005.

Wynne-Jones, M. (2005). "Taking Action in a Suspected Case of Elder Abuse." *Pulse* 65(5): 62–64.

Chuy

GENDER		DISABILITY
Male		■ Congenital deafness

AGE

11

SETTING

■ Deaf school infirmary

ETHNICITY

■ Mother is White American; father is Hispanic American

CULTURAL CONSIDERATIONS

■ Hispanic

PREEXISTING CONDITION

■ Waardenburg Syndrome (WS)
■ Possible Hirschsprung Disease associated with WS

COEXISTING CONDITION

■ Urine infection with low grade fever

COMMUNICATION

■ Congenital deafness; uses American Sign Language

DISABILITY

■ Congenital deafness

SOCIOECONOMIC

■ Upper middle class

SPIRITUAL/RELIGIOUS

■ Catholic

PHARMACOLOGIC

PSYCHOSOCIAL

LEGAL

■ Legal requirements to report suspected child abuse

ETHICAL

■ Unethical to ask questions out of curiosity rather than need to know

ALTERNATIVE THERAPY

PRIORITIZATION

DELEGATION

SEXUAL ABUSE OF A CHILD

Level of difficulty: High

Overview: Requires critical thinking, as well as knowledge of the laws pertaining to reporting of suspected sexual abuse of a child, to determine a course of action to take when a deaf child describes experiences that suggest sexual abuse by his father. Requires knowledge of the communication needs of deaf children and critical thinking to determine how to meet those needs.

DIFFICULT

Client Profile

Chuy, an 11-year-old boy, was born deaf in both ears. At first both eyes looked the same color, but after awhile it was very noticeable that one eye was bright blue and the other brown. His father, a third-generation Hispanic American, blamed the mother for this problem, saying she had bad genes. The paternal grandfather blamed his estranged sister for putting the evil eye on the boy. The neonatologist and the otologist blamed it on Waardenburg Syndrome (WS); their assessments found the father carries the trait, and several members of his family, including the boy's grandfather, have a variety of signs associated with WS, but none are deaf like Chuy.

The father physically and emotionally abused the mother. He was angry with her for producing an imperfect child and angry at the child for not being perfect. The father began to sexually abuse Chuy at about age 4. When the boy went to a residential school for the deaf, the mother went to work, separated from the father, and eventually divorced him. The court decision was joint custody. The mother knew of the sexual abuse, but did not report it or use it in the divorce trial.

Case Study

Chuy is admitted to the school infirmary for observation because he complains of a stomachache and he has a low grade fever. He is found to have urine infection. The infirmary nurse has two other children under her care, and they are isolated with chicken pox. The nurse is able to assess Chuy in a private area of the infirmary. She first plays a game of "Go Fish" and gets him to take turns with her telling "silly jokes." She then takes his vital signs and listens to his heart and lungs and lets him listen to his own heartbeat. The nurse listens for bowel sounds and palpates the stomach, inquiring about pain and about when he had last "pooped." Chuy says maybe three days ago when he was home with his father, but since coming back to school, he is having a hard time pooping. "So it was easier to 'poop' at home," the nurse says. Chuy reveals that his father puts his finger up his "butt" and puts other objects up there to stretch the "butt" and help the "poop" come out. "So he helps you . . ." the nurse says, and Chuy responds: "He helps other people too by taking pictures of how he does this so they will learn to do it, and he sometimes lets them practice on me or do other things with my wee wee and takes pictures. Oh, I am not supposed to tell. My dad told me to keep it secret. He said other people won't understand and they will be jealous. I won't be punished for telling will I, nurse? Dad says I will be punished if I tell and my mom will get real sick and die if I tell. Please don't tell anyone."

Questions and Suggested Answers

1. **Describe Waardenburg Syndrome (WS), including signs and symptoms.** WS is a "group of hereditary conditions (four types of the syndrome have been identified) characterized by deafness and partial albinism (pale skin, hair and eye color)," which can be passed on by one parent. WS affects one in thirty thousand people. The parent who has the gene for WS may have different symptoms than the child or may have no discernable symptoms. Symptoms vary greatly among those with the disorder. (www.shands.org/health/information/article/001428.htm).

   It is estimated that two to three of every one hundred children in the schools for the deaf may have WS. It is thought that for every child with a hearing loss that has WS, there will be four to five people in the family who have the gene but have normal hearing. About 50 percent of people with WS have no hearing loss. About 20 percent have hearing loss requiring some aid to verbal communication. Some people with WS are totally deaf. Some are deaf in one ear and can hear normally in the other ear.

   Some clients with WS have one very blue eye and one very brown eye. Sometimes blue and brown are mixed in the same eye. Some gene carriers have a white patch of hair on the front that can extend toward the back of their head. The space between the eyes is often broader, making it appear the eyes are further apart. The eyebrows growing together in the middle is a symptom, called synophris, in some clients with this syndrome. The client with WS can have cleft lip and/or palate and/or Hirschsprung disease, with its symptoms of constipation, vomiting, distention, and intestinal obstruction (www.medicinenet.com/hirschsprung_disease/article.htm).

2. **What possible reason or reasons did the nurse in this case have for beginning an assessment by first playing "Go Fish" and taking turns telling silly jokes with this client?** Playing games and telling jokes are helpful in putting the child at ease and building some rapport as well as building a trusting relationship with the child. This time of fun and focused activities also provides a chance to observe the client. Some adults have difficulty playing games or telling silly jokes, looking at these activities as a "waste of time." Games do help those playing them to develop concentration and to organize the mind skills, which carry over into more "serious" tasks the person has to do later. Silly jokes help develop a sense of humor and relax a person for more serious things to come.

3. **What do you suppose could be the cause of this child's constipation? What assessments could you do if you were the nurse in this case?** There could be many reasons for this child's constipation. One that comes to mind quickly is dehydration, and you are probably already pushing fluids because of the urinary tract infection. Another reason could be his diet or perhaps not getting exercise. Some children with WS have Hirschsprung Disease, and constipation is a major symptom of this disease. As you palpate the child's stomach, you can check for distention. You can measure the girth with a tape measure at the umbilicus to get a baseline. You can ask the child not to flush if he goes "poop" so you can see the stool and begin to get an idea of what the child's bowel problems are and how to alleviate them.

The nurse, practicing holistic nursing, will consider medical, mental, and sexual abuse factors in an attempt to find and alleviate the causes of constipation and of the urinary tract infection.

4. **What do you think the nurse in this case might think or feel as the child describes his father's behavior associated with his (the client's) genitals? What techniques did the nurse in the case study use in examining the client and why?** Nurses can have any number of feelings such as anger, frustration, or ambivalence—feeling torn between wanting to believe what they are hearing and disbelief that the father would do such a thing to his son and/or confusion about what is sexual abuse and what it not. When a nurse has been abused as a child, this client's description of abuse could arouse old feelings. It is good to think about what your reaction would be in this practice case before being confronted with a real situation since the child will need you to be calm, responsible, composed, in control and "willing to listen without judgment or emotionality and to be concerned for the child's safety" (Webster and Hall, 2004).

In working with this child, the nurse moved slowly with the physical assessment starting with the head, a less threatening area of the body to inspect. She let the boy hear his own heart, making him part of the examination and putting him at ease. She used therapeutic communication tools such as encouraging. She indicated interest and a willingness to listen by using open-ended techniques that did not suggest answers.

5. **How would you define sexual abuse of a child? Are there some gray areas about what is sexual abuse and what is not sexual abuse?** One of the definitions of sexual abuse of a child is "any sexual activity that a child cannot comprehend, give consent to, or that violates the law" (Lahoti et al., 2001). Sexual activity includes touching or fondling of genitals, sodomy, oral genital, genital and anal contact, using objects to penetrate body orifices, and exhibitionism, voyeurism, and exposure to pornography.

Webster and Hall (2004) define sexual abuse of a child as "an adult using a child for sexual gratification with or without physical contact," going on to say that sexual abuse with contact includes the same acts as above "regardless of whether the action is performed on the child or the child performs it." They define noncontact sexual abuse as including "making sexual comments, using a child in pornographic films, and having him view pornographic materials."

Nurses need to review what the law in their state defines as child sexual abuse. There is some confusion about whether adult-child interactions such as sleeping together, showering together, nongenital fondling, or viewing pornography are truly sexual abuse. Some argue that the intent of the adult is a major factor in deciding if this is sexual abuse or not, while others say you also have the child's interpretation, perception, and reaction to the events (Webster and Hall, 2004). The child could later express feelings that he or she was humiliated or coerced into doing something they did not want to do.

6. **Do you need to ask this client questions about the sexual abuse to make sure the child was sexually abused and to get more specific details of the abuse (i.e., take a sexual abuse history)? If yes, what is your rationale? If no, should someone else do this, and if so, who and why?** Once you establish a suspicion of sexual abuse, you must follow your employer's policies and the law. You will report it to the social services agency determined by your state statutes, which is most often Child Protective Services. You will need to alert your supervisor, who will guide you about who in the agency needs to know (e.g., the school health care provider), and the school administrator. You do not want to conduct an in-depth interview to get more details because this case may go to court, and having a skilled, trained child interviewer is critical to having the child's statements carry weight in court. Also, if not done correctly, an interview might cause the child to admit to things that are not true or become fearful and recant his allegations. What are referred to as forensic interviews are usually conducted by Child Protective Services professionals or law enforcement officials (Duncan and Sanger, 2004).

7. **What do you need to do and say in response to the child's request that you tell no one about the things his father did to him? What thoughts do you have about documentation of the child's statements in regard to his treatment by his father? Should you take notes while the child is talking?** You need to stay calm and reassuring and yet let the child know that what his father is doing does not sound safe or comfortable and that you, and the staff of the school, are there to keep him safe and comfortable. Tell the child that you will need to let some helping people know about this. Reassure the child that he did the right thing by telling about what was happening to him.

You probably realize that you need to document carefully the setting, the time, and the statements in quotes, and you need to stay objective in your recording. You should document whom you contacted, such as the health care provider, the administrator, and Child Protective Services. If the child tells his story to the nursing supervisor or the health care provider, they must document also. This lends credibility to the accuracy of your documentation. You may be interviewed by a Child Protective Services caseworker or supervisor, asked to give a deposition, or subpoenaed to appear as a witness in court. Your documentation will help you recall accurately what happened and help support your actions at the time.

Note taking during a disclosure of sexual abuse may inhibit the child from telling his story. It could also keep you from focusing fully on what the child is saying, his affect, behavior, and other observations.

8. **What reasons could the mother have for not reporting the sexual abuse of her son? Should you ask her? Do you need to know the reasons?** Some people don't report a spouse (or significant other) for abusing their child out of fear that the abusers will become angry and be more hurtful or even kill the child and/or themselves. In some cases the nonabusing spouse has become convinced no one will believe her or his word against her or his spouse's word. It is difficult to prove abuse in many cases even if reported. In divorce cases the reporting spouse may be accused of lying for some personal gain such as full custody of the children.

Knowing these possible reasons helps you keep an open mind in working with these individuals and not jump to conclusions that they are bad people. Before questioning the mother or others to get this information, you need to ask yourself if you are asking out of curiosity or if the answers will be helpful in making and carrying out your nursing care plan. It is helpful to build a trusting relationship with the mother and listen to what she has to say, encouraging her, but not questioning her or judging her in regard to her motives in not reporting abuse.

9. **If this client is to have an anogenital examination, what preparation would be helpful to the child? What is usually done in an anogenital examination? What would it mean if the anogenital examination were negative for evidence of sexual abuse?** The preparation for this examination is similar to that for other procedures and includes giving information to the client about what happens during the procedure, how it will feel during the procedure, instructions on anxiety reduction techniques, tour of the exam room, opportunity to talk about fears related to the exam, and a chance to ask questions about the exam (Duncan and Sanger, 2004).

Younger children will tend to seek support and comfort from their parents, or other trusted people, before and during the exam and will be more concrete in their thinking. When calmed by trusted people, they will tend to focus on the equipment in the room and the proceedings of the exam, whereas older children tend to be more concerned about the examiner finding problems such as injury, scarring, or disease, and in the case of girls, the concern extends to worries about pregnancy or infertility. Older children are concerned too about protecting their privacy.

The anogenital examination often follows a medical evaluation. It usually involves the use of a colposcope to look at and photograph the child's anal and genital areas. The external genitalia are manipulated, and the lateral traction is applied to the buttocks so these areas can be visualized. If cultures are indicated, cotton-tipped swab is inserted into the anus. In the case of a girl, there may be a culture taken with a cotton-tip swab inserted into the vagina (Duncan and Sanger, 2004).

A negative finding on anogenital examination only means the examination was negative for evidence. It does not prove that the sexual abuse suspicion is false or untrue.

10. **What behavioral symptoms do sexually abused children display? Will all children who have been sexually abused display behavioral symptoms? What are some thoughts and feelings children have identified in regard to their sexual abuse?** Sometimes (but not always) sexually abused children act out sexually. Valente (2005) writes, "Boys demonstrate some interesting coping skills when they identify with their sexual aggressor or act out their frustrations by abusing other children." Girls may also act out sexually. Some children who have been sexually abused are aggressive to others, and some engage in self-mutilation. Abused children tend to have physical complaints, skip school, have declining grades, become depressed and withdrawn, and/or become attention seeking or become passive.

The victim of childhood sexual abuse can display a wide variety of behavioral changes. Shaw (2004) says, "There is no syndrome or profile of psychological symptoms that is pathonomonic of childhood sexual victimization." He goes on to say that about one-third of sexually abused children are asymptomatic, while 10–25 percent will have delayed onset of symptoms, and two-thirds will have significant abatement of symptoms in the first eighteen months.

Four styles of coping strategies of survivors of sexual abuse described by Dorais and discussed by Valente (2005) include: angry avenger, passive victim, rescuer, and daredevil or conformist.

Some researchers have found that children question who they are and why this happened to them. Valente (2005) reports sexually abused boys feeling they must be flawed to be selected for abuse and "less masculine, more vulnerable, and inadequate" and feeling afraid that anyone observing could tell this.

Loewenstein (2004) describes abused children's need to live in a delusion that their parents are good so they must be bad and have caused the abuse. The abuse feels bad and fills the child with an all-consuming, all-encompassing sense of badness. The child comes to think they are bad, and this is better than feeling helpless. The perpetrator may enforce this by saying the child is "asking for it" or "wanted it."

Boys and girls alike are often scared, frightened, and intimidated, while at the same time they may have experienced sexual pleasure.

11. **What is the incidence of sexual abuse of children? Do you think the incidence is similar or different in other countries? Do you think culture plays any role in this case?** The national Center for the Victims of Crime and the U.S. Department of Health and Human Services (www.acf.dhhs.gov/programs/cb/publications/cm02) reported in 2004 that Child Protective Services found about a million children in this country to be victims of maltreatment. Ten percent of these maltreated children were found to be sexually abused. If this number does not seem sufficiently large enough to represent all the abused children in this country, remember that about three million cases of suspected abuse are reported each year but only about a third are confirmed. Two-thirds of the suspected abuse cases reported are not confirmed for various reasons including the parents quickly moving the family or the fact that abuse is often hard to prove or abuse did not occur. Many cases of abuse are not reported at all. Of the nearly one million proven cases above, 54 percent were white American, 26 percent were black American, and 11 percent were Hispanic.

Lowe (2005), describing a study of white, black, and Hispanic Americans, suggests that Hispanic fathers traditionally view the role of father as "primary protector of his family's dignity and honor," but when the Hispanic father is second- or third-generation American, the cultural influence to protect and honor may be lost.

Shaw (2004) cites the work of Finkelhor, who looked at sexual maltreatment of children in nineteen countries and reported in 1994 that the rates were similar around the world. There may be parts of the world now with more or less child sexual abuse than the United States.

12. **Are sexual abuse rates the same for boys as for girls? Do you think that sexual abuse rates are higher for disabled children? If yes, why do you think this is so?** While boys and girls are nearly equal in experiencing physical abuse and neglect, girls have been found to experience sexual abuse four times as often as boys by some researchers (Massey-Stokes and Lanning, 2004), while others say that sexual abuse of boys is greatly underreported and that "it is believed that boys are abused one to three times less often than girls" (Valente, citing a number of authors, 2005).

The Child Advocate webpage (www.childadvocate.net/child_sexual_abuse.htm) says that boys with disabilities such as blindness, deafness, mental retardation, and other disabilities are overrepresented among sexually abused children,

Sexual abuse rates, in general, are higher for disabled children. Saboe (2002, 1) states that "research suggests children with disabilities are 4–10 times more likely to be abused than children without disabilities" and "in 47% of the cases, workers thought that the disability led to or contributed to the abuse." The Child Advocate webpage (www.childadvocate.net/child_sexual_abuse.htm) points out that the risk of child sexual abuse "is increased for children with physical disabilities, especially those that impair the child's perceived credibility: blindness, deafness, and mental retardation."

Prevent Child Abuse America (www.preventchildabuse.org/learn_more/research_docs/maltreatment. pdf) points out that some researchers have suggested society's response to the disability rather than the disability itself may increase a child's vulnerability to abuse, since children with disabilities may be perceived as less valuable than children without disabilities and they may be given less respect. This webpage also points out that members of society may not consider the reports of these children trustworthy. There is also a tendency for many people, including health professionals, to not want to believe that a child with disabilities could be sexually abused.

Other factors that could increase a disabled child's vulnerability to abuse include families feeling unprepared to deal with their care, being unable to accept a child that is "different," and being unable to meet the financial costs of extra medical care and extra education, and lack of social networks to help. The Prevent Child Abuse America site also points out that the disabled child is often able to "develop more extensive relationships of trust with greater numbers of people, and be unable to distinguish when boundaries are being crossed, resulting in potential sexual abuse."

13. **When children are sexually abused, who is often the perpetrator? Is this the same for other forms of abuse?** The child who is abused almost always knows the perpetrator of sexual abuse whether that child is disabled or not. It is often a family member, a neighbor, a caregiver, or a family friend. In about 45 percent of all cases of sexual abuse of children in the year 2000, the perpetrator was a parent or parents (DHSS National Child Abuse and Neglect Data Systems, 2000, as cited by Saboe, 2002).

14. **What nursing diagnoses and goals would you likely write for this client? What interventions do you think would be helpful for this client?** Possible nursing diagnoses, which may be verified by assessment, include, but are not limited to:

- Anxiety
- Constipation
- Risk for self-harm
- Situationally low self-esteem

Possible goals include:

- Will be free of instances of sexual abuse
- Will verbalize feeling good about self
- Will develop at least one interest
- No evidence of sexual acting out
- No aggressive acts toward others
- Will be free of constipation
- Will be free of urinary tract infection

Interventions that would be helpful include:

- Assign the same nurse each day to care for this client and to facilitate building a trusting relationship. Valente (2005), writing about sexual abuse of boys, states: "Building a therapeutic relationship is essential to the success for treatment."
- Assure client he or she is not to blame and will not be punished. Avoid reinforcing the guilt, blame, and fear of punishment that the client may have.
- Encourage individual therapy such as play therapy and/or a boys group for survivors of sexual abuse.
- Help client identify interests and encourage those interests.
- Encourage fluids and administer medications as ordered for urinary tract infection.
- Monitor bowel habits and chart bowel movements carefully.
- Teach client ways to reduce anxiety.
- Monitor for clues of suicidal ideation and/or self-mutilation.
- Provide interpreter (American Sign Language) when needed and arrange same signer at all times, to increase comfort of child.

References

Duncan, M.K.W. and M. Sanger. (2004). "Coping with the Pediatric Anogenital Exam." *Journal of Child and Adolescent Psychiatric Nursing* 17(3): 126–136.

Lahoti, S.L. et al. (2001). "Evaluating the Child for Sexual Abuse." *American Family Physician* 63(5): 883–892.

Loewenstein, R.J. (2004). "Dissociation of the 'Bad' Parent, Preservation of the 'Good' Parent." *Psychiatry* 67(3): 256–261.

Lowe, M. Jr. (2005). "Ethnicity and Perceptions of Child Sexual Abuse." *Brown University Child and Adolescent Behavior Letter* 21(5): 3.

Massey-Stokes, M. and B. Lanning. (2004). "The Role of CSHPs in Preventing Child Abuse and Neglect." *Journal of School Health* 74(6): 193–194.

Mulryan, K., P. Cathers, and A. Fagin. (2004). "How to Recognize and Respond to Child Abuse." *Nursing* 14(10): 52–56.

Saboe, B.J. (2002). "Sexual Abuse and Children with Disabilities." Available at www.medicine.uiowa.edu/epsdt/win03/sexual_abuse.asp. Accessed June 20, 2005.

Shaw, J. (2004). "The Legacy of Child Sexual Abuse." *Psychiatry* 67(3): 217–221.

Smith, J. (2002). "Evaluation, Diagnosis, and Outcomes of Child Sexual Abuse." www.childadvocate.net/child_sexual_abuse.htm. Accessed June 20, 2006.

Valente, S.M. (2005). "Sexual Abuse of Boys." *Journal of Child and Adolescent Psychiatric Nursing* 18(1): 10–16.

Webster, R.E. and C.W. Hall. (2004). "School-Based Responses to Children Who Have Been Sexually Assaulted." *Education and Treatment of Children* 21(1): 64–81.

www.medicinenet.com/hirschsprung_disease/article.htm. "Hirschsprung Disease." Accessed June 20, 2006.

www.preventchildabuse.org/learn_more/research_docs/maltreatment.pdf. Accessed June 2005.

www.shands.org/health/information/article/001428.htm. "Waardenburg Syndrome." Accessed June 20, 2006.

Notes

Notes

Notes

Notes

Notes

Notes

Notes

Notes

Notes

Notes

Notes

Notes

Notes

Notes

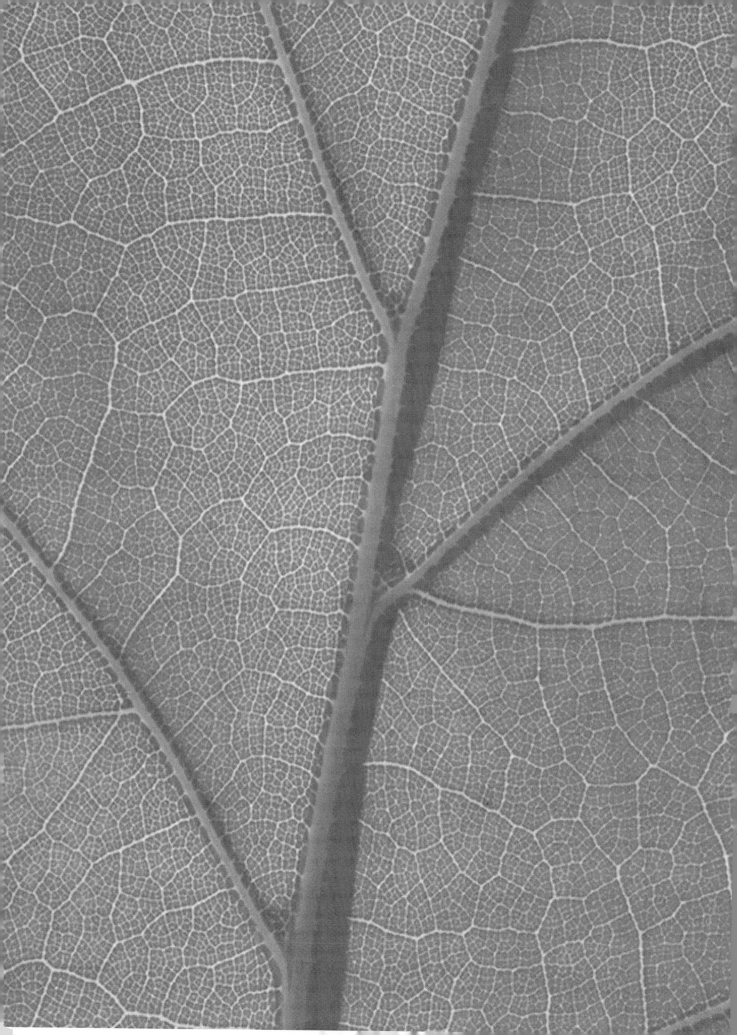